The Clinician's Gui... t
and Managemen...
Tourette Syndron... ers

The Clinician's Guide to Treatment and Management of Youth with Tourette Syndrome and Tic Disorders

Edited by

Joseph F. McGuire
Department of Psychiatry and Behavioral Sciences, Johns Hopkins University School of Medicine, Baltimore, MD, United States

Tanya K. Murphy
Rothman Center for Pediatric Neuropsychiatry, University of South Florida, St. Petersburg, FL, United States

John Piacentini
Department of Psychiatry and Biobehavioral Sciences, David Geffen School of Medicine, University of California, Los Angeles, CA, United States

Eric A. Storch
Menninger Department of Psychiatry and Behavioral Sciences, Baylor College of Medicine, Houston, TX, United States

ELSEVIER

ACADEMIC PRESS
An imprint of Elsevier

Academic Press is an imprint of Elsevier
125 London Wall, London EC2Y 5AS, United Kingdom
525 B Street, Suite 1650, San Diego, CA 92101, United States
50 Hampshire Street, 5th Floor, Cambridge, MA 02139, United States
The Boulevard, Langford Lane, Kidlington, Oxford OX5 1GB, United Kingdom

Notices

Knowledge and best practice in this field are constantly changing. As new research and experience broaden our understanding, changes in research methods, professional practices, or medical treatment may become necessary.

Practitioners and researchers must always rely on their own experience and knowledge in evaluating and using any information, methods, compounds, or experiments described herein. In using such information or methods they should be mindful of their own safety and the safety of others, including parties for whom they have a professional responsibility.

To the fullest extent of the law, neither the Publisher nor the authors, contributors, or editors, assume any liability for any injury and/or damage to persons or property as a matter of products liability, negligence or otherwise, or from any use or operation of any methods, products, instructions, or ideas contained in the material herein.

British Library Cataloguing-in-Publication Data
A catalogue record for this book is available from the British Library

Library of Congress Cataloging-in-Publication Data
A catalog record for this book is available from the Library of Congress

ISBN: 978-0-12-811980-8

For Information on all Academic Press publications
visit our website at https://www.elsevier.com/books-and-journals

Publisher: Nikki Levy
Acquisition Editor: Emily Ekle
Editorial Project Manager: Karen Miller
Production Project Manager: Mohana Natarajan
Designer: Christian Bilbow

Typeset by MPS Limited, Chennai, India

Dedications

To the children and families struggling with tics and Tourette disorder and the clinicians who serve them. It is my hope that this book will make a difference in their lives. And also to my mentors, for their unwavering support and guidance.

Joseph F. McGuire

To my mother who has taught me more about patient advocacy than I ever learned in medical school.

Tanya K. Murphy

To my family for their support and to the Tourette's community for their inspiration.

John Piacentini

To my father and mother for teaching me the importance of helping others. To my mentors for their support and guidance. And, finally, to my family (Jill, Noah, Ellie, and Maya) for making all of my dreams come true.

Eric A. Storch

Contents

List of Contributors

Kaushalendra Amatya, PhD Department of Psychiatry and Behavioral Sciences, Division of Child and Adolescent Psychiatry, The Johns Hopkins Hospital, Baltimore, MD, United States

Alicia A. Barnes, DO, MPH Department of Psychiatry, Saint Louis University School of Medicine, St. Louis, MO, United States

Christopher C. Bauer, MS Department of Psychology, Marquette University, Milwaukee, WI, United States

Renae Beaumont, PhD Weill Cornell Medicine, NY, United States

Shannon M. Bennett, PhD Weill Cornell Medicine, NY, United States

Emilie J. Bertschinger, BA Child Study Center, Yale School of Medicine, New Haven, CT, United States

Cathy L. Budman, MD Long Island Center for Tourette & Associated Disorders, Great Neck, NY, United States; Zucker School of Medicine at Hofstra-Northwell, Hempstead, NY, United States

Corinne Catarozoli, PhD Weill Cornell Medicine, NY, United States

Christine A. Conelea University of Minnesota, Minneapolis, MN, United States

Jack Dempsey Department of Pediatrics, Psychology Service, Baylor College of Medicine, Texas Children's Hospital, Houston, TX, United States

Allison G. Dempsey Department of Pediatrics, University of Texas Health Science Center, Houston, TX, United States

Kim R. Edwards, PhD Department of Psychiatry and Behavioral Neurosciences, McMaster Children's Hospital and McMaster University, Hamilton, ON, Canada

Flint M. Espil, PhD Department of Psychiatry and Behavioral Sciences, Stanford University School of Medicine, Stanford, CA, United States

S. Evelyn Stewart University of British Columbia, Vancouver, BC, Canada; British Columbia Children's Hospital,Vancouver, BC, Canada; Massachusetts General Hospital, Boston, MA, United States; Harvard Medical School, Boston, MA, United States

Rachel Fein Department of Pediatrics, Psychology Service, Baylor College of Medicine, Texas Children's Hospital, Houston, TX, United States

Anjali Gera, MD Department of Neurological Sciences, Rush University Medical Center, Chicago, IL, United States

Kathy Giordano Tourette Association of America, New York, NY, United States

Loran P. Hayes Department of Psychology, University of Utah, Salt Lake, UT, United States

Meme Hieneman Positive Behavior Support Applications, Tampa, FL, United States

Michael B. Himle Department of Psychology, University of Utah, Salt Lake, UT, United States

David C. Houghton, MS Department of Psychology, Texas A&M University, College Station, TX, United States

Tara Jukes British Columbia Children's Hospital,Vancouver, BC, Canada

Katie Kompoliti, MD Department of Neurological Sciences, Rush University Medical Center, Chicago, IL, United States

Alexandra M. Kushman, BA Tufts University School of Medicine, Boston, MA, United States

Ashlie V. Llorens Department of Crisis Intervention, Houston Independent School District, Houston, TX, United States

Melanie McConnell University of British Columbia, Vancouver, BC, Canada; British Columbia Children's Hospital,Vancouver, BC, Canada

Joseph F. McGuire, PhD Department of Psychiatry and Behavioral Sciences, Johns Hopkins University School of Medicine, Baltimore, MD, United States

Tanya K. Murphy, MD, MS Department of Pediatrics, University of South Florida, Tampa, FL, United States; Department of Psychiatry and Behavioral Neurosciences, University of South Florida, Tampa, FL, United States; All Children's Hospital, Johns Hopkins Medicine, St. Petersburg, FL, United States

Joshua M. Nadeau Department of Pediatrics, University of South Florida, Tampa, FL, United States; Rogers Behavioral Health—Tampa Bay, Tampa, FL, United States

Carisa Perry-Parrish, PhD Department of Psychiatry and Behavioral Sciences, Division of Child and Adolescent Psychiatry, The Johns Hopkins Hospital, Baltimore, MD, United States

John Piacentini, PhD Semel Institute for Neuroscience and Human Behavior, University of California, Los Angeles, Los Angeles, CA, United States

Justyna Piasecka, MD Child Study Center, Yale School of Medicine, New Haven, CT, United States

Hannah E. Reese, PhD Department of Psychology, Bowdoin College, Brunswick, ME, United States

Emily J. Ricketts, PhD Department of Psychiatry, University of California, Los Angeles, CA, United States

Babar M. Saggu, MD Department of Psychiatry, Butler Hospital, Providence, RI, United States

Meghan C. Schreck McLean Hospital, Harvard University Medical School, Belmont, MA, United States

Robert R. Selles University of British Columbia, Vancouver, BC, Canada; British Columbia Children's Hospital,Vancouver, BC, Canada

Sana Shad, MA Long Island Center for Tourette & Associated Disorders, Great Neck, NY, United States

Matthew W. Specht, PhD Weill Cornell Medical College/NewYork-Presbyterian Hospital-Westchester, White Plains, NY, United States

Eric A. Storch, PhD Menninger Department of Psychiatry and Behavioral Sciences, Baylor College of Medicine, Houston, TX, United States

Denis G. Sukhodolsky, PhD Child Study Center, Yale School of Medicine, New Haven, CT, United States

Megan E. Tudor, PhD Child Study Center, Yale School of Medicine, New Haven, CT, United States

Brianna C.M. Wellen Department of Psychology, University of Utah, Salt Lake, UT, United States

Monica S. Wu, PhD UCLA Semel Institute for Neuroscience and Human Behavior, Los Angeles, CA, United States

Chapter 1

Introduction to Treatment and Management of Youth With Tourette Disorders and Tic Disorders

Joseph F. McGuire, PhD[1], Tanya K. Murphy, MD, MS[2,3,4], John Piacentini, PhD[5] and Eric A. Storch, PhD[6]

[1]Department of Psychiatry and Behavioral Sciences, Johns Hopkins University School of Medicine, Baltimore, MD, United States, [2]Department of Pediatrics, University of South Florida, Tampa, FL, United States, [3]Department of Psychiatry and Behavioral Neurosciences, University of South Florida, Tampa, FL, United States, [4]All Children's Hospital, Johns Hopkins Medicine, St. Petersburg, FL, United States, [5]Semel Institute for Neuroscience and Human Behavior, University of California, Los Angeles, Los Angeles, CA, United States, [6]Menninger Department of Psychiatry and Behavioral Sciences, Baylor College of Medicine, Houston, Texas, United States

MANAGEMENT OF TIC DISORDERS

Tourette syndrome and other tic disorders (TDs) are neuropsychiatric conditions characterized by the presence of motor and/or vocal tics (American Psychiatric Association, 2013). Although tics are the hallmark feature of TDs, youth with TDs commonly suffer from co-occurring psychiatric conditions like anxiety disorders, attention deficit hyperactivity disorder (ADHD), and obsessive–compulsive disorder (OCD) (Freeman et al., 2000). Together, tics and these co-occurring psychiatric symptoms can contribute to a wide range of physical (e.g., bodily harm to tics), social (e.g., poor self-perception, peer teasing), emotional (e.g., symptoms of anxiety, depression, suicidal ideations), and behavioral problems (e.g., aggressive and/or disruptive behaviors). As such, it is not surprising that youth with TD have been reported to experience impairment across multiple domains (e.g., school, social, home) (Storch, Lack, et al., 2007) and a diminished quality of life (Conelea et al., 2011; Storch, Merlo, et al., 2007). Therefore, effective treatments are needed to efficiently manage tics and associated problems.

The Clinician's Guide to Treatment and Management of Youth with Tourette Syndrome and Tic Disorders.
DOI: https://doi.org/10.1016/B978-0-12-811980-8.00001-7

Two principle evidence-based interventions exist for youth with TD: pharmacotherapy and behavior therapy. Historically, psychotropic medications such as antipsychotics (e.g., haloperidol, pimozide, risperidone, ziprasidone, and aripiprazole), and more recently alpha-2 agonists (e.g., clonidine, guanfacine) have been used to managed tic symptom severity (Scahill, Erenberg, et al., 2006). Antipsychotic medications have been found to produce moderate sized reductions in tic symptom severity, with no significant difference noted between medication types in terms of efficacy (Weisman, Qureshi, Leckman, Scahill, & Bloch, 2013). Meanwhile, alpha-2 agonists have been found to produce more modest reductions in tic symptom severity on the whole, but appear to have larger treatment effects among youth who present with both TD and ADHD (Weisman et al., 2013). Although pharmacotherapy significantly reduces tic symptom severity, many troublesome tics remain even among treatment responders. Moreover, these medications are often accompanied by side effects that can limit long-term tolerability (e.g., weight gain, sedation, etc.) (Scahill, Erenberg, et al., 2006).

Behavior therapy serves as the other evidence-based intervention for reducing tic symptom severity. Behavior therapy is a broad term for behavioral interventions that use behavioral strategies to minimize the expression of tics. Multiple types of behavioral interventions have been evaluated in randomized controlled trials: habit reversal training (HRT), mass negative practice, awareness training, exposure response prevention, and comprehensive behavior intervention for tics (CBIT) (McGuire, Ricketts, et al., 2015). However, only HRT and CBIT have consistently demonstrated efficacy across these clinical trials and meta-analyses, with moderate-to-large effects (McGuire et al., 2014; Piacentini et al., 2010; Wilhelm et al., 2012). HRT is a multi-component intervention that can consist of psycho-education, awareness training, competing response training, generalization training, self-monitoring, relaxation training, behavioral rewards, motivational procedures, and social support (McGuire, Ricketts, et al., 2015). Despite containing multiple components, the core therapeutic skills of HRT are suggested to be awareness training, competing response training, and social support (Woods, Miltenberger, & Lumley, 1996). Meanwhile, CBIT utilizes these core HRT components in combination with relaxation training and behavioral rewards, and incorporates functional assessments and function-based interventions to mitigate daily life factors that can exacerbate tic symptoms (Woods et al., 2008). While behavior therapy produces significant reductions in tic symptom severity, a considerable percentage of youth do not achieve a clinically significant response, with tics persisting even among treatment responders (Piacentini et al., 2010). Moreover, youth may have difficulty consistently refraining from tic engagement due to age, comorbid conditions, and/or experience difficulty recognizing premonitory urges.

THE NEED FOR COMPREHENSIVE INTERVENTION

Practice parameters recommend behavior therapy for youth with moderate tic symptom severity, with the combination of behavior therapy and pharmacotherapy recommended when tics are severe (Murphy, Lewin, Storch, & Stock, 2013). Despite reducing tic symptom severity, these two treatment options are predicated on the assumption that tics and tic symptom severity are entirely responsible for the problems, impairment, and poor quality of life that youth with TD experience. While this may be true for some, it is not representative of all youth with TD. Moreover, even when receiving evidence-based treatment individually or in combination with pharmacotherapy, the efficacy of these interventions is not sustained indeterminately and symptom remission is rare. Thus youth have to learn to manage the more obvious tic symptoms at least on an intermittent basis, even when receiving evidence-based care.

While current evidence suggests that tic symptom severity substantially subsides in youth with TD by early adulthood (Bloch et al., 2006), experts acknowledge that tics can have adverse psychosocial consequences that may endure even after tics diminish and/or remit (Scahill et al., 2013). These psychosocial consequences may manifest in a variety of ways. For instance, youth with TD may become overly dependent on parents and/or family accommodation due to tics (Storch et al., 2017). Additionally, youth with TD may develop a poor sense of self-concept due to personalization of the illness (e.g., "I have Tourette's") or focus on negative self-attributes related to the illness state (e.g., "I'm odd", "I have few friends") (Hanks, McGuire, Lewin, Storch, & Murphy, 2016), rather than on areas of strength and resilience (e.g., "I am unique", "the friends I have are quality"). Furthermore, youth with TD may become reliant on maladaptive coping strategies developed early in life for the physical, social, and emotional problems associated with tics (e.g., avoidance, withdrawal, substance abuse)—which can persist into adulthood even if tics subside or remit. Indeed, when adults with TD were surveyed about their experiences, many reported that they continued to feel different from peers because of their tics, used social avoidance to manage their tics, experienced social impairment, and believed that tics had contributed to other psychological problems (Conelea et al., 2013). In short, adults with TD continue to experience the adverse psychosocial consequences associated with tics that likely began in childhood. Thus in almost every circumstance, youth must have to endure tics and their psychosocial consequences for many years to come.

LIVING WITH TICS

There has been limited research on helping youth with tics develop skills to efficiently and effectively cope with adverse psychosocial consequences and manage co-occurring problems. Specifically, there is a need for interventions that not only reduce tic symptom severity, but also provide the skills to manage the adverse psychosocial consequences of tics and common co-occurring problems. While a few treatment protocols have attempted to target the specific cooccurring problems among youth with TD (i.e., aggression and/or disruptive behaviors, Scahill, Sukhodolsky, et al., 2006; Sukhodolsky et al., 2009), only two studies directly addressed the psychosocial challenges associated with tics themselves (McGuire, Arnold, et al., 2015; Storch et al., 2012). Storch et al. (2012) developed a modular cognitive behavioral therapy (CBT) intended to promote resiliency and coping skills to manage the psychosocial consequences of tics among youth with TD. In this adaptive intervention, the clinician conducts a thorough assessment to identify the specific problems youth experience due to tics. Afterward, clinicians select the most appropriate CBT modules to reduce the identified impairment related to tics. In this preliminary evaluation, the eight participating youth exhibited significant reductions in tic symptom severity and tic impairment on the Yale Global Tic Severity Scale (YGTSS), and also experienced improved self-concept and quality of life (Storch et al., 2012). McGuire, Arnold, et al. (2015) extended these initial findings in a randomized controlled trial and incorporated additional therapeutic modules into the intervention. In this study, 24 youth with TD were randomly assigned to either the modular CBT or a waitlist condition of equal duration. Youth in the intervention group exhibited significantly reduced tic impairment and improved quality of life compared to the waitlist condition. There were also large clinically meaningful improvements in tic symptoms severity and obsessive–compulsive symptom severity relative to the waitlist condition, which did not achieve statistical significance due to the small sample size. However, all acute treatment gains were maintained at a one-month follow-up assessment.

PURPOSE OF THIS BOOK

This book serves as a synthesis and extension of the two studies by Storch et al. (2012) and McGuire, Ricketts, et al. (2015), McGuire, Arnold, et al. (2015). It uses the CBT modules developed for these studies as a basis for chapters, and incorporates the clinical experience of veteran tic clinicians to expand upon and further refine these CBT modules. It takes a comprehensive approach to the management of TDs by providing clinicians with expert guidance on managing tics with pharmacotherapy and behavior therapy, as well as managing the common cooccurring problems and the adverse psychosocial consequences of tics using empirically informed strategies. Thus the ultimate goal of this treatment guide is not necessarily to make tics "go away." Rather, this intervention seeks to minimize tic impairment and improve quality of life by reducing tic symptom severity, addressing cooccurring problems, developing effective coping strategies for tics, and cultivating resiliency among patients with TD. As noted above, this comprehensive approach to managing TD in youth may play a key role in preventing a negative developmental trajectory that can lead to poor self-concept, result in maladaptive coping strategies (e.g., avoidance, accommodation, withdrawal, and substance abuse), and lead to an overall poor quality of life.

PRESENTING THE TREATMENT APPROACH TO YOUTH AND PARENTS

The goal of treatment is to reduce tic symptom severity, minimize tic impairment, manage distress, develop effective coping skills, and improve quality of life of youth with TD. This modular adaptive intervention works toward this goal by providing psychoeducation to youth and families about TD (Chapter 2: Psychoeducation About Tic Disorders and Treatment), evidence-based approaches to manage tic symptom severity (Chapters 3: Habit Reversal Training and 4: Pharmacological Management of Tic Disorders in Youth), strategies to overcome maladaptive cognitions/perceptions (Chapters 5: Cognitive Restructuring About Tics and 6: Improving Self-Esteem for Youth With Tourette Syndrome and Tic Disorders), management of social and educational concerns (Chapters 7: Talking about Tics With Peers and Coping in Social Interactions, 8: Tourettes in the Classroom: Support and Guidance on Education Issues for Clinicians, and 9: Overcoming Tic-Related Avoidance), difficulties with executive functioning (Chapter 10: Problem Solving Strategies to Overcome Common Challenges Associated With Tourette Syndrome), managing anger/disruptive behaviors (Chapters 11: Brief Trans-Diagnostic Parent Training: A Strengths-Based, Parent-Centered Treatment for Youth With Tourette Syndrome and 12: Assessing and Treating Emotion Dysregulation and Anger Management), creating healthy lifestyles and habits (Chapters 13: Mindfulness for Tics and 15: Promoting Healthy Behaviors), and coping with family issues (Chapter 14: Family Issues Associated With Tics). The book concludes with a discussion of relapse prevention and strategies to move forward in the patients care depending on their response to intervention (Chapter 16: Relapse Prevention Strategies and Guidance on Refractory Cases).

When presenting this approach to treatment to youth and families, a clinician might state the following:

The goal of this treatment is to help you (and your family) cope with having tics, so that they don't get in the way and bother you so much. This means helping you manage your tics with medication (if needed) and behavioral strategies that have helped many others just like you. We will also figure out when and where tics are getting in the way and give you tools to help deal with those situations. For example, you mentioned that you often avoid going to sleepovers because you are worried about your friends asking questions about your tics, since they happen a lot during the evening. So we'll work together to help you feel okay about going to sleepovers, and practicing ways to talk to people about having tics, and how to handle situations in which you might get teased because of tics at a sleep over. We'll also talk about other stuff to help you too. Overall, I want to make sure you have the skills to overcome any challenge that tics might cause you. This way, if different problems come up at another point in the future, you will have the knowledge, skills, and experience on how to deal with them.

This sample language should be tailored to the particular patient, and modified as developmentally appropriate. For instance, the sample text is appropriate for a child who avoided sleeping over at friends' houses, but should be individualized to fit a problem area identified by the youth and/or parents. This is important to help youth recognize the benefit and relevance of treatment, rather than to just "get rid of tics" which they may not always perceive as bothersome. For parents, a more detailed explanation should be provided. During this explanation, the clinician should emphasize that the approach to treatment is comprehensive. Therefore, "success" of treatment is not entirely contingent upon whether the number or severity of tics are decreased. Rather, treatment is intended to reduce tic symptom severity, minimize tic impairment and distress, and develop effective coping skills to improve overall quality of life. Thus a patient may often continue to exhibit tics at the end of treatment, but these tics may no longer cause interference in daily activities or impact quality of life due to effective intervention and coping strategies.

Next, clinicians should describe a "typical course" of treatment that involves collaboratively identifying problem areas using a thorough assessment and selecting specific treatment targets based on impairment and patient/parent preference. When explaining what treatment might look like to parents and children, a clinician might say the following:

Many families often ask what treatment will look like for my child. Typically, we'll begin with a detailed assessment to identify the severity of tics and where and how tics are getting in the way for your child. Next, we'll begin with psychoeducation about tics and common co-occurring problems to help you, [patient's name], and family members better understand tics and answer questions you may have about them. Then, we'll collaboratively discuss and prioritize which challenges [patient's name] and you want to work on first. After which, we'll work on helping [patient's name] develop skills and strategies to overcome these challenges. While we will focus on providing [patient's name] with behavioral skills to manage his tics (and incorporate pharmacotherapy if needed), the emphasis of treatment is to help [patient's name] develop the skills and strategies to minimize impairment from tics, and improve quality of life. As tics will infrequent remit even with the most robust treatment, developing these skills and strategies is very important to learn to effectively cope with tics in any situation or at any point in life.

Youth and parents may have more specific questions about the ordering of the treatment modules, and seek clarification about the parent's role in treatment. The specific ordering and individualization of the treatment modules is discussed in greater detail in the below section, but needless to say treatment typically begins with psychoeducation to provide background on TD to the patient and family. Next, youth and families are often interested to immediately learn behavioral skills to manage tics and/or initiate a trial of pharmacotherapy to get tics "under control." As tic specific interventions are implemented, treatment typically turns toward addressing the tic-related impairment identified during the assessment using empirically informed strategies. In response, a clinician might say the following:

While treatment is individualized for each patient, a typical course begins with psychoeducation about TD and then proceeds on to the management of tics with behavior therapy (sometimes called habit reversal training) and pharmacotherapy if needed. Behavior therapy and pharmacotherapy have been shown to be helpful in managing tics. This way, we start to reduce [patient's name]'s tic severity first. As the behavioral strategies are implemented and appropriate doses of pharmacotherapy reached, treatment can shift towards addressing impairment from persistent tics, and developing appropriate coping skills to overcome related difficulties. This portion of therapy might include helping [patient's name] develop and effectively implement coping skills in challenging situations. It could also consist of learning strategies to manage aggressive outbursts and/or frustration, or perhaps learning to change thoughts about situations that bring up negative feelings, or even practicing communicating about tics to other.

In addition to explaining the "typical" course of treatment, it is also important to clarify the role of parents in the context of treatment. Unless contraindicated, parents (or other relevant caregivers) should be involved in treatment as they can play a key role in behavior therapy and other aspects of the intervention. However, it is important to balance this with protecting patient autonomy, especially for adolescent patients. Thus a clinician might state to the parents:

We have found that it is best to work together as a team. This does not mean that I share everything with you that [patient's name] shares with me. Instead, it means that I might ask you to participate in sessions to learn the skills that I'm introducing, so that you can help [patient's name] practice using the skill outside of the clinic. It might also mean that I spend part of each session with your child alone, and part of it with you and your child together, to make sure that we are all on the same page.

CONDUCTING THE INITIAL ASSESSMENT

A comprehensive evidence-based assessment is the cornerstone of evidence-based treatment. Prior to initiating any intervention, it is important to characterize tic symptom severity, identify the areas of impairment caused by tics in youth, and evaluate quality of life. The characterization of tic symptom severity is critical to monitor treatment progress, whereas the identification of tic-related impairment is important to specifically identifying how and where tics are causing interference so that appropriate skills can be provided in treatment. In terms of selecting assessments to evaluate and monitor tic symptom severity, there are several options available (see McGuire et al., 2012 for a comprehensive review). The YGTSS a semi-structured clinical interview that serves as the gold standard to evaluate tic symptom severity and impairment over the past week (Leckman, Riddle, Hardin, & Ort, 1989). The YGTSS is comprised of a Symptom Checklist, Severity Scale, and Impairment Scale. The Symptom Checklist consists of common tics separately categorized as simple motor, complex motor, simple vocal, and complex vocal. The Symptom Checklist can be used to help clinicians complete the YGTSS Severity Scale, in which the clinician rates motor and phonic tics separately across five dimensions: number, frequency, intensity, complexity, and interference. These ratings are summed to produce a Total Tic Score (range: 0–50). Clinicians also provided an Impairment score that reflected overall tic-related impairment (range: 0–50). The YGTSS has demonstrated reliability, validity, and treatment sensitivity (Leckman et al., 1989; Piacentini et al., 2010; Storch et al., 2005), with 25–35% reductions in the Total Tic Score (or 6–7 raw reductions in the Total Tic Score) associated with a treatment response in clinical trials (Jeon et al., 2013; Storch et al., 2011). Although widely used in clinical research, the YGTSS may sometimes be challenging to administer in clinical practice for multiple reasons (e.g., requires training, time burden).

Comparatively, brief self-report rating scales offer some advantages in evaluating tic symptom severity in an efficient manner. Self-report measures are cost-effective, require minimal training to administer and interpret, and have the advantage of removing potential interviewer bias. The Parent Tic Questionnaire (PTQ) is a brief parent-report scale of tic symptom presence and tic severity over the past week (Chang, Himle, Tucker, Woods, & Piacentini, 2009). It consists of individual ratings of tic presence or absence of 14 common motor tics and 14 common vocal tics, which are then rated on the dimensions of frequency and intensity on a 1–4 scale. While frequency and intensity items are summed to produce a severity score for each individual tic (range: 0–8), all items are summed to produce a Total Score. The PTQ has demonstrated reliability, validity, and treatment sensitivity (Chang et al., 2009; Ricketts et al., 2018), with 55% reductions in the Total Score (or 10 point raw reductions in the Total Score) associated with a treatment response in clinical trials (Ricketts et al., 2018).

When considering evaluating impairment from tics, there are at least two options. The YGTSS includes an Impairment Scale that is commonly used in clinical research. Although providing a global rating of tic-related impairment, this scale does not provide descriptive detail about the specific domains and/or impairment caused by the tics. In comparison, the Child Tourette Impairment Scale (CTIM) is a brief parent-report scale that assesses the impairment from tics and related co-occurring psychopathology across multiple domains (e.g., school, home, social activities) (Storch, Lack, et al., 2007). It consists of 37-items that are rated on a 0 ("not at all") to 3 ("very much") scale, with items summed to produce an overall impairment score. The CTIM had demonstrated excellent reliability, validity, and treatment sensitivity (Storch, Lack, et al., 2007; Storch et al., 2012).

Lastly, it is important to monitor the impact of intervention on a patient's quality of life. Although not traditionally incorporated in treatment outcome studies or clinical trials of youth with TD, evaluating and monitoring patients' quality of life is particularly relevant for chronic conditions like TD as reductions in symptoms severity may be more modest. For example, while intervention may reduce tic symptom severity and minimize impairment, tics and tic-related impairment often still persist. However, patients may experience a marked improvement in the quality of life, despite the persistence of tic symptoms and some impairment. There have been several measures that have been used to capture quality of life among youth with TD in research studies. These include more general quality of life measures such as the Pediatric Quality of Life Inventory (PedsQL) (Varni, Seid, & Rode, 1999) and the Youth Quality of Life Instrument-Research Version (YQOL-R) (Edwards, Huebner, Connell, & Patrick, 2002), as well as a more disorder specific measures like the Gilles de la Tourette Syndrome—Quality of Life Scale (GTS-QOL) (Cavanna et al., 2013). The PedsQL (23 items), YQOL-R (56 items), and GTS-QOL (27 items) are all child-rated measures that assess quality of life, with the GTS-QOL providing more specific focus on TD quality of life.

Beyond using quantitative rating scales to assess and track tic symptom severity, tic-related impairment, and quality of life, it is important to conduct a thorough clinical interview to assess tic-related impairment. While clinicians can use the completed rating scales to inform the interview, the interview should broadly cover the domains of tic-related impairment in school, peer relationships, extracurricular activities, family life, as well as assess the impact of tics on physical, emotional, and behavioral domains. For example, a clinician may have the parent complete the PTQ and CTIM to assess tic symptom severity and impairment, respectively, and have the youth complete the PedsQL or GTS-QOL to ascertain youth's quality of life. Afterwards, the clinician would review the forms and identify that youth had some tic-related impairment (from the parent's perspective) in school, home, and social activities. The clinician might use this information and say the following:

I know that you and your parent completed some paperwork asking about how bad your tics have been (tic symptom severity), how tics have been getting in the way (tic-related impairment), and how tics might impact your life (quality

> *of life). I'm just going to ask some follow-up questions about some things your parent put down here, so I have a better understanding of how tics have been getting in the way. I'm going to ask you about how tics might get in the way at school, with friends, when you're other activities, and also at home. I'm also going to ask you how tics impact your body, might influence your emotions such as making you feel more anxious or sad, and also ask about other difficulties related to tics like controlling your frustration and behavior.*

School Impairment

When asking about school-related impairment, the clinician should begin broadly and also have prepared sample follow-up questions. For example, broad questions might be "*how do you feel that tics have gotten in the way of school?*" For youth who are less responsive to open ended questions, more specific questions may be useful to help guide school-related dialog. Thus a clinician may follow-up with specific questions about school such as any of the following:

> *For example, do tics ever get in the way while you are taking tests or doing your homework? Is there anything you avoid doing at school because of your tics? This might include raising your hand to answer questions, giving a class presentation, going to the library (or other public places), or even participating in specific classes (e.g., physical education, music class)? Do you have trouble talking to teachers about your tics? Or have you ever gotten into trouble at school because teachers or peers didn't understand your tics?*

Social Impairment

Similarly, when asking about impairment in peer relationships, the clinician should begin broadly and also have prepared sample follow-up questions. For instance, a broad opening question might be "*In what ways have tics gotten in the way with friends or caused problems with peers?*" Specific follow-up questions for less responsive youth might include: *For example, what is it like to meet new people or peers for you? Is it difficult to make or keep friends because of your tics? Do peers often ask about your tics, and if so, how does that make you feel? Have you ever been teased or bullied because of your tics?* For adolescents, clinicians may inquire if tics have interfered with dating or driving.

Clinicians should also inquire about impairment in social and extracurricular activities. For example, clinicians may ask whether youth "*Have ever avoided going to certain places or doing certain activities because of your tics?*" More specific follow-up questions may include: *Have tics ever gotten in the way of you participating in extracurricular activities like playing sports, playing an instrument, being involved in a club? Are there places you will not go because of your tics like to the mall, movies, or to school functions?* For adolescents, clinicians may inquire as to whether tics have interfered with employment and/or employment opportunities.

Family Impairment

Clinicians should also inquire about the impact of tics on family functioning. For example, a clinician may open with a general question such as "*Do tics ever cause problems at home and/or get in the way with family?*" Follow-up questions may include: "*For example, do tics ever make it harder for you to get along with your parents or siblings? Do others in your family complain about your tics, or complain that you are treated differently because of your tics? Do your tics ever get in the way of spending time with your family (e.g., going to church/religious services, going out to eat, going on vacation, etc.)?*"

Physical, Emotional, and Behavioral Problems Related to Tics

Clinicians should also inquire about whether youth experience any physical, emotional, and/or behavioral problems related to tics. For example, a clinician might ask youth the following to assess physical impact of tics, "*have you ever experienced any physical discomfort due to tics?*" Follow-up prompts could include: "*For example, some people tell me that certain tics cause them pain, or make it difficult for them to fall or stay asleep at night?*" Clinicians should ask about emotional difficulties related to tics. For example a clinician might open with the question, "*Do you ever feel that you have trouble controlling your emotions more so than others?*" Follow-up prompts may include: "*Do you often get angry or frustrated over some of the smallest things? Do you ever have a hard time controlling your temper at school, with friends, or at home? Do you worry that your tics will get in the way in the future (e.g., driving, going to college, getting married, having a roommate, etc.)? Do you ever worry that tics may make things harder for you than for other individuals?*" In regards to behavioral problems associated with tics, a clinician might ask whether youth "*experience any difficulty controlling their behavior compared to their peers?*" As some youth (especially younger children) may have difficulty distinguishing emotions from behavior, a clinician could clarify that "*I don't mean that you get more frustrated or angry than other peers, rather that you have more trouble controlling your behavior or response to a situation that gets you angry or frustrated?*" For younger children, a clinician could also direct the question to the parent such as, "*Is your child ever disruptive or aggressive towards others? Does your child have difficultly managing their behavior?*"

In summary, the goal of the assessment is to characterize tic symptom severity, tic-related impairment, and quality of life using quantitative rating scales. Meanwhile, the goal of the interview is to identify the specific areas and challenges that tics cause so that appropriate treatment components can be determined and utilized.

PERSONALIZING TREATMENT

After completing a comprehensive evidence-based assessment described above, intervention should be initiated. First, it is critical to provide the patient and family with psycho-education about TD to help them understand and contextualize the difficulties they may be experiencing related to TD (see Chapter 2). This is often completed within a single session. In most cases, patients and families will want to start a course of behavior therapy and/or initiate a trial of pharmacotherapy to reduce tic symptom severity. Practice parameters recommend behavior therapy when tics are moderate in severity, with pharmacotherapy reserved for moderate-to-severe tics (Murphy et al., 2013). Thus the quantitative rating scales and qualitative interview should be used to guide determination of tic symptom severity and impairment. After selecting the appropriate course of intervention, Chapters 3, Habit Reversal Training, and 4, Pharmacological Management of Tic Disorders in Youth, can be used to implement behavior therapy and/or guide pharmacotherapy selection (if appropriate). While the duration and course of pharmacotherapy is well covered in Chapter 4, Pharmacological Management of Tic Disorders in Youth, there are more ambiguities concerning the duration of behavior therapy. In clinical trials, a "standard" course of behavior therapy has been 7–14 sessions (McGuire et al., 2014). However, the number of sessions will vary on the number of bothersome tics and the patient's (and parent's) ability to master/implement the behavioral strategies. Thus some youth may only need a few sessions of behavior therapy due to few bothersome tics and quick skill mastery; whereas others may require a longer course of behavior therapy due to many bothersome tics and difficulties implementing behavioral strategies. Although comorbid ADHD may attenuate reductions in tic symptom severity, youth with co-occurring ADHD still continue to exhibit a clinically (and statistically) significant benefit to behavior therapy (McGuire et al., 2014). As youth (and parents) demonstrate mastery over behavioral skills and exhibit reductions in tic symptoms severity, the emphasis of treatment can transition toward tic-related impairment and quality of life. This does not mean that behavioral therapy skills should not be discussed at any further point in treatment. Rather, competing responses and behavioral strategies can be reviewed at subsequent sessions, but may no longer serve as the emphasis of any single session.

After providing psychoeducation and targeted interventions to reduce tic symptom severity, information obtained from the quantitative rating scales and qualitative interview should be utilized to guide the selection of subsequent therapy modules. Specifically, the clinician should use the collective child and parent reports and clinical judgment to identify primary problems caused by tics, and select appropriate therapy skills to address these problems. Several examples are provided below to help guide clinicians in selecting therapy skills in treatment. Keep in mind that each therapy chapter/ module will likely require more than a single session, so please plan accordingly.

Primarily Tics

Consider the case of a young adolescent who experiences moderate-to-severe tics, but denies impairment in any other domains. After concluding an evidence-based assessment, a clinician might begin treatment with psychoeducation about TD (Chapter 2: Psychoeducation About Tic Disorders and Treatment). Next, habit reversal training (Chapter 3: Habit Reversal Training) and medication management (Chapter 4: Pharmacological Management of Tic Disorders in Youth) could be initiated as appropriate. Given that some youth experience difficulties implementing competing responses due to increased distress related to premonitory urges, mindfulness skills may be helpful to reduce distress associated with tics and/or competing responses (Chapter 13: Mindfulness for Tics). Additionally, youth may benefit from general discussion of promotion of healthy behaviors and lifestyles, if indicated during the course of treatment (Chapter 15: Promoting Healthy Behaviors). Finally, as the patient begins to exhibit reduced tic symptom severity and improved quality of life, relapse prevention strategies can be utilized (Chapter 16: Relapse Prevention Strategies and Guidance on Refractory Cases).

Tics and Social Impairment

Take for example, a child who had moderate tic symptom severity and who reports getting picked on at school (because of tics) and feeling different from their peers. A clinician might start off with psychoeducation (Chapter 2: Psychoeducation About Tic Disorders and Treatment) and habit reversal training (Chapter 3: Habit Reversal Training) to provide background on TD and skills to manage tics respectively. Given the specific tic-related impairment reported by the child, the patient may benefit from learning different ways to talk about tics with peers and cope with tics in social interactions (Chapter 7: Talking About Tics With Peers and Coping in Social Interactions), and strategies to improving self-esteem and self-concept (Chapter 6: Improving Self-Esteem for Youth With Tourette Syndrome and Tic Disorders). Additionally, given concerns related to feeling different, youth may benefit from cognitive restructuring about tics to address feeling different from peers (Chapter 5: Cognitive Restructuring About Tics). If the child was also experiencing declining grades in school and/or other academic problems, it could be worthwhile to discuss with parents whether educational interventions are warranted and how to manage tics in a school setting (Chapter 8: Tourettes in the Classroom: Support and Guidance on Education Issues for Clinicians). Furthermore, as treatment progresses, if the youth avoids specific social situations and/or other activities due to tics, then the clinician could consider utilizing skills to help youth overcome tic-related avoidance (Chapter 9: Overcoming Tic-Related Avoidance). As tic symptom severity and tic-related impairment are reduced, there will likely be an increase in youth's quality of life. As youth feel comfortable managing their tics, talking to peers at school, and feel better about themselves, relapse prevention strategies can be discussed (Chapter 16: Relapse Prevention Strategies and Guidance on Refractory Cases).

Tics and Academic/School Problems

Consider the case of a child who has moderate-to-severe tics and reports experiencing considerable impairment in school functioning in both academic and social domains. A clinician would start off with psychoeducation (Chapter 2: Psychoeducation About Tic Disorders and Treatment) followed by habit reversal training (Chapter 3: Habit Reversal Training) and/or pharmacotherapy (Chapter 4: Pharmacological Management of Tic Disorders in Youth) as appropriate. Given that impairment is primarily experienced in school, the clinician may provide the youth with skills to talk about tics with peers and cope with tics in social interactions (Chapter 7: Talking About Tics With Peers and Coping in Social Interactions). From a parent perspective, the clinician should also cover strategies to manage tics in a school setting and discuss potentially relevant accommodations and/or modifications (Chapter 8: Tourettes in the Classroom: Support and Guidance on Education Issues for Clinicians). Additionally, as many youth with TD may experience challenges in executive functioning domains, problem solving strategies to overcome executive functioning and other related challenges associated with tics could prove useful (Chapter 10: Problem Solving Strategies to Overcome Common Challenges Associated With Tourette Syndrome). As appropriate coping skills are established and school-based interventions implemented, relapse prevention strategies can be incorporated (Chapter 16: Relapse Prevention Strategies and Guidance on Refractory Cases).

Tics and Emotional Problems

Take the case of an adolescent with moderate tic symptom severity, who experiences significant problems with emotion regulation related to tics that may manifest as either anxiety, depression, and/or anger/frustration. The clinician would start off with psychoeducation (Chapter 2: Psychoeducation About Tic Disorders and Treatment) followed by habit reversal training

(Chapter 3: Habit Reversal Training) to provide skills to manage tics. Next, a clinician may consider utilizing emotion regulation and anger management strategies (Chapter 12: Assessing and Treating Emotion Dysregulation and Anger Management) to help the adolescent better manage their emotions. Similarly, mindfulness strategies (Chapter 13: Mindfulness for Tics) may also prove useful to manage the distress associated with tics, competing responses, and/or other daily stressors. If youth are particularly disruptive and/or aggressive, the clinician may consider providing parent training strategies for disruptive behaviors, if developmentally appropriate (Chapter 11: Brief Trans-Diagnostic Parent Training: A Strengths-Based, Parent-Centered Treatment for Youth With Tourette Syndrome). The clinician may also consider discussing the ways in which tics and emotion regulation may influence (or be exacerbated) by family functioning (Chapter 14: Family Issues Associated With Tics). If the youth was engaging in any avoidance of social situations due to tics, and/or engaging in any unhealthy behaviors as coping strategies, then the clinician may consider employing strategies on overcoming tic-related avoidance (Chapter 9: Overcoming Tic-Related Avoidance), and/or discuss healthy behaviors and lifestyles associated with tics (Chapter 15: Promoting Healthy Behaviors). As the patient demonstrates mastery over behavioral strategies to manage tics and competency over related skills to reduce tic-related impairment, relapse prevention strategies can be initiated to support therapeutic gains (Chapter 16: Relapse Prevention Strategies and Guidance on Refractory Cases).

THE IMPORTANCE OF HOMEWORK COMPLIANCE

Compliance with out-of-session homework and practice assignments is an important aspect of treatment. Empirical research has shown that homework assignments have a moderate effect on treatment outcome in psychosocial interventions (Kazantzis, Deane, & Ronan, 2000). Although many youth will be engaged and interested in treatment, they may struggle to complete out-of-session therapeutic activities for a variety of reasons. Therefore, it is important to explain to youth early in treatment that you will be asking them to complete homework assignments between sessions. You should let them and their parents know that their commitment to following through with recommendations for between-session activities (i.e., practicing behavioral strategies, making modifications to school, and practicing talking about tics) can play an influential role in therapeutic outcomes. For instance, a clinician might say:

We will be working on a lot of different skills here at the clinic. To help you to practice using these skills, I will give you assignments to complete at home. These are not the kind of homework assignments that you get from your teacher at school; I will not grade them, I don't care about your spelling or handwriting. The homework is your chance to try out what you learn in therapy, so that you can let me know what is easy or hard for you, and what you find most helpful. We have found that kids who do their homework each week make the most progress.

Often times, it helps to use an age-appropriate analogy that incorporates the youth's interests (e.g., learning to play a sport or a musical instrument). A clinician might describe how assignments and skills initially seem challenging and require considerable practice, but over time, become much easier. In this instance, the clinician might be seen as a "coach," the patient as "a player," in-session activities as "practice" and out-of-session activities as "games." Another common strategy is to suggest that the child (or parent) purchase a notebook to keep track of homework assignments. Younger children might also enjoy decorating the notebook, which may increase the likelihood that they will use it and remember to bring it to session. Beyond these suggestions, there are also several empirically supported strategies for maximizing homework compliance. These include: (1) collaborating with the patient to generate homework assignments, (2) matching assignments to the patient's ability level, (3) providing a rationale for how the assignment can promote change, (4) describing assignments in detail, (5) providing written prompts, and (6) preemptively discussing potential barriers to completing assignments.

IMPLEMENTATION OF A REWARD SYSTEM

In-session and out-of-session activities can definitely be challenging for even the most interested and motivated patients. Many youth will be motivated in treatment to participate in-session and complete out-of-session assignments due to the physical, emotional, and social impairment of tics. However, some younger children or children with specific co-occurring conditions (e.g., ADHD) may have greater difficulty with in-session and out-of-session assignments. Thus, a behavioral reward system may be implemented to encourage and reinforce therapeutic compliance. The clinician should first collaboratively discuss the potential for a reward system with the parent (or caregiver), consider appropriate rewards based on a patient's interest, and discuss an appropriate system to reinforce compliance. After obtaining parent support for the implementation of the reward system, a clinician can introduce the topic of using rewards for compliance to the patient. "*I know that therapy can be hard work. To help you stay motivated, it might be good for us to work with your parents to come up with a list of rewards and/or prizes that you can earn for coming to therapy and completing homework assignments. Does that sound good to you?*" While a discussion of a reward system can happen at any point when compliance is diminishing, it is often brought up following the initial habit reversal training session as this is when out-of-session therapy assignments are initially introduced.

CONCLUSION

In summary, this intervention takes a comprehensive approach to the clinical care of youth with TD. It seeks to minimize tic impairment and improve quality of life by reducing tic symptom severity, addressing co-occurring problems, developing effective coping strategies for tics, and cultivating resiliency among youth with TD. This comprehensive approach is critical to help youth (and families) navigate the challenging periods of childhood and adolescence, and develop adaptive skills that can support youth into and throughout adulthood. When these skills are applied effectively, they possess the potential to transform a patient's life trajectory. Indeed, as shown in the artwork and description from a young person with TD, living with TD can be difficult. Youth (and families) can experience numerous challenges and setbacks due to the waxing/waning nature of tics and unanticipated life events. At times, youth (and families) may feel despair and begin to believe that things will never get better. However, comprehensive treatment approaches that address impairment and quality of life can help youth (and families) overcome daily challenges and bring strength, hope, and renewal. As youth (and families) learn to implement these skills, some may even feel a new person or given a new lease on life. We are grateful to the young person with TD who shared his work with us, and offer the drawing and his description as a reminder to clinicians (and patients and families) of transformative change that can come from comprehensive and compassionate care.

Importantly, this intervention should be personalized to a patient's specific clinical presentation based on a thorough evidence-based assessment that includes both quantitative measures and a qualitative interview to assess specific areas of impairment. Monitoring of tic symptom severity, tic-related impairment, and quality of life should be completed throughout the intervention. Through this intervention, it is anticipated that a patient will experience reductions in tic symptom severity, develop skills to overcome tic-related impairment, and develop effective and efficient coping strategies to manage the adverse psychosocial consequences of tics in short-term and develop resiliency to manage tics and associated difficulties in the long-term.

REFERENCES

American Psychiatric Association. (2013). *Diagnostic and statistical manual of mental disorders (DSM-5®)*. American Psychiatric Pub.

Bloch, M. H., Peterson, B. S., Scahill, L., Otka, J., Katsovich, L., Zhang, H., & Leckman, J. F. (2006). Adulthood outcome of tic and obsessive–compulsive symptom severity in children with Tourette syndrome. *Archives of Pediatric and Adolescent Medicine*, *160*, 65–69.

Cavanna, A. E., Luoni, C., Selvini, C., Blangiardo, R., Eddy, C. M., Silvestri, P. R., ... Cardona, F. (2013). The Gilles de la Tourette Syndrome-Quality of Life Scale for children and adolescents (C&A-GTS-QOL): Development and validation of the Italian version. *Behavioural Neurology*, *27*, 95–103.

Chang, S., Himle, M. B., Tucker, B. T. P., Woods, D. W., & Piacentini, J. (2009). Initial psychometric properties of a brief parent-report instrument for assessing tic severity in children with chronic tic disorders. *Child & Family Behavior Therapy, 31*, 181–191.

Conelea, C. A., Woods, D. W., Zinner, S. H., Budman, C., Murphy, T., Scahill, L. D., ... Walkup, J. (2011). Exploring the impact of chronic tic disorders on youth: Results from the Tourette Syndrome Impact Survey. *Child Psychiatry and Human Development, 42*, 219–242.

Conelea, C. A., Woods, D. W., Zinner, S. H., Budman, C. L., Murphy, T. K., Scahill, L. D., ... Walkup, J. T. (2013). The impact of Tourette syndrome in adults: Results from the Tourette Syndrome Impact Survey. *Community Mental Health Journal, 49*, 110–120.

Edwards, T. C., Huebner, C. E., Connell, F. A., & Patrick, D. L. (2002). Adolescent quality of life, part I: Conceptual and measurement model. *Journal of Adolescence, 25*, 275–286.

Freeman, R. D., Fast, D. K., Burd, L., Kerbeshian, J., Robertson, M. M., & Sandor, P. (2000). An international perspective on Tourette syndrome: Selected findings from 3500 individuals in 22 countries. *Developmental Medicine and Child Neurology, 42*, 436–447.

Hanks, C. E., McGuire, J. F., Lewin, A. B., Storch, E. A., & Murphy, T. K. (2016). Clinical correlates and mediators of self-concept in youth with chronic tic disorders. *Child Psychiatry & Human Development, 47*, 64–74.

Jeon, S., Walkup, J. T., Woods, D. W., Peterson, A., Piacentini, J., Wilhelm, S., ... Scahill, L. (2013). Detecting a clinically meaningful change in tic severity in Tourette syndrome: A comparison of three methods. *Contemporary Clinical Trials, 36*, 414–420.

Kazantzis, N., Deane, F. P., & Ronan, K. R. (2000). Homework assignments in Cognitive and Behavioral Therapy: A meta-analysis. *Clinical Psychology: Science and Practice, 7*, 189–202.

Leckman, J. F., Riddle, M. A., Hardin, M. T., & Ort, S. I. (1989). The Yale Global Tic Severity Scale: Initial testing of a clinician-rated scale of tic severity. *Journal of the American Academy of Child & Adolescent Psychiatry, 28*, 566–573.

McGuire, J. F., Arnold, E., Park, J. M., Nadeau, J. M., Lewin, A. B., Murphy, T. K., & Storch, E. A. (2015). Living with tics: Reduced impairment and improved quality of life for youth with chronic tic disorders. *Psychiatry Research, 225*, 571–579.

McGuire, J. F., Ricketts, E. J., Piacentini, J., Murphy, T. K., Storch, E. A., & Lewin, A. B. (2015). Behavior therapy for tic disorders: An evidenced-based review and new directions for treatment research. *Current Developmental Disorders Reports, 2*, 309–317.

McGuire, J. F., Kugler, B. B., Park, J. M., Horng, B., Lewin, A. B., Murphy, T. K., & Storch, E. A. (2012). Evidence-based assessment of compulsive skin picking, chronic tic disorders and trichotillomania in children. *Child Psychiatry & Human Development, 43*, 855–883.

McGuire, J. F., Piacentini, J., Brennan, E. A., Lewin, A. B., Murphy, T. K., Small, B. J., & Storch, E. A. (2014). A meta-analysis of behavior therapy for Tourette syndrome. *Journal of Psychiatric Research, 50*, 106–112.

Murphy, T. K., Lewin, A. B., Storch, E. A., & Stock, S. (2013). Practice parameter for the assessment and treatment of children and adolescents with tic disorders. *Journal of the American Academy of Child and Adolescent Psychiatry, 52*, 1341–1359.

Piacentini, J., Woods, D. W., Scahill, L., Wilhelm, S., Peterson, A. L., Chang, S., ... Walkup, J. T. (2010). Behavior therapy for children with Tourette disorder: A randomized controlled trial. *Journal of the American Medical Association, 303*, 1929–1937.

Ricketts, E. J., McGuire, J. F., Chang, S. W., Bose, D., Rasch, M. M., Woods, D. W., ... Piacentini, J. (2018). Benchmarking treatment response in Tourette syndrome: A psychometric evaluation and signal detection analysis of the parent tic questionnaire. *Behavior Therapy, 49*, 46–56.

Scahill, L., Erenberg, G., Berlin, C. M., Jr., Budman, C., Coffey, B. J., Jankovic, J., ... Walkup, J. (2006). Contemporary assessment and pharmacotherapy of Tourette syndrome. *NeuroRx: The Journal of the American Society for Experimental NeuroTherapeutics, 3*, 192–206.

Scahill, L., Sukhodolsky, D. G., Bearss, K., Findley, D., Hamrin, V., Carroll, D. H., & Rains, A. L. (2006). Randomized trial of parent management training in children with tic disorders and disruptive behavior. *Journal of Child Neurology, 21*, 650–656.

Scahill, L., Woods, D. W., Himle, M. B., Peterson, A. L., Wilhelm, S., Piacentini, J. C., ... Mink, J. W. (2013). Current controversies on the role of behavior therapy in Tourette syndrome. *Movement Disorders, 28*, 1179–1183.

Storch, E. A., De Nadai, A. S., Lewin, A. B., McGuire, J. F., Jones, A. M., Mutch, P. J., ... Murphy, T. K. (2011). Defining treatment response in pediatric tic disorders: A signal detection analysis of the Yale Global Tic Severity Scale. *Journal of Child and Adolescent Psychopharmacology, 21*, 621–627.

Storch, E. A., Johnco, C., McGuire, J. F., Wu, M. S., McBride, N. M., Lewin, A. B., & Murphy, T. K. (2017). An initial study of family accommodation in children and adolescents with chronic tic disorders. *European Child & Adolescent Psychiatry, 26*, 99–109.

Storch, E. A., Lack, C. W., Simons, L. E., Goodman, W. K., Murphy, T. K., & Geffken, G. R. (2007). A measure of functional impairment in youth with Tourette's syndrome. *Journal of Pediatric Psychology, 32*, 950–959.

Storch, E. A., Merlo, L. J., Lack, C., Milsom, V. A., Geffken, G. R., Goodman, W. K., & Murphy, T. K. (2007). Quality of life in youth with Tourette's syndrome and chronic tic disorder. *Journal of Clinical Child and Adolescent Psychology, 36*, 217–227.

Storch, E. A., Morgan, J. E., Caporino, N. E., Brauer, L., Lewin, A. B., Piacentini, J., & Murphy, T. K. (2012). Psychosocial treatment to improve resilience and reduce impairment in youth with tics: An intervention case series of eight youth. *Journal of Cognitive Psychotherapy, 26*, 57–70.

Storch, E. A., Murphy, T. K., Geffken, G. R., Sajid, M., Allen, P., Roberti, J. W., & Goodman, W. K. (2005). Reliability and validity of the Yale Global Tic Severity Scale. *Psychological Assessment, 17*, 486.

Sukhodolsky, D. G., Vitulano, L. A., Carroll, D. H., McGuire, J., Leckman, J. F., & Scahill, L. (2009). Randomized trial of anger control training for adolescents with Tourette's syndrome and disruptive behavior. *Journal of the American Academy of Child & Adolescent Psychiatry, 48*, 413–421.

Varni, J. W., Seid, M., & Rode, C. A. (1999). The PedsQL: Measurement model for the Pediatric Quality of Life Inventory. *Medical Care, 37*, 126–139.

Weisman, H., Qureshi, I. A., Leckman, J. F., Scahill, L., & Bloch, M. H. (2013). Systematic review: Pharmacological treatment of tic disorders—efficacy of antipsychotic and alpha-2 adrenergic agonist agents. *Neuroscience & Biobehavioral Reviews, 37*, 1162–1171.

Wilhelm, S., Peterson, A. L., Piacentini, J., Woods, D. W., Deckersbach, T., Sukhodolsky, D. G., ... Walkup, J. T. (2012). Randomized trial of behavior therapy for adults with Tourette syndrome. *Archives of General Psychiatry, 69*, 795–803.

Woods, D. W., Miltenberger, R. G., & Lumley, V. A. (1996). Sequential application of major habit-reversal components to treat motor tics in children. *Journal of Applied Behavior Analysis, 29*, 483–493.

Woods, D. W., Piacentini, J., Chang, S. W., Deckersbach, T., Ginsburg, G. S., Peterson, A. L., ... Wilhelm, S. (2008). *Managing Tourette syndrome: A behavioral intervention for children and adolescents*. New York: Oxford University Press.

ARTIST'S NOTE

The idea behind the drawing revolves around the feeling of rebirth, strength and victory one feels when their treatment is successful. Living with Tourettes is often very difficult. There were times when [this artist] felt despair and fear that he would never feel better. With the right therapies, he is like a new person- more confident, happy, and proud. The drawing symbolizes this through the language of flowers: as you may know certain flowers and plants have a meaning and symbolize a particular thought or feeling. The large teal figure represents all who are struggling with Tourette Syndrome. The figure is before an oak tree which symbolizes strength and endurance. In the picture are these additional flowers/plants: palm leaves—victory and success; nasturtium—victory in battle; cactus—endurance; iris—hope; white heather—wishes will come true, protection; gladiolus—strength; holly—hope; coriander—hidden worth—Tank James, age 19.

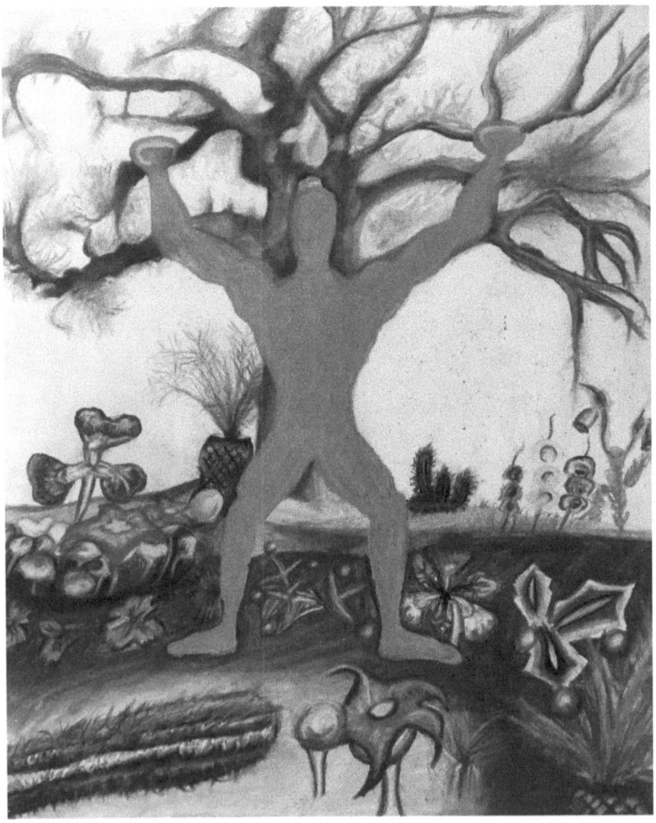

Chapter 2

Psychoeducation About Tic Disorders and Treatment

Monica S. Wu, PhD[1] and Joseph F. McGuire, PhD[2]
[1]UCLA Semel Institute for Neuroscience and Human Behavior, Los Angeles, CA, United States,
[2]Department of Psychiatry and Behavioral Sciences, Johns Hopkins University School of Medicine, Baltimore, MD, United States

When patients, parents, and families first present to a clinician's office, they often have many questions about tics and tic disorders. These questions can cover a variety of topics such as etiology ("*What is a tic and what causes them?*"), clinical course ("*What can we expect now for my child?*"), prognosis ("*Will my child's tics ever go away?*"), and treatment ("*How can we help our child manage the tics so they can have a normal life?*"). Psychoeducation plays an important role in treatment as it serves to educate the patient and family about tic disorders, provides important information to answer their questions, and can address misconceptions about the condition and its treatment. It also presents the opportunity to reduce stigma by normalizing the difficulties the patient and family may be experiencing. Indeed, practice parameters from professional organizations recommend psychoeducation as the primary intervention when tics are mild in severity, and consider it an important aspect of treatment for any tic disorder regardless of severity (Murphy, Lewin, Storch, Stock, & AACAP Committee on QualityIssues, 2013). For those youth and families requiring intervention beyond psychoeducation, it also presents the chance to orient the patient and family to the treatment model and to address any treatment concerns. This chapter provides an overview of psychoeducation on tic disorders and offers a practical approach with examples of how to convey this information to patients and families. For those youth with tic disorders requiring habit reversal training (HRT) and/or pharmacotherapy to reduce tic symptom severity, the chapter outlines the neurobehavioral treatment model of tic disorders. Finally, the chapter concludes with guidance on addressing common myths and misconceptions related to treatment.

The Clinician's Guide to Treatment and Management of Youth with Tourette Syndrome and Tic Disorders.
DOI: https://doi.org/10.1016/B978-0-12-811980-8.00002-9

PSYCHOEDUCATION ABOUT TICS AND TIC DISORDERS

What are tics and what is a Tic Disorder? When patients and families first arrive in a clinician's office, there may be considerable confusion as to what constitutes a "tic." Indeed, patients and parents may refer to certain actions and/or behaviors as "tics" when in fact they are better characterized as ritualized behaviors associated with obsessive–compulsive disorder (OCD; e.g., "handwashing tic," "evening up tic"), body-focused repetitive behaviors (BFRBs; e.g., hair pulling, nail biting, or skin picking), or a stereotypic movement (e.g., hand flapping). A tic is a sudden, recurrent, nonrhythmic motor movement or vocalization (American Psychiatric Association, 2013). Although there is some shared phenomenology with "not just right sensations" associated with OCD (Mansueto & Keuler, 2005), tics are largely different from ritualized behaviors of OCD that are performed to alleviate obsession-induced distress. Tics are also notably different from BFRBs, which are obsessive–compulsive-related disorders that involve compulsively damaging one's physical appearance in a way that can cause physical, social, and emotional injury. Similarly, tics are different from stereotypies, which are stereotyped motor movements that are often more fixed, rhythmic, and prolonged in duration (American Psychiatric Association, 2013). Common bothersome motor tics include eye blinking, head jerks, shoulder shrugs, and hand movements, with common bothersome vocal tics including sniffing, throat clearing, animal noises, and coughing (McGuire, Piacentini, et al., 2015). This presentation is different from OCD rituals (e.g., handwashing, rereading, or checking behaviors), common BFRBs that include hair pulling, nail biting, and skin picking, or even common stereotypies that include hand flapping, finger licking, body rocking, self-biting, and head banging. Given that co-occurring BFRBs and/or stereotypic movements may be present, it is important to accurately differentiate between these symptoms as their clinical course and response to intervention can differ. Moreover, as the interventions and therapeutic skills described in this book are focused on tics and tic-related phenomenon, their treatment response may not adequately generalize to these other psychiatric symptoms due to the phenomenological distinction. Although there are shared features between evidence-based treatments for tics and BFRBs like hair pulling (McGuire, Ung, et al., 2014), the therapeutic components that are emphasized in treatment are different. When clarifying the difference between tics and other related psychiatric symptoms, a clinician might say the following for a patient with tics and OCD symptoms:

> *I know that we've covered a lot of information today, but I just want to take some time to discuss the difference between tics and some of the other behaviors you mentioned. A tic is a sudden, rapid, and recurrent motor movement or vocalization. To help illustrate this point, let us think about some of the behaviors we have discussed today. Your eye blinking, neck rolling, shoulder*

shrugs and sniffing seem to all fit this description. We also talked about some other behaviors that you do, in which you feel the need to repeat things over and over again, such as repetitive hand washing and showering multiple times a day. You said that you did these behaviors when you touched something that you were worried was contaminated. These repetitive behaviors do not seem to fit the description of tics, but are called compulsions. While many children with tics also have compulsive behaviors, it is important to understand the difference because the way that we think about them and will treat them in therapy will be different.

Tics are relatively common among children and adolescents, with up to 20% of school-aged youth reported to have a tic for some period of time (Kurlan et al., 2002). In most cases, tics that emerge during this period will fade away just as they came within 6 months. However, when tics persist longer than a year, the diagnosis of a tic disorder should be considered. The term "tic disorders" is a broad umbrella term that reflects the myriad ways that tics can manifest in youth. Especially for youth and parents who are learning about the diagnosis for the first time, it is helpful to differentiate between the various types of tic typology and tic disorders. Tics are categorized by type (motor or vocal) and complexity, such as simple or complex (Tourette Syndrome Classification Study Group, 1993). Motor tics require some type of physical movement or kinetics (e.g., toe curling or arm tensing), whereas vocal tics are characterized by the passage of air in some capacity that typically produces an audible noise (e.g., sniffing, throat clearing, chirping). Meanwhile, tic complexity is characterized by its automatic/purposeful nature. For example, simple tics are brief, repetitive, meaningless movements (e.g., eye blinking, nose movements, head jerk) or vocalizations (e.g., coughing, throat clearing, sniffing). Comparatively, complex tics are often involve larger muscle groups (for motor tics) and appear more purposeful in nature. Complex motor tics could include a purposeful head-rolling motion, running fingers through hair, or copropraxia (i.e., obscene gestures), whereas complex phonic tics could include syllables, words, short phrases (e.g., "oh boy," "you bet"), coprolalia (i.e., saying obscene words), or echolalia (i.e., repeating sounds/words).

Given that many youth and parents may be unaware (or confused) by various tic disorder diagnoses, discussion of the diagnostic criteria surrounding tic disorders can be clarifying. Indeed, Tourette syndrome (TS) is often used colloquially as a catch-all for any tic disorder, and can sometimes be perceived by patients and families as having greater severity. Thus, informing parents that a diagnosis of TS only conveys that both motor *and* vocal tics are present for a year or more can be helpful (American Psychiatric Association, 2013). Meanwhile, when only one type of tic (motor or vocal) is present for a year or more, then a persistent tic disorder should be considered. However, when tics (motor, vocal, or both) have been present for less than a year, a provisional tic disorder is most applicable. Persistent tic disorders and Tourette disorder are not entirely uncommon among youth, with well-controlled studies suggesting that 4–8 youth out of every 1000 have a persistent tic disorder or Tourette disorder (Scahill, Specht, & Page, 2014). Thus, the type, timeline, and duration of tics are considered in establishing the diagnosis, and not the severity per se. Through clarification regarding the various tic diagnoses, parents will be better equipped to use the correct terminology and minimize any confusion.

What causes tics? After characterizing tics and establishing the appropriate tic disorder diagnosis, patients and families will often inquire into the cause of tics and tic disorders. Parents presenting to a clinician's office commonly convey perplexity regarding the source of these behaviors in hopes of better understanding the etiology and subsequent interventions. Similar to other disorders, there are multiple components that contribute to the etiology of tics. First, existing literature has demonstrated some genetic associations (Tarnok et al., 2007) as well as familial risks of tic disorders (Mataix-Cols et al., 2015). Second, tic expression has also been shown to be influenced by neurotransmitters in the brain (e.g., dopamine; Singer, Hahn, & Moran, 1991), specifically in brain circuits (cortico-striatal-thalamo-cortical loop (CSTC); Kates et al., 2002; Rauch et al., 2001). Third, there is substantive evidence regarding the influence of internal and external factors in tic expression, which will be discussed at length later in the chapter, as it is an important part of behavioral interventions for tic disorders. Given the confluence of factors that contribute to the etiology and expression of tic disorders, families can display some confusion about the multiple reasons for why their child has tics. As such, a simplified dialogue about the purported causes of tics may be helpful to provide psychoeducation about the etiology and alleviate uncertainty about the disorder:

> *It can be confusing and sometimes frightening to see a child's tics if there is some uncertainty about where they are coming from or what causes them. Based on the research that we know so far, it appears that there are a number of different factors that can contribute to tics and impact how the tics are expressed. There are some genetic components, in which we see certain genes and familial lineage in the passage of tic disorders. There are also some brain-based factors, where certain chemicals and connections in the brain can influence tics. Lastly, environmental factors that are observed within the child and around the child can definitely influence how the tics present as well. In sum, there is no specific answer for what causes tic disorders, but the aforementioned components work together in various ways to influence how tics are developed and how they manifest in your child.*

By providing this psychoeducation, it can also help reduce stigma and allow family members to better understand tic disorders. Indeed, this component of treatment can be utilized to ameliorate any blame that might be perceived, particularly if there is not a good understanding of what causes tics.

In these cases, directly addressing this with families can help set a positive precedent for moving forward and facilitate a better appreciation for what the child is experiencing. Example dialogue may be approached in the following way:

Parent: *"I do not understand why he can't just stop it. I really feel like he is doing it on purpose just to annoy us!"*

Clinician: *"I understand that the tics can be quite startling and bothersome at times. Indeed, it is highly likely that Billy is quite bothered by them as well! It unfortunately isn't something that Billy can stop all together at once if he simply 'wishes to.' Tic disorders have genetic, neurobiological, and environmental factors that make it hard for him to control these behaviors on his own. As all of these factors work together to influence the expression of his tics, we can understand how it can be more complex than simply willing himself to cease all of his vocal sounds and motor tics."*

What is the clinical course of tic disorders? Parents often inquire about the clinical course of tic disorders and the waxing/waning nature of the symptoms. The tics associated with tic disorders typically emerge in early childhood (e.g., 4–6 years of age), with the number, frequency, and intensity of tics reportedly peaking in early adolescent years (Bloch & Leckman, 2009; Leckman et al., 1998). Thereafter, many youth are observed to have their tic symptom severity greatly attenuate by early adulthood (with some individuals still exhibiting tics, but much decreased in frequency and related interference), but approximately a quarter of youth will still experience significant tic symptoms (Bloch & Leckman, 2009). Thus, the long-term outcome can be positive for many children who exhibit tics at a young age and even those with a tic disorder. While elevated tic symptom severity can persist into adulthood for some, many adults with tic disorders lead productive lives and make valuable contributions to society (e.g., Tim Howard, the US soccer goalkeeper, or possibly Wolfgang Amadeus Mozart, the classical composer). However, an important consideration in the long-term prognosis is how the child or adolescent copes with having tics, as the youth may rely upon maladaptive coping strategies that could lead to a negative developmental trajectory and a poor quality of life later.

Throughout the course of the disorder, tics exhibit a waxing and waning nature typically over a period of weeks (Lin et al., 2002). As a result, parents commonly wonder if tics will remit on their own or if intervention is indicated for their child. Tic symptom severity, tic impairment, and developmental considerations are all important aspects to consider with the family to determine the necessity and intensity of intervention needed. For instance, if a child's tics are nascent, sporadic, and occur without any distress or impairment, then there may be no need to implement intervention beyond psychoeducation. Alternatively, if the child has had tics for several years, the tics are increasing in intensity and complexity, and the tics are causing physical distress, then direct intervention is recommended. Indeed, practice parameters recommend behavior therapy such as HRT when tics cause impairment or are moderate in severity, with the incorporation of pharmacotherapy recommended only when patients have moderate to severe tics that cause severe impairment (Murphy et al., 2013).

Some parents may present with heightened anxiety about their child's tics and demand overt attention on these behaviors and intensive intervention, despite the lack of impairment and mild severity of the tics. In these cases, it may be helpful to provide more intensive psychoeducation with these families, supplemented with validation of the caregiver's desire to help their child and careful assessment of the interference/distress related to these behaviors.

Parent: *"Billy started displaying these really weird behaviors 2 months ago. I feel like all the kindergarteners are going to look at him weird when he's blinking excessively and then he's going to get made fun of! I really feel that we need to tackle this immediately, since I don't want him to get made fun of or have this get out of hand."*

Clinician: *"I hear your concern and can definitely understand why these behaviors may seem strange to you. Billy is right around the age where tics may first start manifesting in children, as we previously discussed regarding the typical timeline of the development of tics. It seems like these behaviors are still pretty early on in their development. Has Billy mentioned anything or have you seen anything about how it may be bothering him, bothering others, or making it hard for him to do anything he wants to do? For instance, does he complain that he wants them to stop or does he avoid certain things because of his tics?"*

Parent: *"Well, no, he doesn't even seem to care that he has these tics and when I ask other people, they say that they don't even notice these behaviors. It seems like I'm the only one that cares right now, but I just feel like if I don't do something about it now, it's going to get worse and go on forever."*

Clinician: *"Your concerns are completely understandable. I think it is quite telling and important to consider Billy's point of view, as well as others that are in close contact with him. From what I am hearing, it seems like Billy isn't experiencing much distress or impairment from it, and none of his teachers, friends, or relatives have paid particular attention to it. This is not uncommon, as many kids may experience tics at some point in their lives, but they also have been observed to go away on their own without any treatment. Given the low impairment and distress that it's causing right now, he may very well fall into that category. Why don't we monitor his tics from afar for the time being to see if there are any changes in his tic frequency, severity, or complexity? If things change, we can reassess and potentially begin intervening then."*

What are the factors that influence tic expression? When discussing clinical course and the waxing/waning nature of tic symptoms, parents (and youth) often have questions about the factors that influence tic expression. Indeed, parents often describe a flare-up of tics "out of nowhere," also reporting the occurrence of a supposedly inexplicable attenuation in tic frequency and severity. As such, it is helpful for parents to learn about the role of various internal and external factors in influencing tic expression.

Internal factors are factors that are influenced by the internal experiences of the child. For instance, common internal factors influencing tic expression are anxiety, stress, as well as premonitory urges. With an increase of these internal factors, it is likely that an increase in tics will be observed. Conversely, with a decrease of these internal factors (e.g., lower stress or anxiety), an abatement of tics often occurs. External factors, on the other hand, are factors that occur in the child's environment and subsequently influence tic expression. For instance, environments that elicit high stress (e.g., high family conflict at home, low social support, stressful life events such as the loss of a loved one), represent undesirable activities (e.g., homework), or cause anxiety (e.g., novel social situations) are likely to increase tics. On the other hand, certain external factors can also contribute to decreased tics, such as engaging in motor activities (e.g., sports), a relaxing stress-free environment, engaging in positive social supports, as well as good sleeping/eating/exercise habits.

To facilitate this discussion with families, it can be helpful to start off with an assessment of what types of factors have been observed to make their child's tics better or worse. Once the parents are able to provide certain examples, the clinician can use this information to place it within the context of internal/external factors influencing tic expression and normalize this experience.

Clinician: *"So you just told me that when Billy gets really stressed about doing well at school, his tics seem to 'flare up' quite a bit. However, when he's doing something active, like soccer, you really don't see any tics at all. I can appreciate why it has been confusing for you, as it seems like his tics appear to come and go in certain situations. That is completely normal, and it is indeed the case that certain factors can influence the expression of his tics. Specifically, there are certain things that happen internally and externally that often impact the frequency and severity of tics. Let's talk a bit about some common factors..."*

What are the common problems youth with tics experience? When providing psychoeducation about tics and tic disorders, it is important to remember that tics are often the overt behavioral symptoms that are noticed. However, youth with tic disorders experience a wide range of difficulties and challenges. For instance, given the high preponderance of comorbidities in these youth (Bloch & Leckman, 2009), these youth may also struggle with other disorders such as attention-deficit hyperactivity disorder (ADHD) and OCD (Freeman & Tourette Syndrome International Database Consortium, 2007; Sheppard, Bradshaw, Purcell, & Pantelis, 1999). Psychosocial interference may also be observed, with youth exhibiting difficulties in the social, behavioral, and emotional domains. Socially, these youth can have poorer self-perception, lower self-concept, and increased peer teasing (Cutler, Murphy, Gilmour, & Heyman, 2009; Hanks, McGuire, Lewin, Storch, &

Murphy, 2016; McGuire, Hanks, Lewin, Storch, & Murphy, 2013; Stokes, Bawden, Camfield, Backman, & Dooley, 1991). Secondary to the tics, these youth may experience some consequent anxiety, depressive symptoms, and suicidal ideation (Bloch & Leckman, 2009; Johnco et al., 2016; Storch et al., 2015). Behavioral difficulties can also co-occur, including rage, aggression, and/or disruptive behaviors (Budman, Bruun, Park, & Olson, 1998; Chen et al., 2013). Collectively, it is evident that tics are not the entire problem, but may be the most noticeable difficulty. As such, clinicians and parents should be watchful of co-occurring difficulties in youth with tic disorders.

PSYCHOEDUCATION ABOUT INTERVENTIONS FOR TICS AND TIC DISORDERS

There are two primary evidence-based treatment options for tic disorders, namely pharmacotherapy and behavior therapy. As previously mentioned, behavior therapy (e.g., HRT, comprehensive behavioral intervention for tics) is recommended when tics are moderate in severity or cause impairment, with the combination of pharmacotherapy and behavior therapy recommended for moderate to severe tics causing severe impairment (Murphy et al., 2013). In either case, it is important to clearly explain the treatment model so that parents and youth understand the rationale and approach to intervention.

Orientation to the Neurobehavioral Treatment Model

Although genetic, environmental, and neurobiological factors have been associated with the emergence of tics and tic disorders (see earlier sections), tics themselves are neurological in origin and are suggested to come from dysregulation in cortico-striato-thalamo-cortical (CSTC) pathways in the brain (Mink, 2001). Several neurotransmitters have been implicated within the CTSC pathway (dopamine, glutamate, serotonin, GABA, acetylcholine), but no one specific neurotransmitter has been suggested to account for the pathophysiology of tics and tic disorders. Several psychotropic medications that target neurotransmitters have been investigated in randomized controlled trials and found to influence tic symptom severity in youth and adults with tic disorders. These medications include antipsychotics (e.g., haloperidol, pimozide, risperidone, ziprasidone, aripiprazole), alpha agonists (e.g., clonidine, guanfacine), anticonvulsants (e.g., topiramate, levetiracetam, baclofen), and many others (see Egolf and Coffey (2014) for a comprehensive review), with the best available evidence for antipsychotic and alpha agonists classes of medication (see Chapter 4: Pharmacological Management of Tic Disorders in Youth for further discussion of tic medication management). While several other pharmacological and/or novel neurotherapeutics have been explored for tic disorders (e.g., deep brain stimulation, delta-9-tetrahydrocannabinol, biofeedback, nutritional supplements), these interventions either have limited evaluation in youth, demonstrated minimal efficacy in controlled clinical trials, or are intended only for refractory cases.

In addition to the neurobiological contributions (Felling & Singer, 2011; Leckman, Bloch, Smith, Larabi, & Hampson, 2010), environmental factors play an influential role in the exacerbation and maintenance of tic symptoms (Silva, Munoz, Barickman, & Friedhoff, 1995). Specifically, different antecedents and consequences (both internal and external) can influence the expression of tics, and these environmental factors serve as the crux of the behavioral treatment of tic symptoms (Woods, Piacentini, et al., 2008). To understand the maintaining forces acting upon the tics, the antecedents, behaviors, and consequences need to be considered. Antecedents are factors that occur before the behavior (tics). Common internal antecedents include anxiety, stress, and/or premonitory urges. Premonitory urges are a somatosensory sensation that youth and adults describe as an internal discomfort, "itchiness," or "pressure," which occurs right before the tic and is relieved by the performance of the tic (Leckman, Walker, & Cohen, 1993). However, younger children may have difficulty identifying and/or recognizing premonitory urges. External antecedents are considered to be the settings or actions that precede a tic, such as being in certain contexts (e.g., home, school, being alone), engaging in certain activities (e.g., playing sports, video games), or experiencing an event (e.g., teasing). To help illustrate the salience of internal/external factors in impacting tic expression, it can be helpful to use the specific factors that are known to influence the expression of tics in that particular child in the discussion. For instance, if a child has previously mentioned that playing soccer tends to make his tics go away, a sample dialogue could be: "*So Billy, I know you told me earlier that your tics seem to be better when you're playing at a soccer game. We actually see this quite a lot in kids with tics, in which certain activities or emotional states affect how their tics are. Can you think of other activities or times when your tics are better or worse?*"

After the tic occurs, there are internal and external consequences that follow. Internally, youth and adults with tics report that the tic alleviates the premonitory urge and its associated distress. This creates a negative reinforcement cycle whereby tic symptoms are reinforced due to the alleviation of the associated urge/distress (Capriotti, Brandt, Turkel, Lee, & Woods, 2014; Woods, Piacentini, Himle, & Chang, 2005). External consequences can also occur, maintaining and/or exacerbating the tics (Conelea & Woods, 2008b). For instance, parents may provide extra attention during bouts of tics, which subsequently reinforces tic symptoms as the youth receives additional parental time. Alternatively, allowing the child to avoid homework or undesirable tasks because of the tics can also be reinforcing, as it is facilitating avoidance of an otherwise boring activity (Storch et al., 2016).

Collectively, these aforementioned factors and processes can be placed within a conditioning model. As tics occur, the internal/external factors become associated with the tics and functionally "conditioned" with one another. Therefore, the focus of behavioral interventions is to develop new associations whereby internal/external factors do not become continually associated with the tic. Indeed, this association serves to compete with and inhibit the initially learned association.

The Neurobehavioral Model in Practice

When considering medications, pharmacotherapy works by increasing neurotransmitters in the brain to counter the CTSC dysregulation. As multiple neurotransmitters may be in play, it may require finding the right medication (if needed) for the patient. See Chapter 4, Pharmacological Management of Tic Disorders in Youth, for further guidance regarding selecting the appropriate medications for the child.

When consider behavioral interventions, HRT is a multicomponent treatment for tics, with the primary components being (Woods, Miltenberger, & Lumley, 1996): (1) awareness training, (2) competing response training, and (3) social support.

All components of HRT are used to break the negative reinforcement cycle and create new learning associations to compete with initial associations. Building awareness into the occurrence of tics is an important first step for children to follow (Himle, Woods, Piacentini, & Walkup, 2006), as independent use of the competing responses will be dependent on whether or not the child realizes when the tics occur. Once awareness has been built for specific tics, the child and the family segue into competing response training (Himle et al., 2006; Piacentini & Chang, 2005). Competing responses are generally characterized as behaviors that are physically incompatible with the tic itself (e.g., clenching their hand into a fist if they have tapping tics). Ideally, competing response should also be relatively inconspicuous when compared to the tic and should also be able to be sustained for a period of time to promote generalizability of these skills in various settings. Social supports can be considered within the familial context, such as having family members help the child achieve treatment goals (Piacentini et al., 2010). As children are expected to be practicing HRT-related tasks at home, caregivers are in a unique position to help implement these techniques outside of therapy sessions, praising the child for the correct implementation of the techniques, and also gently (and neutrally) reminding the child to remember to use the skills. Relaxation training can also be used as an adjunct to reduce stress/anxiety (other internal triggers), and generalization training will be used to generalize learning across challenging environments (external factors). See McGuire, Ricketts, et al. (2015) for a detailed discussion of the components of HRT.

When considering the use of pharmacotherapy and behavioral interventions together, they can synergistically target the tics in an effective manner. As the optimal medication is identified for the child and titrated to an appropriate dose, the "volume" of the tics can be turned down as well, making the tics easier to manage. The skills acquired in the behavioral interventions will help target tics and break the aforementioned associations, so that new ones that are formed become more natural. It is noted that habituation to the unpleasant premonitory urge is not necessary during the treatment of tics, but can be helpful to reduce patient distress.

Therapeutic Outcomes With the Neurobehavioral Model

While often examined individually in the context of clinical trials, these therapeutic components (pharmacotherapy and HRT) significantly reduce tic symptom severity. For instance, meta-analytic investigations of clinical trials of antipsychotic medications found a significant moderate-sized reduction in tic symptom severity relative to placebo (effect size = 0.58), with no significant difference between medication types (Weisman, Qureshi, Leckman, Scahill, & Bloch, 2013). Meanwhile, a meta-analysis of alpha-2 agonist medications found a small reduction in tic symptom severity on the whole (effect size = 0.31) that was considerably larger when circumscribed to only youth who presented with both tic disorders and ADHD (effect size = 0.68; Weisman et al., 2013). Although able to reduce tic symptom severity, these medications are often accompanied by side effects that may limit the long-term tolerability. Moreover, these medications reduce tic symptom severity, but many tics continue to persist despite continued pharmacotherapy.

When considering the efficacy of behavioral interventions like HRT and comprehensive behavioral intervention for tics (CBIT) for youth with tic disorders, significant decreases in tic symptom severity have been observed immediately following eight sessions of treatment (Piacentini et al., 2010). Additionally, treatment gains are noted to be maintained 6 months after therapy for the large majority of children with no decrease in academic or psychosocial functioning (Woods et al., 2011). A meta-analytic investigation of behavior therapy clinical trials (HRT and CBIT) found a medium-to-large reduction in tic symptom severity (effect size = 0.67–0.94) in comparison to control conditions (McGuire, Piacentini, et al., 2014). This investigation found several factors to influence the therapeutic benefit of behavioral interventions. Increased age and therapeutic contact were found to be associated with larger treatment effects (i.e., greater reductions in tic symptom severity), whereas the increased presence of co-occurring ADHD was associated with smaller treatment effects (i.e., less reductions in tic symptom severity; McGuire, Piacentini, et al., 2014). However, it should be noted that this does not suggest that youth with tic disorders and ADHD would not benefit from behavior therapy, rather that the reductions after a "standard course" may be smaller. Irrespective of these enhancing or attenuating factors, it is important to consider that few tics remit in response to a standard course of behavior therapy (McGuire, Piacentini, et al., 2015).

In summary, whether the patient receives behavior therapy, pharmacotherapy, or their combination, tics will continue to persist and likely continue to cause adverse psychosocial consequences. Thus, the skills outlined in this book play a key role in not only helping to reduce tic symptom severity, but also in developing skills to overcome tic-related impairment, establish effective and efficient coping strategies to manage the adverse psychosocial consequences of tics in the short term, and develop resiliency to manage tics and associated difficulties in the long term.

THE FIRST STEP TOWARD INTERVENTION

Consistent with the neurobehavioral model and considering the impact of contextual influences, parents are encouraged to create and maintain a "tic-neutral environment" that prevents the tics from being inadvertently reinforced (Capriotti, Himle, & Woods, 2014; Franklin, Harrison, & Benavides, 2013; Woods, Piacentini, et al., 2008). It is helpful to clarify that parental responses, whether positive or negative, are reinforcing; any attention paid to the tics may be strengthening tic expression. Examples should be provided to help illustrate the types of relevant behaviors, including but not limited to: (1) asking if the child had any tics at school, (2) comforting the child every time he/she has a tic, (3) yelling at the child to stop when seeing tics, and (4) nonverbal attention such as purposefully "watching like a hawk." It is important to clarify that parents can still monitor a patient's tics without becoming intrusive, and can engage with the child when needing to prompt the use of therapeutic skills. In the spirit of maintaining a tic-neutral environment, clinicians should conscientiously review the appropriate expectations and potentially restrict the number of reminders from the caregiver by either frequency or time blocks (e.g., five reminders maximum per hour) as indicated.

COMMON MYTHS AND MISCONCEPTIONS ABOUT TIC DISORDERS AND TREATMENT

Many youth, parents, and family members (and even clinicians, sometimes!) have misconceptions about tic disorders and/or interventions to manage them. These myths and misperceptions can perpetuate stigma and even impede the utilization of evidence-based treatments for tic disorders (Scahill et al., 2013; Woods, Conelea, & Walther, 2007). Several common myths and misconceptions are reviewed here, with corrective feedback provided on how to address them.

I thought all children with TS curse? Although often believed to be prototypic of TS, coprophenomena is not all that frequent among youth with TS. Coprophenomena include copropraxia (making obscene gestures), coprolalia (saying obscene words), and bouts of uncontrolled cursing. It affects an estimated 19% of patients with TS at some point in their lives (Freeman et al., 2009), with point-prevalence estimates from treatment-seeking samples of youth (3%–4%) and adults (3%–8%) reported to be even lower (McGuire, Nyirabahizi, et al., 2013). Corprolalia (i.e., saying obscene words, cussing, etc.) has been found to occur more frequently than copropraxia (obscene gestures), with an average age of onset occurring around 11 years old (Freeman et al., 2009). However, in approximately 11%–12% of cases in which coprophenomena were present, it was reported to be one of the initial tic symptoms (Freeman et al., 2009). For those youth who do experience coprophenomena as the first tic symptoms, there is no evidence that early coprophenomena serves as a harbinger of a longer persistence of tic symptoms. When patients, parents, or clinicians present concerns related to coprophenomena, it is important to inform them that there is actually a limited chance that youth with tic disorders will exhibit coprophenomena at some point in their lives. However, when it is present, providing parents with the knowledge that early-onset coprophenomena does not serve as an indicator of its prolonged persistence can be reassuring.

Talking about tics or focusing attention on tics makes tics worse. There is a belief among some patients, parents, and health-care providers that talking about tics (Marcks, Woods, Teng, & Twohig, 2004) or focusing attention on tics will make them worse (Shimberg, 1995). As a result, some youth and/or parents may not wish to pursue treatment because it will involve talking about tics, which "makes them worse." When patients or parents raise these questions, it is important to validate their concern. Indeed, there is evidence to suggest that tic-related discussions and direct attention can momentarily increase tic frequency (Piacentini et al., 2006; Woods, Twohig, Flessner, & Roloff, 2003). However, awareness training (a core component of HRT) and self-monitoring of tics has actually been shown to produce modest reductions in tics (Woods et al., 1996). Thus, while there may be a momentary increase, talking about tics and utilizing evidence-based strategies actually reduces tic symptom severity over the long term.

Tic suppression leads to an increase in tic frequency. Patients, parents, and clinicians will sometimes express concern that strategies which suppress tics (i.e., tic suppression, competing responses) inadvertently produce increased tic frequency when suppression strategies are discontinued, often called a "tic rebound" effect. Indeed, many parents will report that after their child has "suppressed" tics all day at school, they will come home and have a surge or explosion of tic symptoms. Accordingly, many parents and youth may be wary to implement the competing responses included in HRT. Therefore, it is helpful to assuage this fear by explaining to parents and youth that this phenomenon has been examined in various studies in both research laboratory and treatment, with no evidence in support of this fear (Himle & Woods, 2005; Specht et al., 2013; Verdellen, Hoogduin, & Keijsers, 2007). Indeed, these studies have found that the return of tics typically do not exceed the child's average baseline number of tics.

If my child can suppress his/her tics, then he/she should be able to do it all the time. Many youth are able to suppress their tics (either partially or entirely) for some period of the time (Conelea & Woods, 2008a; Specht et al., 2013; Woods, Himle, et al., 2008). However, little is known about the precise neurobiological mechanism of tic suppression (in the absence of behavioral strategies), with evidence suggesting that differential reinforcement enhances youth's ability to suppress tics (Conelea & Woods, 2008b; Greene et al., 2015; Himle, Woods, & Bunaciu, 2008; Woods & Himle, 2004). This is consistent with anecdotal reports from youth and parents that tics are minimal at school due to active tic suppression efforts. Naturally, many parents have raised the question why children cannot suppress their tics all the time, and engage in tic suppression at both home and school. Indeed, one type of behavioral intervention for tics specifically instructs youth to practice tic suppression as the primary therapeutic component (Verdellen, Keijsers, Cath, & Hoogduin, 2004). Although youth have been found to successfully engage in tic suppression for up to 40 minutes when differentially reinforced (Woods, Himle, et al., 2008), there can be consequences. While there is no empirical evidence for "tic rebounds" following suppression (as noted earlier), evidence suggests that performance on attention-demanding tasks can be negatively impacted if a child is simultaneously suppressing tics (Conelea & Woods, 2008a). On the other hand, there has been no negative impact on academic performance, neuropsychological functioning, or other psychosocial outcomes for youth who successfully utilize HRT strategies (Chang et al., 2018; Woods et al., 2011). Therefore, youth and their parents be encouraged to utilize behavior therapy skills rather than relying upon tic suppression.

Targeting tics with behavior therapy will make other tics or symptoms worse. Some parents and mental health providers have a misconception that behavior therapy can lead to symptom substitution. Specifically, parents express concerns that treating some tics will worsen other tic symptoms, cause new tics to develop as initial tics are managed, or lead to a worsening of other psychiatric symptoms overall. Although symptom substitution was initially identified in a few anecdotal case reports (Burd & Kerbeshian, 1987, 1988), systematic empirical evaluations have found no evidence that treating tics with behavior therapy causes other tic symptoms to worsen, leads to the development of new tics, or worsens psychosocial symptoms in comparison to the nontargeted interventions (Peterson et al., 2016; Woods et al., 2003). Thus, the anecdotal reports of new tic symptom onset or tic symptom worsening are likely attributed to the normal waxing and waning nature of tic disorders. In short, there does not appear to be any significant evidence that treating tics with behavior therapy will worsen other psychiatric symptoms or create new ones.

In line with this concern, some youth and/or parents may also be confused by the difference between the "tic" and the "competing response." Indeed, some youth and parents may inquire whether behavior therapy just replaces the initial tic (e.g., an arm jerk), with a "new tic" (e.g., folded arms as the competing response). It is important to help the patient and parent understand that the competing response is not a tic, with the primary distinction being that the competing response is voluntary whereas the tic is not. If youth or parents continue to struggle to discern the difference, it may be helpful to review the definition of the tic covered earlier in the chapter with them to help them recognize the distinction.

Behavior therapy and pharmacotherapy will make tics go away. As mentioned earlier, behavior therapy and pharmacotherapy are the two primary evidence-based interventions for reducing tic symptom severity (Murphy et al., 2013). While 53% of youth receiving behavior therapy were found to exhibit a treatment response in a controlled clinical trial (Piacentini et al., 2010), treatment response rates are less definitive for pharmacotherapy trials due to multiple types and classes of medication. In either case, a treatment response among youth with tic disorders corresponds with a 25%–35% reduction in tic symptom severity on semi-structured clinician-administered scales (Jeon et al., 2013; Storch et al., 2011). While some tics have been found to remit in response to behavior therapy (McGuire, Piacentini, et al., 2015), tics on the whole do not. Therefore, it is important to temper the expectations of youth and parents who are receiving evidence-based interventions for tics about appropriate reductions in tic symptom severity to minimize any confusion.

Once the tics go away, my child will no longer have any more problems. Tics are the overt symptom of tic disorders and garner much attention. As such, some parents and youth enter treatment with the perception that when tics go away (or are under better control), any associated problems will also resolve. Although this may be true for some youth, it is not the case for every child. When evaluating the acute (10-week) and long-term (6-month) outcomes of a standard course of behavior therapy, youth who responded to treatment continued to exhibit reductions in tic symptom severity at the 6-month follow-up (Woods et al., 2011). However, there was no significant change in ADHD symptom severity, depressive symptoms, internalizing problems, externalizing problems, or any measure of psychosocial functioning (Woods et al., 2011). Meanwhile, there was significant reduction in disruptive behaviors, obsessive–compulsive symptom severity, and child-reported anxiety symptoms, with improvement observed in caregiver strain and social adjustment with friends (Woods et al., 2011). Taken together, this suggests that behavior therapy reduces tic symptom severity efficaciously but largely has minimal impact on other psychiatric or psychosocial difficulties. Thus, while some youth may only need a tic-specific intervention to reduce tic symptom severity, many others may require a more comprehensive treatment approach covered in this book. An evidence-based assessment (covered in Chapter 1: Introduction to Treatment and Management of Youth With Tourette Disorders and Tic Disorders) can help inform the magnitude of tic symptom severity, tic-related impairment, and quality of life to help inform treatment selection.

CONCLUSION

Given the complex etiology and variations in the topography of tic disorders, psychoeducation is an important first step of treatment. Information regarding the etiology, presentation, and treatment of tic disorders in youth is pertinent to helping families achieve a better understanding about the disorder; it is hoped to mitigate confusion and subsequent maladaptive responses to these behaviors as well. Depending on the severity of the tics, psychoeducation may be the only necessary intervention at the time for the family, or it may be a first step of a more comprehensive behavioral/pharmacological intervention for tics. Through the review of the typical components of psychoeducation and the inclusion of practice-friendly dialogue, this chapter is purposed to help clinicians discuss childhood tic disorders in a more accessible and comprehensible manner for families.

REFERENCES

American Psychiatric Association. (2013). *Diagnostic and statistical manual of mental disorders* (5th ed.). Arlington, VA: American Psychiatric Publishing.

Bloch, M. H., & Leckman, J. F. (2009). Clinical course of Tourette syndrome. *Journal of Psychosomatic Research*, *67*(6), 497–501. Available from https://doi.org/10.1016/j.jpsychores.2009.09.002.

Budman, C. L., Bruun, R. D., Park, K. S., & Olson, M. E. (1998). Rage attacks in children and adolescents with Tourette's disorder: A pilot study. *The Journal of Clinical Psychiatry*, *59* (11), 576–580.

Burd, L., & Kerbeshian, J. (1987). Treatment-generated problems associated with behavior modification in Tourette disorder. *Developmental Medicine and Child Neurology*, *29*(6), 831–833.

Burd, L., & Kerbeshian, J. (1988). Symptom substitution in Tourette disorder. *Lancet*, *2*(8619), 1072.

Capriotti, M. R., Brandt, B. C., Turkel, J. E., Lee, H. J., & Woods, D. W. (2014). Negative reinforcement and premonitory urges in youth with Tourette syndrome: An experimental evaluation. *Behavior Modification*, *38*(2), 276–296. Available from https://doi.org/10.1177/0145445514531015.

Capriotti, M. R., Himle, M. B., & Woods, D. W. (2014). Behavioral treatments for Tourette syndrome. *Journal of Obsessive–Compulsive and Related Disorders*, *3*(4), 415–420. Available from http://dx.doi.org/10.1016/j.jocrd.2014.03.007.

Chang, S., Deckersbach, T., McGuire, J.F., Walkup, J.T., Woods, D.W., Scahill, L., ... Piacentini, J. Neurocognitive correlates of treatment response in children with Tourette's disorder. *Psychiatry Research 261*, 2018. Available from https://doi.org/10.1016/j.psychres.2017.12.066.

Chen, K., Budman, C. L., Diego Herrera, L., Witkin, J. E., Weiss, N. T., Lowe, T. L., ... Mathews, C. A. (2013). Prevalence and clinical correlates of explosive outbursts in Tourette syndrome. *Psychiatry Research, 205*(3), 269–275. Available from https://doi.org/10.1016/j.psychres.2012.09.029.

Conelea, C. A., & Woods, D. W. (2008a). Examining the impact of distraction on tic suppression in children and adolescents with Tourette syndrome. *Behaviour Research and Therapy, 46* (11), 1193–1200. Available from https://doi.org/10.1016/j.brat.2008.07.005.

Conelea, C. A., & Woods, D. W. (2008b). The influence of contextual factors on tic expression in Tourette's syndrome: A review. *Journal of Psychosomatic Research, 65*(5), 487–496. Available from https://doi.org/10.1016/j.jpsychores.2008.04.010.

Cutler, D., Murphy, T., Gilmour, J., & Heyman, I. (2009). The quality of life of young people with Tourette syndrome. *Child: Care, Health and Development, 35*(4), 496–504. Available from https://doi.org/10.1111/j.1365-2214.2009.00983.x.

Egolf, A., & Coffey, B. J. (2014). Current pharmacotherapeutic approaches for the treatment of Tourette syndrome. *Drugs Today (Barc), 50*(2), 159–179. Available from https://doi.org/10.1358/dot.2014.50.2.2097801.

Felling, R. J., & Singer, H. S. (2011). Neurobiology of Tourette syndrome: Current status and need for further investigation. *Journal of Neuroscience, 31*(35), 12387–12395. Available from https://doi.org/10.1523/jneurosci.0150-11.2011.

Franklin, M. E., Harrison, J., & Benavides, K. (2013). Treatment of childhood tic disorders with comorbid OCD. In E. A. Storch, & D. McKay (Eds.), *Handbook of treating variants and complications in anxiety disorders* (pp. 135–148). New York: Springer New York.

Freeman, R. D., & Tourette Syndrome International Database Consortium. (2007). Tic disorders and ADHD: Answers from a world-wide clinical dataset on Tourette syndrome. *European Child & Adolescent Psychiatry, 16*(1), 15–23. Available from https://doi.org/10.1007/s00787-007-1003-7.

Freeman, R. D., Zinner, S. H., Muller-Vahl, K. R., Fast, D. K., Burd, L. J., Kano, Y., ... Berlin, C. M., Jr. (2009). Coprophenomena in Tourette syndrome. *Developmental Medicine and Child Neurology, 51*(3), 218–227. Available from https://doi.org/10.1111/j.1469-8749.2008.03135.x.

Greene, D. J., Koller, J. M., Robichaux-Viehoever, A., Bihun, E. C., Schlaggar, B. L., & Black, K. J. (2015). Reward enhances tic suppression in children within months of tic disorder onset. *Developmental Cognitive Neuroscience, 11*, 65–74. Available from https://doi.org/10.1016/j.dcn.2014.08.005.

Hanks, C. E., McGuire, J. F., Lewin, A. B., Storch, E. A., & Murphy, T. K. (2016). Clinical correlates and mediators of self-concept in youth with chronic tic disorders. *Child Psychiatry & Human Development, 47*(1), 64–74. Available from https://doi.org/10.1007/s10578-015-0544-0.

Himle, M. B., & Woods, D. W. (2005). An experimental evaluation of tic suppression and the tic rebound effect. *Behaviour Research and Therapy, 43*(11), 1443–1451. Available from https://doi.org/10.1016/j.brat.2004.11.002.

Himle, M. B., Woods, D. W., & Bunaciu, L. (2008). Evaluating the role of contingency in differentially reinforced tic suppression. *Journal of Applied Behavior Analysis, 41*(2), 285–289.

Himle, M. B., Woods, D. W., Piacentini, J. C., & Walkup, J. T. (2006). Brief review of habit reversal training for Tourette syndrome. *Journal of Child Neurology, 21*(8), 719–725.

Jeon, S., Walkup, J. T., Woods, D. W., Peterson, A., Piacentini, J., Wilhelm, S., ... Scahill, L. (2013). Detecting a clinically meaningful change in tic severity in Tourette syndrome: A comparison of three methods. *Contemporary Clinical Trials, 36*(2), 414–420. Available from https://doi.org/10.1016/j.cct.2013.08.012.

Johnco, C., McGuire, J. F., McBride, N. M., Murphy, T. K., Lewin, A. B., & Storch, E. A. (2016). Suicidal ideation in youth with tic disorders. *Journal of Affective Disorders, 200* (Suppl. C), 204–211. Available from https://doi.org/10.1016/j.jad.2016.04.027.

Kates, W. R., Frederikse, M., Mostofsky, S. H., Folley, B. S., Cooper, K., Mazur-Hopkins, P., ... Kaufmann, W. E. (2002). MRI parcellation of the frontal lobe in boys with attention deficit hyperactivity disorder or Tourette syndrome. *Psychiatry Research, 116*(1-2), 63–81.

Kurlan, R., Como, P. G., Miller, B., Palumbo, D., Deeley, C., Andresen, E. M., ... McDermott, M. P. (2002). The behavioral spectrum of tic disorders: A community-based study. *Neurology, 59*(3), 414–420.

Leckman, J. F., Bloch, M. H., Smith, M. E., Larabi, D., & Hampson, M. (2010). Neurobiological substrates of Tourette's Disorder. *Journal of Child and Adolescent Psychopharmacology, 20*(4), 237–247. Available from https://doi.org/10.1089/cap.2009.0118.

Leckman, J. F., Walker, D. E., & Cohen, D. J. (1993). Premonitory urges in Tourette's syndrome. *American Journal of Psychiatry, 150*(1), 9.

Leckman, J. F., Zhang, H., Vitale, A., Lahnin, F., Lynch, K., Bondi, C., ... Peterson, B. S. (1998). Course of tic severity in Tourette syndrome: The first two decades. *Pediatrics, 102* (1 Pt 1), 14–19.

Lin, H., Yeh, C. B., Peterson, B. S., Scahill, L., Grantz, H., Findley, D. B., ... Leckman, J. F. (2002). Assessment of symptom exacerbations in a longitudinal study of children with Tourette's syndrome or obsessive–compulsive disorder. *Journal of the American Academy of Child and Adolescent Psychiatry, 41*(9), 1070–1077. Available from https://doi.org/10.1097/00004583-200209000-00007.

Mansueto, C. S., & Keuler, D. J. (2005). Tic or compulsion? It's Tourettic OCD. *Behavior Modification, 29*(5), 784–799. Available from https://doi.org/10.1177/0145445505279261.

Marcks, B. A., Woods, D. W., Teng, E. J., & Twohig, M. P. (2004). What do those who know, know? Investigating providers' knowledge about Tourette's syndrome and its treatment. *Cognitive and Behavioral Practice, 11*(3), 298–305. Available from https://doi.org/10.1016/S1077-7229(04)80044-0.

Mataix-Cols, D., Isomura, K., Perez-Vigil, A., Chang, Z., Ruck, C., Larsson, K. J., ... Lichtenstein, P. (2015). Familial risks of Tourette syndrome and chronic tic disorders. A population-based cohort study. *JAMA Psychiatry, 72*(8), 787–793. Available from https://doi.org/10.1001/jamapsychiatry.2015.0627.

McGuire, J. F., Hanks, C., Lewin, A. B., Storch, E. A., & Murphy, T. K. (2013). Social deficits in children with chronic tic disorders: phenomenology, clinical correlates and quality of life. *Comprehensive Psychiatry, 54*(7), 1023–1031. Available from https://doi.org/10.1016/j.comppsych.2013.04.009.

McGuire, J. F., Nyirabahizi, E., Kircanski, K., Piacentini, J., Peterson, A. L., Woods, D. W., ... Scahill, L. (2013). A cluster analysis of tic symptoms in children and adults with Tourette syndrome: Clinical correlates and treatment outcome. *Psychiatry Research, 210*(3), 1198–1204. Available from https://doi.org/10.1016/j.psychres.2013.09.021.

McGuire, J. F., Piacentini, J., Brennan, E. A., Lewin, A. B., Murphy, T. K., Small, B. J., & Storch, E. A. (2014). A meta-analysis of behavior therapy for Tourette syndrome. *Journal of Psychiatric Research, 50*, 106–112. Available from https://doi.org/10.1016/j.jpsychires.2013.12.009.

McGuire, J. F., Piacentini, J., Scahill, L., Woods, D. W., Villarreal, R., Wilhelm, S., ... Peterson, A. L. (2015). Bothersome tics in patients with chronic tic disorders: Characteristics and individualized treatment response to behavior therapy. *Behaviour Research and Therapy, 70*, 56–63. Available from https://doi.org/10.1016/j.brat.2015.05.006.

McGuire, J. F., Ricketts, E. J., Piacentini, J., Murphy, T. K., Storch, E. A., & Lewin, A. B. (2015). Behavior therapy for tic disorders: An evidenced-based review and new directions for treatment research. *Current Developmental Disorders Reports, 2*(4), 309–317. Available from https://doi.org/10.1007/s40474-015-0063-5.

McGuire, J. F., Ung, D., Selles, R. R., Rahman, O., Lewin, A. B., Murphy, T. K., & Storch, E. A. (2014). Treating trichotillomania: A meta-analysis of treatment effects and moderators for behavior therapy and serotonin reuptake inhibitors. *Journal of Psychiatric Research, 58*, 76–83. Available from https://doi.org/10.1016/j.jpsychires.2014.07.015.

Mink, J. W. (2001). Neurobiology of basal ganglia circuits in Tourette syndrome: Faulty inhibition of unwanted motor patterns? *Advances in Neurology, 85*, 113–122.

Murphy, T. K., Lewin, A. B., Storch, E. A., Stock, S., & AACAP Committee on QualityIssues. (2013). Practice parameter for the assessment and treatment of children and adolescents with tic disorders. *Journal of the American Academy of Child & Adolescent Psychiatry, 52* (12), 1341–1359.

Peterson, A. L., McGuire, J. F., Wilhelm, S., Piacentini, J., Woods, D. W., Walkup, J. T., ... Scahill, L. (2016). An empirical examination of symptom substitution associated with behavior therapy for Tourette's disorder. *Behavior Therapy, 47*(1), 29–41. Available from https://doi.org/10.1016/j.beth.2015.09.001.

Piacentini, J., & Chang, S. (2005). Habit reversal training for tic disorders in children and adolescents. *Behavior Modification, 29*(6), 803–822. Available from https://doi.org/10.1177/0145445505279385.

Piacentini, J., Himle, M. B., Chang, S., Baruch, D. E., Buzzella, B. A., Pearlman, A., & Woods, D. W. (2006). Reactivity of tic observation procedures to situation and setting. *Journal of Abnormal Child Psychology, 34*(5), 649–658. Available from https://doi.org/10.1007/s10802-006-9048-5.

Piacentini, J., Woods, D. W., Scahill, L., Wilhelm, S., Peterson, A. L., Chang, S., ... Walkup, J. T. (2010). Behavior therapy for children with Tourette disorder: A randomized controlled trial. *JAMA, 303*(19), 1929–1937. Available from https://doi.org/10.1001/jama.2010.607.

Rauch, S. L., Whalen, P. J., Curran, T., Shin, L. M., Coffey, B. J., Savage, C. R., ... Jenike, M. A. (2001). Probing striato-thalamic function in obsessive–compulsive disorder and Tourette syndrome using neuroimaging methods. *Advances in Neurology, 85*, 207–224.

Scahill, L., Specht, M., & Page, C. (2014). The prevalence of tic disorders and clinical characteristics in children. *Journal of Obsessive–Compulsive and Related Disorders, 3*(4), 394–400. Available from https://doi.org/10.1016/j.jocrd.2014.06.002.

Scahill, L., Woods, D. W., Himle, M. B., Peterson, A. L., Wilhelm, S., Piacentini, J. C., ... Mink, J. W. (2013). Current controversies on the role of behavior therapy in Tourette syndrome. *Movement Disorders, 28*(9), 1179–1183. Available from https://doi.org/10.1002/mds.25488.

Sheppard, D. M., Bradshaw, J. L., Purcell, R., & Pantelis, C. (1999). Tourette's and comorbid syndromes: Obsessive compulsive and attention deficit hyperactivity disorder. A common etiology? *Clinical Psychology Review*, *19*(5), 531–552. Available from https://doi.org/10.1016/S0272-7358(98)00059-2.

Shimberg, E. F. (1995). *Living With Tourette syndrome*. New York: Fireside Books.

Silva, R. R., Munoz, D. M., Barickman, J., & Friedhoff, A. J. (1995). Environmental factors and related fluctuation of symptoms in children and adolescents with Tourette's disorder. *Journal of Child Psychology and Psychiatry*, *36*(2), 305–312.

Singer, H. S., Hahn, I., & Moran, T. H. (1991). Abnormal dopamine uptake sites in postmortem striatum from patients with Tourette's syndrome. *Annals of Neurology*, *30*(4), 558–562. Available from https://doi.org/10.1002/ana.410300408.

Specht, M. W., Woods, D. W., Nicotra, C. M., Kelly, L. M., Ricketts, E. J., Conelea, C. A., … Walkup, J. T. (2013). Effects of tic suppression: Ability to suppress, rebound, negative reinforcement, and habituation to the premonitory urge. *Behaviour Research and Therapy*, *51* (1), 24–30. Available from https://doi.org/10.1016/j.brat.2012.09.009.

Stokes, A., Bawden, H. N., Camfield, P. R., Backman, J. E., & Dooley, J. M. (1991). Peer problems in Tourette's disorder. *Pediatrics*, *87*(6), 936–942.

Storch, E. A., De Nadai, A. S., Lewin, A. B., McGuire, J. F., Jones, A. M., Mutch, P. J., … Murphy, T. K. (2011). Defining treatment response in pediatric tic disorders: a signal detection analysis of the Yale Global Tic Severity Scale. *Journal of Child and Adolescent Psychopharmacology*, *21*(6), 621–627. Available from https://doi.org/10.1089/cap.2010.0149.

Storch, E. A., Hanks, C. E., Mink, J. W., McGuire, J. F., Adams, H. R., Augustine, E. F., … Murphy, T. K. (2015). Suicidal thoughts and behaviors in children and adolescents with chronic tic disorders. *Depression and Anxiety*, *32*(10), 744–753. Available from https://doi.org/10.1002/da.22357.

Storch, E. A., Johnco, C., McGuire, J. F., Wu, M. S., McBride, N. M., Lewin, A. B., & Murphy, T. K. (2016). An initial study of family accommodation in children and adolescents with chronic tic disorders. *European Child & Adolescent Psychiatry*, *26*(1), 99–109.

Tarnok, Z., Ronai, Z., Gervai, J., Kereszturi, E., Gadoros, J., Sasvari-Szekely, M., & Nemoda, Z. (2007). Dopaminergic candidate genes in Tourette syndrome: Association between tic severity and 3′ UTR polymorphism of the dopamine transporter gene. *American Journal of Medical Genetics Part B: Neuropsychiatric Genetics*, *144B*(7), 900–905. Available from https://doi.org/10.1002/ajmg.b.30517.

Tourette Syndrome Classification Study Group. (1993). Definitions and classification of tic disorders. *Archives of Neurology*, *50*(10), 1013–1016.

Verdellen, C. W., Hoogduin, C. A., & Keijsers, G. P. (2007). Tic suppression in the treatment of Tourette's syndrome with exposure therapy: The rebound phenomenon reconsidered. *Movement Disorders*, *22*(11), 1601–1606. Available from https://doi.org/10.1002/mds.21577.

Verdellen, C. W., Keijsers, G. P., Cath, D. C., & Hoogduin, C. A. (2004). Exposure with response prevention versus habit reversal in Tourettes's syndrome: A controlled study. *Behaviour Research and Therapy*, *42*(5), 501–511. Available from https://doi.org/10.1016/s0005-7967(03)00154-2.

Weisman, H., Qureshi, I. A., Leckman, J. F., Scahill, L., & Bloch, M. H. (2013). Systematic review: Pharmacological treatment of tic disorders—efficacy of antipsychotic and alpha-2 adrenergic agonist agents. *Neuroscience and Biobehavioral Reviews*, *37*(6), 1162–1171. Available from https://doi.org/10.1016/j.neubiorev.2012.09.008.

Woods, D. W., Conelea, C. A., & Walther, M. R. (2007). Barriers to dissemination: Exploring the criticisms of behavior therapy for tics. *Clinical Psychology: Science and Practice, 14*(3), 279–282. Available from https://doi.org/10.1111/j.1468-2850.2007.00088.x.

Woods, D. W., & Himle, M. B. (2004). Creating tic suppression: Comparing the effects of verbal instruction to differential reinforcement. *Journal of Applied Behavior Analysis, 37*(3), 417–420. Available from https://doi.org/10.1901/jaba.2004.37-417.

Woods, D. W., Himle, M. B., Miltenberger, R. G., Carr, J. E., Osmon, D. C., Karsten, A. M., ... Bosch, A. (2008). Durability, negative impact, and neuropsychological predictors of tic suppression in children with chronic tic disorder. *Journal of Abnormal Child Psychology, 36*(2), 237–245. Available from https://doi.org/10.1007/s10802-007-9173-9.

Woods, D. W., Miltenberger, R. G., & Lumley, V. A. (1996). Sequential application of major habit-reversal components to treat motor tics in children. *Journal of Applied Behavior Analysis, 29*(4), 483–493. Available from https://doi.org/10.1901/jaba.1996.29-483.

Woods, D. W., Piacentini, J., Himle, M. B., & Chang, S. (2005). Premonitory urge for tics scale (PUTS): Initial psychometric results and examination of the premonitory urge phenomenon in youths with tic disorders. *Journal of Developmental and Behavioral Pediatrics, 26*(6), 397–403.

Woods, D. W., Piacentini, J. C., Chang, S. W., Deckersbach, T., Ginsburg, G. S., Peterson, A. L., & Wilhelm, S. (2008). *Managing Tourette syndrome: A Behavioral Intervention for Children and Adults (Therapist Guide)*. New York: Oxford University Press.

Woods, D. W., Piacentini, J. C., Scahill, L., Peterson, A. L., Wilhelm, S., Chang, S., ... Walkup, J. T. (2011). Behavior therapy for tics in children: Acute and long-term effects on psychiatric and psychosocial functioning. *Journal of Child Neurology, 26*(7), 858–865. Available from https://doi.org/10.1177/0883073810397046.

Woods, D. W., Twohig, M. P., Flessner, C. A., & Roloff, T. J. (2003). Treatment of vocal tics in children with Tourette syndrome: Investigating the efficacy of habit reversal. *Journal of Applied Behavior Analysis, 36*(1), 109–112. Available from https://doi.org/10.1901/jaba.2003.36-109.

Chapter 3

Habit Reversal Training for Tics

Emily J. Ricketts, PhD[1] and Christopher C. Bauer, MS[2]
[1]*Department of Psychiatry, University of California, Los Angeles, CA, United States,*
[2]*Department of Psychology, Marquette University, Milwaukee, WI, United States*

HABIT REVERSAL TRAINING DESCRIPTION

Habit reversal training (HRT) is a behavioral treatment package originally developed by Azrin and Nunn (1973) to address body-focused repetitive behaviors and tics. The treatment consisted of 14 different components, including awareness training, self-monitoring, relaxation training, competing response training, generalization training, an inconvenience review, and behavioral rewards (Azrin & Nunn, 1973; Azrin & Peterson, 1990). Since its initial development, researchers have worked to simplify the treatment through identification of the key therapeutic components. As a result, the current iteration of HRT, referred to as simplified HRT consists of three major components including awareness training, competing response training, and social support (Himle, Woods, Piacentini, & Walkup, 2006; Woods & Miltenberger, 1996; Woods et al., 2008), with awareness and competing response training considered the most active treatment components (Azrin & Peterson, 1989; Miltenberger, Fuqua, & McKinley, 1985). However, although not considered to be core components of simplified HRT, many of the other components of the original HRT package (Azrin & Nunn, 1973) have demonstrated some therapeutic benefit (Finney, Rapoff, Hall, & Christophersen, 1983). The present chapter provides procedures and clinical insights into HRT as further developed by Woods et al. (2008), in addition to relaxation training (diaphragmatic breathing and progressive muscle relaxation (PMR)). Behavioral rewards and the inconvenience review are discussed elsewhere in this book (see Chapters 1: Introduction to Treatment and Management of Youth With Tourette Disorders and Tic Disorders and 14: Family Issues Associated With Tics).

The Clinician's Guide to Treatment and Management of Youth with Tourette Syndrome and Tic Disorders.
DOI: https://doi.org/10.1016/B978-0-12-811980-8.00003-0

TREATMENT STRUCTURE

HRT sessions are typically conducted once weekly for approximately 45–60 minutes per session. However, length of HRT course may vary greatly depending on the number and severity of tics, with more intensive treatment courses providing sessions across 1 or 2 week periods showing positive outcomes (Blount, Raj, & Peterson, 2017; Kennedy et al., 2016). Generally, one tic is targeted each session; however, more may be treated at one time if they are similar in topography or would involve similar treatment procedures. The first session should begin with a psychosocial interview regarding patient medical and psychiatric history, including tic developmental course and features, as described earlier in this book (see Chapters 1: Introduction to Treatment and Management of Youth With Tourette Disorders and Tic Disorders and 2: Psychoeducation About Tic Disorders and Treatment). Next, a comprehensive list of the patient's tics should be developed. Following the development of this list, the clinician and patient should work together to determine the first tic to target for the following week's session when HRT procedures will begin. Homework for this first session will include monitoring the first selected tic from the list. The beginning of the second session should start with a review of self-monitoring homework, and an update of the tic list. Then, HRT procedures should be implemented for the first targeted tic. Homework will include practicing the competing response for the first tic during planned times, in addition to implementing it during unplanned times in everyday settings, to promote generalization; and monitoring the next tic selected for intervention.

TIC SYMPTOM TRACKING

Tracking tic symptoms over the course of treatment provides an assessment of how well treatment is working. This will allow the clinician to address potential reemergence of tics that have already been targeted in treatment, or note sudden improvement in particular tic symptoms (e.g., improvement in several tics following competing response training for only one tic). Tracking tics also provides the patient with a visual log of their treatment progress, which may boost treatment motivation and indicate whether more targeted effort is needed for particular tics. Tic symptom tracking is also used to make decisions regarding which tics to target in treatment first, which is an important consideration as one of the factors used to establish the order of tics addressed in treatment is how bothersome the patient perceives a particular tic to be.

In addition to using weekly tic questionnaires as described in Chapter 1, Introduction to Treatment and Management of Youth With Tourette Disorders and Tic Disorders, it is recommended that clinicians complete the tic list at the beginning of each treatment session to track how bothersome the patient's tics have been in the past week. The list would include the name and description of the tic (e.g., *jaw movement: teeth clenching with mouth closed*), and multiple columns to track bothersomeness ratings across the sessions. "Bothersomeness" of tics refers to the degree to which tics interfere with daily living, cause distress, or lead to physical pain for the patient. The patient should rate bothersomeness using a 0 (not at all bothersome) to 10 (extremely bothersome) scale.

SELECTING TICS TO TARGET

Treatment will typically begin with the most bothersome tic for which HRT is likely to lead to successful outcomes. Tics perceived as bothersome by the patient are often associated with greater impairment, which may serve as a motivating factor to adhere to treatment procedures, especially if the patient's quality of life improves the following reduction of such tics. When selecting tics to target first, bothersomeness should be weighed against the responsiveness of specific tics to treatment procedures. Research suggests that eye blinking, head jerking/nodding, sniffing, throat clearing, complex head, shoulder, and neck tics, and other complex tics—all rated as bothersome—responded well to HRT relative to psychoeducation and supportive psychotherapy (McGuire et al., 2015). Nevertheless, addressing eye blinking, in particular, may pose a challenge for some patients due to the degree to which individuals blink naturally throughout the day. Therefore if the patient rates eye blinking as most bothersome, it may be best to begin with the next most bothersome tic on the list. An additional consideration when selecting tics to treat is the strength of the premonitory urge (i.e., feeling or sensation occurring just prior to a tic, which may be temporarily relieved following tic occurrence; Woods, Piacentini, Himle, & Chang, 2005). The presence of a premonitory urge can aid treatment success, as it can act as a cue or warning sign for the impending tic (McGuire et al., 2015). However, if the urge for a given tic is experienced as particularly strong, it may help to begin with a tic associated with a milder urge.

AWARENESS TRAINING

The first major component in HRT is awareness training, which involves teaching the patient to enhance the degree to which he/she notices the occurrence of tics, premonitory urges, or earliest tic movements or sounds. Some patients may not initially be aware of their tics even as they are happening. Additionally, patients vary in their awareness of premonitory urges. Awareness of urges or ability to report on urges is generally lacking in young children but increases with age (Woods et al., 2005), with 90% of individuals with tics ages 16 and above endorsing the presence of an urge to some degree (Reese et al., 2014). Nevertheless, the presence of a premonitory urge may boost awareness training, which can in turn aid treatment success (McGuire et al., 2015). Therefore it is helpful to work on increasing awareness for all tics during treatment. As awareness training exercises are practiced regularly, the patient may even begin to notice a premonitory urge that was previously unnoticed.

The following is an example of how to introduce awareness training to the patient:

Now that we've selected the first tic you will work on, we're ready to move on to awareness training. The goal of awareness training is to increase your ability to notice your tics, urges, and any tic warning signs. This will be helpful because we want to improve your ability to manage your tics, and the first step to learning to better manage your tics is knowing when they are occurring or are about to occur.

The first step in awareness training is defining the tic—meaning describing the specific muscle movements and/or sounds involved. The best way to do this is for the clinician to collaborate with the patient to form a detailed description of the tic, dividing the tic into small ordered components as much as possible. For example, if a patient has a head jerking tic, the clinician should ask the patient to describe the very first movement involved. Does the head fling backward? Does it move from the center to the right? Is the tic complex, involving multiple movements? Are there two or more variations of the tic? Next, the clinician should proceed onward to defining the subsequent movements. It may be the case that the patient has not thought about the tics to this degree of detail before, so the clinician should feel free to ask him/her to demonstrate the tic to provide a better sense of its appearance or sound. Once the clinician has established this detailed description, it should be recorded for future reference (see Table 3.1, for example).

TABLE 3.1 Example of Tic, Urge and Competing Response Record

Description of Tic	Premonitory Urge or Earliest Tic Movement or Sound	Competing Response
Shoulder roll with head jerk: Shoulder slowly raises towards ear then rolls backward then downwards; then head jerks quickly from center to right	Premonitory urge: tension in right shoulder and neck	Sit/stand up straight; draw shoulders downward and pull head and neck backwards
Arm extension: Left arm quickly moves outward with bent elbow, forearm punches outward with relaxed hand	Earliest movement: elbow begins to move outward away from body	Press left elbow into side of torso

Next, the clinician should ascertain whether the patient experiences a premonitory urge associated with the targeted tic. As individuals vary in their awareness of premonitory urges, not all patients will report having one for each tic or generally for any tics (Leckman, King, & Bloch, 2014; Woods et al., 2005). If the patient does report experiencing an urge, the clinician should ask the patient to describe it. First, the clinician should determine which part of the body he/she feels the urge in and the sensation or feelings experienced. While premonitory urges often occur in the muscles of the body region involved in tic occurrence (McGuire et al., 2016), they may also be experienced as nonlocalized feelings or sensations. Descriptions will vary, but may include a feeling of pressure, tension, anxiety, an ache, tingling, energy, burning, or even a feeling that things are *not just right* (Neal & Cavanna, 2013; Woods et al., 2005). If the patient does report awareness of an urge for a particular tic, but has difficulty describing this urge, it may be helpful for the clinician to provide some of the previous examples of urge descriptions to help the patient define it. Once the patient has described the urge, this information should be listed (see Table 3.1).

Finally, the clinician should ask the patient to identify the very first muscle twitch, movement, or sound occurring in the tic sequence. This information is especially useful for patients who do not report experiencing a premonitory urge for the targeted tic. Any earliest movements or sounds involved in the tic should be recorded (see Table 3.1).

Once the clinician has worked with the patient to describe the tic, any premonitory urges, and/or earliest tic movements or sounds, the patient should practice noticing the tic as it occurs during session. To do this, the clinician should spend 10–15 minutes having a conversation with the patient while the patient practices tic awareness. The conversation may vary in content, but might include mention of school, work, the events of the past week, hobbies, travel plans, and upcoming events. During this conversation, the clinician should ask the patient to acknowledge each time a tic has occurred by raising an index finger in the air. The conversational aspect reinforces the importance of the patient learning to multitask while noticing and responding to tics. The clinician will also raise a finger in the air each time he/she notices the patient exhibiting the targeted tic. Parents and/or other support persons present in session can also join in with this activity. This helps to ensure that everyone agrees on the nature of the tic and is able to identify it. It is important for the clinician to praise the patient's success in noticing tic occurrence, and gently point out to the patient when he/she misses an occurrence of the tic. This will model for the parent or social support person appropriate ways to express support to the patient. Below is an example of how to explain this awareness training activity to the patient and parent/support person:

Now that we have agreed upon what your tic is, let's spend the next few minutes trying to catch your tic. So for the next 10-to-15 minutes we'll have a chat, and when you notice you've had your tic I want you to raise your pointer finger in the air. I will also raise my finger if I see that you've had your tic. [To the parent/support person] And if you notice the tic, I want you to help me out and raise your finger too.

For children, you can make this activity a "tic catching game," in which the child receives a point for every tic he/she notices, and the clinician receives a point for noticing a tic that the patient misses. The clinician can keep a running tally of the points and whoever has the most at the end of the timeframe wins the game.

If the patient masters noticing the tic, then ask him/her to practice noticing the premonitory urge/earliest tic movement or sound by raising a finger each time he/she experiences the premonitory urge to tic or notices the first movement or sound involved in the tic sequence. This may be completed during an additional 10–15 minute conversation, or other tic eliciting activity as discussed below. The clinician and parent/support person may also join in this activity if the patient has described an earliest tic movement or sound that is visible/audible to others. However, it would be difficult for the clinician and parent/support person to help the patient detect premonitory urges due to their internal nature. In any case, if the patient is able to identify signs that the tic is coming prior to its occurrence, this increases the likelihood of successful implementation of the competing response.

What Happens if the Tic Does not Occur During the 10-Minute Conversation?

If the tic occurs at a low frequency, and has not yet occurred or is not likely to occur during the 10–15 minutes conversation, the clinician may ask the patient to continue attempting to notice tic occurrences throughout the remainder of the treatment session while the clinician moves forward with competing response training (described below). Additionally, the clinician can work to elicit tic occurrences. There are a number of ways to do this. Discussion of tics can increase their likelihood of occurrence (Woods, Watson, Wolfe, Twohig, & Friman, 2013). Furthermore, determining the contexts under which the tic is more likely to occur and mimicking those contexts when possible may also boost success with awareness training. For example, if the patient reports that the tic occurs more often when walking or standing, then the clinician and patient could leave the office and walk around the building or outside to help elicit tics. If the patient reports that the tic happens more often when reading or doing homework, then the clinician can ask him/her to read a book or complete homework for part of the session in order to elicit the tic.

What Happens if the Patient is not Successful at Noticing the Tics?

If the clinician notices many more occurrences of the targeted tic than the patient, then the patient may need further awareness training. If awareness continues to be poor (e.g., the patient is only able to detect 50% of tic occurrences), then it is best for the clinician to spend the majority of the session working on awareness training, and refrain from initiating competing response training until awareness improves. Strategies that may boost awareness are having the patient look into a mirror, view a recording of him/herself, or perform self-monitoring homework (described later). Alternatively, the clinician may select a different tic to target that may be more frequent and/or easier for the patient to identify in session. The clinician should praise the patient's efforts and reassure him/her that awareness should improve with increased practice.

Awareness Training Overview

- Develop a detailed description of the tic and any premonitory urges/earliest tic movements or sounds.
- Record descriptions for later reference (as shown in Table 3.1).
- Ask the patient to practice raising a finger for each targeted tic occurrence with the patient and parent/support person joining in when available.
- Ask the patient to practice raising a finger for each premonitory urge/earliest tic movement or sound. (Clinician and parent/support person should join in when appropriate.)

COMPETING RESPONSE TRAINING

Competing response training involves teaching the patient to use muscle movements or breathing patterns that are incompatible with or opposite of the tic; and is implemented contingent upon the occurrence of the tic, premonitory urge, or earliest tic movement or sound. Over time, this may help the patient learn to tolerate the premonitory urge while performing this physically incompatible behavior instead of the tic. Generally, it is helpful for competing responses to be discreet, so as not to draw more attention to the patient from others than that created by the tics. The competing response also needs to be comfortable enough to be able to be held for 1 minute or until the patient feels he/she can tolerate the urge without ticcing.

The following is an example of how to introduce competing response training to the patient:

> *Now that you've practiced noticing when the tic (and premonitory urge/earliest tic movement or sound) has occurred, we're ready to move on to competing response training. The goal of competing response training is to teach you to*

use an exercise that is opposite of the tic, or physically blocks the tic whenever it occurs, or whenever you feel an urge to tic or the earliest movement or sound of the tic. Learning to use a competing response takes practice, but over time, this should help you to manage your tics better. [For children: Just like playing a sport, or taking dance or music lessons takes practice in order to get better, it also takes practice to learn to use your exercises].

There are a few key points to know about these exercises. As I was just saying, they should involve body movements or breathing patterns that are opposite to the tic or block the tic. Also, competing responses should be able to be used for 1 minute or until you are able to tolerate the premonitory urge while using the competing response instead of ticcing. They should not be too noticeable to others. Certainly, they should not be more noticeable than the tics themselves. This is because we don't want you to feel uncomfortable or awkward when using them, or for the exercises to distract you or others. It is best if they do not draw unnecessary attention to you. And remember, these exercises are meant to be used whenever the tic occurs, or whenever you notice a premonitory urge or first movement or sound of the tic occurring. It is important to remember that this competing response may be used before, during or even after the tic occurs. It might seem odd to use the exercise after the tic happens, but tics often happen one after the other, or in bouts, so even if you do not catch the first tic, using the exercise right after may block the next tics from occurring.

The clinician should use the examples of competing responses (see Table 3.2) to help the patient create a competing response that adheres to the previous guidelines. It is important to maintain flexibility and creativity in establishing a competing response. As stated above, it is generally beneficial for the competing response to engage opposing muscle movements or breathing patterns to the tic. This can be achieved by considering the detailed description of the order of movements and sounds in a given tic. For complex motor tics involving multiple tics in a chain, forming a competing response for the first one or two tics in the chain may be enough to manage the complex tic. For vocal tics, the competing response will consist of variations of diaphragmatic breathing (see section on "Relaxation Training" described later in this chapter). The patient should begin the competing response with an inhale or exhale using the mouth or nose depending on whichever is opposite of the breathing pattern involved in the vocal tic. For example, for a patient with a sniffing tic involving a quick breath in through the nose, the patient would first breathe out through the nose and then in through the mouth. For a "hah" sound involving a quick exhale, the competing response would involve inhaling through the mouth and out through the nose. Before addressing any vocal tics, diaphragmatic breathing should be taught first. This will allow the patient to become comfortable with the basic skill before applying it to specific tics. The clinician should note that in some cases, diaphragmatic

TABLE 3.2 Examples of Competing Responses

Competing Response	Description
Arm extending	Press arms/elbows into sides; fold arms
Eye rolling or darting	Focus eyes on a still object and blink every 3–5 (or predetermined number of) seconds
Eyebrow raising	Subtly furrow brow
Eye widening	Subtly squint eyes
Foot raising while seated	Bend knees, bring feet closer towards you, press ball of one foot into floor, and cross the other foot behind at ankle
Head jerking	Hold good posture (sit up straight), look straight ahead and pull neck and head back
Jumping/kicking leg back	Stand with weight on heels (or stand with balls of feet on ground and pads of toes slightly raised) with knees locked
Knee/heel raising while seated	Press heel into floor and squeeze thighs together
Knuckle cracking	Make fist; clasp hands together; press palms into sides or onto lap
Mouth widening	Close lips and gently press teeth together
Nostril flaring or Nose scrunching	Press upper lip (where upper lip meets bottom of the nose) downward
Shoulder raising or rolling	Draw shoulders downward and press arms or elbows into side of torso
Stomach tensing	Hold good posture (sit up); deep breathing
Toe clenching	Press ball of foot into ground, spread and raise toes upward

breathing may be used as a competing response for a motor tic, such as a stomach tensing tic (see competing response examples below). Once the clinician has worked with the patient to identify a competing response, the clinician should check to make sure performing the competing response feels physically comfortable to him/her. For instance, the patient should not perform the competing response too intensely, so as to avoid risk of pain or injury. Additionally, the patient should feel at ease socially while performing the movement, and the competing response should not be more intense in nature than the tic. The clinician should model the competing response for the patient and have the patient try to use it as a check to ensure it meets these guidelines. Once the clinician and patient have agreed on the competing response, it should be recorded (see Table 3.1, for example).

The next step is to have the patient practice using the competing response during session. As previously stated, the patient should use it contingent upon the occurrence of the premonitory urge, first movement or sound in the tic sequence, or occurrence of the tic. With respect to tics, the patient may implement the competing response before, during, or even after the tic has occurred. In order for the patient to practice using the competing response, the clinician should have a 10–15-minute conversation with the patient as described in awareness training. The goal is for the patient to practice as much as possible, so the clinician should ask the patient to practice using the competing response contingent upon tic or premonitory urge/earliest tic movement or sound occurrence concurrently during the conversation. The parent/support person may also be involved in this conversation. The clinician should be sure to praise the patient for each successful use of the competing response contingent upon occurrence of the tic or premonitory urge/first movement or sound of tic. However, the clinician should gently let the patient know if a targeted tic occurred and the patient failed to use a contingent competing response. The clinician may do this verbally or by raising a finger (as was performed during awareness training). However, the clinician should ensure the patient does not become discouraged during this exercise.

What if the Tic Does not Occur During Session?

As described previously, if the targeted tic does not occur frequently during session, the clinician has several options. These include spending a long time conversing with the patient; spending time eliciting the tic by talking about tics; or asking the patient to engage in activities that typically serve as antecedents to ticcing. As a last resort, if the tic does not occur at all during session, the clinician may ask the patient to fake having the tic a few times followed by immediate use of the competing response. Although less ideal, this will allow the patient to get a sense of what it feels like to use the competing response appropriately.

What if the Tic is Occurring During Session, but the Patient is not Using the Competing Response?

If the patient has several occurrences of the tic in session and fails to use the competing response, the clinician will need to do some troubleshooting to identify the cause. This may be due to the competing response feeling uncomfortable, or perhaps failing to be physically incompatible with the tic, and/or some other reason (e.g., inattention, boredom). If the patient reports not being aware of targeted tic occurrence, then more awareness training is needed before continuing on with competing response training. If the patient reports that it is too challenging to perform the competing response because the tic is occurring too frequently (or the premonitory urge is too strong), then the clinician can try to reinforce the patient's success incrementally. One strategy is to award tokens for successively increasing durations of time (beginning with seconds) that the patient is able to hold the competing response. For example, a clinician may begin by awarding the patient with a token for every 10 seconds he/she is able to hold the competing response, regardless of whether a tic occurs during this exercise. The duration may increase to 15 seconds, then 30, 45, and 60 seconds. What is important is that the patient practices implementing the competing response contingent upon occurrences of the tic or premonitory urge/earliest tic movement or sound in order to help form an association between use of the competing response and tic occurrence. These tokens may be turned in for a reward at the end of the session. However, if the patient struggles to use the competing response because the tic is too intense, an alternative option to consider is to have the patient perform the tic in a way that camouflages it or makes it seem like an intentional movement (e.g., making an arm extending tic look like stretching). There are some reports suggesting that a competing response may still be beneficial even if it does not engage opposing movements or breathing patterns to the tic (Sharenow, Fuqua, & Miltenberger, 1989).

For homework, the patient should practice using the competing response contingent on occurrence of the targeted tic, premonitory urge, or earliest tic movement or sound both during planned and unplanned times as much as possible for all occurrences of the targeted tic. With respect to planned practice, the patient should practice for three-to-four 30-minute periods over the week. During these planned periods, the patient and support person should attend to how frequently tics are occurring, but formal written monitoring is not necessary. During this time, the support person should encourage appropriate use of competing responses as described later in the "Social Support" section of this chapter. Ideally, it is helpful if these periods of time set for planned practice are different than the time windows set for self-monitoring new tics (see "Self-Monitoring" section below for details) for which competing responses have not yet been developed. This is so that the child is able to focus on correct implementation of the competing responses without other demands for his/her attention. However, when it makes sense, planned practice may overlap with self-monitoring of new tics. As the patient targets new tics with competing responses each week, homework will include formal practice of all competing responses learned up until that point.

When possible, it is helpful if planned practice occurs during times when the targeted tic is most likely to occur. The clinician should work with the patient to identify two to three situations during which the tic occurs more frequently. Results of function-based assessment can aid this process (see Chapter 14: Family Issues Associated With Tics for details on function-based assessment).

The goal is for use of the competing response to generalize to all contexts (i.e., places, moods, activities) in which the tic is likely to occur. Therefore from the outset of treatment, the patient should practice using the competing response for each occurrence of the targeted tic or associated urge/earliest tic movement or sound across all settings during homework. It is possible that following homework practice the patient may return to the next session stating that he/she had difficulty focusing on other activities while performing the competing response. This is a common observation; however, this should reside as the patient continues to practice, and becomes more comfortable multitasking while using the competing response. The goal is for use of these competing responses to become natural and fluid over time without too much effort and concentration. It is also possible that the patient may report difficulty implementing the competing response for all instances of the tic due to the tic occurring too frequently. In the event that it is challenging for the patient to implement the competing response consistently across all settings, the goal should be for the patient to focus his/her efforts on the planned practice—using the competing response for as many instances of the tic or urge/earliest tic movement or sound as possible in situations when the tic is most likely to occur, as explained above.

In some instances, the patient may lack motivation to practice implementing the competing response, and return to the next session having not completed any practice. If such is the case, the clinician should work with the patient and support person to identify the barriers to practicing. There could be any number of reasons why a patient fails to practice. However, there are several strategies detailed in this text that may increase adherence. First, "Social Support" discussed below in the present chapter directly encourages use of the competing responses through prompting and praising by the support person. Another strategy to encourage treatment engagement is to discuss with the patient, the bothersome aspects of having tics (e.g., physical pain, teasing, occupational/school challenges). This may serve as a means of reminding the patient the reasons why he/she had initially decided to work on managing tics. In some instances when working with children, there may be family barriers (e.g., schedules, parental involvement) that need to be addressed to ensure that homework practice takes place. Chapter 14, Family Issues Associated With Tics provides information on family interventions for tic disorders. Another strategy for children is to use a behavioral reward system, for which the patient can earn points for completion of treatment-related activities (e.g., attending session, participating in session, completing treatment-related homework assignments). These points can be tracked and exchanged for tangible rewards (see Chapter 1: Introduction to Treatment and Management of Youth With Tourette Disorders and Tic Disorders).

The following example leads the reader through competing response development and practice. This example will involve developing a competing response for a complex tic.

Clinician: *Now that you know the general rules about competing responses, let's try to make a competing response for your shoulder movement-arm straightening-head jerking-stomach tensing tic.*

Patient: *Okay*

Clinician: *First, let's refresh our memories on your description of the tic, urge and earliest tic movement. Going by what we previously wrote, the first part of your tic involves a quick movement of your right shoulder forward with a straightening of your right arm and spreading of the fingers on your right hand.*

Patient: *Yeah and then my head moves. And my stomach tenses after that.*

Clinician: *Yes, we did write about the head movement and stomach tensing too, but we are only going to focus on the first part of your tic for just this moment. Tics like this one, which include multiple movements across the body, sometimes respond well to a competing response that blocks just the first one or two movements in the chain. So we will first try having you practice using only the first one or two competing responses that block the first one or two movements involved in your tic. So let's begin with the shoulder, arm, and finger movements. If we find that this helps you manage all parts of the tic as we are practicing in session today, then we will stop there. If not, we'll work on adding a competing response for the head movement and stomach tensing tics.*

Patient: *Okay. That makes sense.*

Clinician: *So what do you think would be an opposite movement for this first part of your tic? Remember it should also be something that is not too noticeable to others, and something you can hold for 1 minute or until you feel you are able to tolerate or manage the feeling of the premonitory urge without ticcing.*

Patient: *Hmm...well my arm straightens outward a little bit when the tic happens so maybe I could hold it against the side of my leg to try to block it.*

Clinician: *Great idea! That's a good start. Pressing your hands and fingers flat into your sides as well might also help. What do you think?*

Patient: *Yeah that could help too.*

Clinician: *Now what about your shoulder? It might still move in this position. See. [Clinician tries using movement as suggested by patient and shows shoulder can still move back and forth].*

Patient: *Well I could try pushing my right shoulder back.*

Clinician: *Okay, that would definitely be an opposite movement. Maybe you could sit up straight and push both your shoulders back and hold your arms by your side. Let's try it.*

Patient: *Yeah I think that would work.*

Clinician: *How does it feel? Do you feel comfortable?*

Patient: *Yeah it feels fine.*

Clinician: *Great! The next movement is the head jerking movement. According to our definition, your head first moves to the right towards your right shoulder and then rolls backwards in a circle once.*

Patient: *Yeah that's right.*

Clinician: *Okay, which movement do you think would help with managing this part of the tic?*

Patient: *Maybe I could look down and press my chin into my chest.*

Clinician: *Well, we want this to be a movement that allows you to carry on with your day normally. It would be hard to see where you are going if you were looking down. Also others might think it was odd if they saw you doing this. How about pulling your head and neck inwards towards you while tensing your neck slightly and looking straight ahead? Watch me do it. What do you think of that?*

Patient: *I can do that.*

Clinician: *Ok, let's put this together with the first part of the competing response. So all together you will sit up straight and push both your shoulders back and press your arms, hands, and fingers into your side; and then you will pull your head and neck backwards towards you while tensing your neck slightly and looking straight ahead. So try using these movements at the same time and see how it feels. See if you can hold the position for a minute.*

Patient: *Okay [patient holds it for 1 minute].*

Clinician: *How did that feel?*

Patient: *Argh, my back is starting to ache.*

Clinician: *Which part?*

Patient: *The upper-middle part. I think it's from sitting up straight. I don't usually sit up very straight throughout the day so it kind of aches. Can we try something else?*

Clinician: *We don't want the movement to feel uncomfortable or cause you pain. So, let's see if we can do it without you sitting up. Go ahead and relax your back. Sit back in your chair. Act as if you are sitting on the couch watching TV while using your competing responses. Hold the position for 1 minute to see if it feels okay.*

Patient: *That feels better. I think this will work better for me.*

Clinician: *Good! I will record this description so we can return to it later for adjustment if needed. Now let's practice having you use it. Remember you'll use it any time you notice the tic, premonitory urge, or earliest tic movement or sound. And you'll hold it for 1 minute or until you feel you can handle the feeling of the urge without having the tic. You had said your urge feels like a tightness and tingling in your right shoulder, and the earliest tic movement is when your right shoulder begins to move forward so keep that in mind during practice.*

Patient: *Okay*

Clinician: *For the next 10 to15 minutes, we are going to have a casual chat. At the same time, I would like you to practice using your competing response whenever you notice the tic, premonitory urge, or earliest sign that the tic is occurring. If I notice you did not use the competing response for a particular tic, I will let you know by raising a finger. Alright, let's begin. So how was your weekend?*

Clinician: *Good! My mom took me, my little brother, and my friend to a waterpark. It was pretty awesome. I hadn't been in years.*

Clinician: *That sounds like a lot of fun! [raises finger]*

Patient: *Oops, I got distracted.*

Clinician: *That's okay. Remember you can still use the competing response just after the tic has happened, so go ahead and start it right now. Hold it for 1 minute or until you feel you can manage the urge without ticcing.*

Patient: *One minute feels kind of long.*

Clinician: *Holding it for one minute allows you to get used to using the movement, but later on when using the competing response becomes more automatic you probably won't need to hold it that long.*

Patient: *Okay.*

Clinician: *So what rides did you go on at the theme park?*

Patient: *We got in this raft thingy and went down a really twisty slide. It was really scary. My little brother started crying. He's such a baby.*

Clinician: *Aww, well it sounds pretty scary. I think my stomach would drop if I went on that ride. [raises finger]*

Patient: *Yeah it was fun though.*

Clinician: *[Raises finger] Remember to use your competing response.*

Patient: *Oh yeah. This is harder than I thought it would be.*

Clinician: *Which part makes it hard?*

Patient: *The feeling in my shoulder is really strong, and it's hard to focus on using the competing response while we're talking.*

Clinician: *That's understandable and pretty common. At first, it may feel like it's hard to do anything else when you are using the competing response, but over time as you get used to using it, it will begin to get easier and feel more automatic like you don't have to think about it as much. As for the feeling in your shoulder – your urge, at first you may feel like it keeps getting stronger and stronger until it becomes so bothersome that the tic will happen know matter what you do, but the more you practice handling the urge being that strong without having the tic the better you will be able to manage your tics in the long run. So let's keep at it.*

Patient: *Okay.*

Clinician: *What other rides did you go on?*

Patient: *I went on the biggest waterslide in the park. It was so fast. And we all went... [trails off and begins using the competing response after experiencing earliest tic movement – shoulder beginning to move forward].*

Clinician: *Wow! Nice work using the competing response! And you caught it just as the tic was starting. I only saw your shoulder slightly twitch. Well done! Go ahead and hold it for 1 minute or until you can manage the urge. I'll use the clock to keep track of the time for you and we can stay silent if it's easier for you to concentrate.*

Patient: *[patient nods]*

Clinician: *Okay, the minute is up. Do you feel like you can handle the feeling of the urge without ticcing?*

Patient: *Yeah I think I can. I finally caught one!*

Clinician: *Yes, you did a great job! Next time, we'll try to keep the conversation going while you're using the competing response. So you said you went on a waterslide, and then you were about to tell me what you all did next.*

Patient: *Oh yeah. I was about to say we all went in the lazy river.*

Clinician: *That sounds very relaxing. Did anything else happen this weekend?*

Patient: *Yeah, my friend slept over and we...[patient experiences earliest tic movement and then immediately begins using the competing response]*

Clinician: *You caught another one! Nice work! Remember to keep trying to talk while using it. So your friend slept over...and what did you do?*

Patient: *[patient speaks while using competing response] We stayed up really late playing video games and watching movies.*

Clinician: *What kind of video games did you play and which movies did you watch?*

Patient: *[patient speaks while using the competing response] We watched some scary movies. My mom said we shouldn't watch them because we'd get scared and have a hard time going to sleep but we did it anyway. She was right. Afterwards we were kind of scared so we played some of my racing videogames before going to sleep. We stayed up until 3 in the morning, and didn't wake up until 11.*

Clinician: *Wow! That sounds like a fun night. I love scary movies myself. Okay, the minute is up. Great job keeping the conversation going while using the competing response. How did it feel?*

Patient: *It was easier to talk and use it at the same time this time.*

Clinician: *Good! And I wanted to check, the last two times when you used the competing response, did you notice your stomach tighten up?*

Patient: *Actually, the stomach tensing didn't happen both times.*
Clinician: *Okay, that's great! It seems like the competing response may have blocked the stomach tensing part of the tic for now without you needing to use a specific competing response to directly target it. So for this week we'll have you practice using this version of the competing response at home and when I see you next week we'll figure out if we need to adjust it.*

Competing Response Overview

- Use list of competing responses in addition to detailed descriptions of tic and premonitory urge/earliest tic movement or sound to develop a competing response.
- Competing response should engage muscles that are incompatible with or opposite to the tic, discreet, and able to be held for 1 minute or until the patient feels he/she can tolerate the urge without ticcing.
- The competing response should be used contingent upon occurrence of tic or premonitory urge/earliest tic movement or sound. It may be used before during or just after the tic occurs.
- Model competing response for patient and have the patient try performing it to ensure it feels physically and socially comfortable.
- Record description of competing response for later adjustment if needed.
- Patient practices using the competing response, preferably contingent upon occurrence of tic or premonitory urge/earliest tic movement or sound.
- For homework, the patient practices using the competing response, contingent upon the occurrence of the tic or premonitory urge/earliest tic movement or sound for three to four 30-minute planned periods when the tic is most likely to occur, in addition to any other times the tic occurs across settings.

SOCIAL SUPPORT

Social support within the context of HRT refers to prompting or reminding the patient to use competing responses to target tics when he/she fails to, and praising the patient for appropriate use of competing responses. Social support is helpful as it serves to reinforce the patient's treatment adherence by validating the patient's efforts. It also promotes increased awareness of tics as they occur throughout the day. The first step in social support is to identify a social support person. For children, it will most likely be a parent. The goal should not be for the parent to overwhelm the child by becoming a constant "tic monitor," so it may be helpful to have only one designated parent to play this role within a given household. For those who divide their time between two households, a designated parent may fulfill this position at each home. For children with tics occurring at severe rates in settings outside of the home, it may be helpful for another adult (e.g., a teacher or a coach) to serve as a supplemental social support person. Should the decision be made to use a supplemental support person, there should be a discussion between the selected individual, child, and parent regarding how best to carry out the procedure so as not to draw unnecessary social attention to the child from peers. For older teens who are experiencing increasing autonomy, the social support component may need to be minimized so it is not experienced as "nagging." For example, it may be helpful for the parent to provide prompts only when tics are at their most severe. Additionally, the social support person should focus on their delivery of the prompt. It should be a gentle reminder to use the competing response when the parent sees the child has ticced or begun to tic without using it. This reminder may be as simple as stating "*Remember to use your exercise(s).*" The statement should be delivered in a pleasant tone and should not result in yelling, blaming, or arguments, which could potentially draw more attention to the tics (see Chapter 14: Family Issues Associated With Tics for more details). After witnessing the child engage in appropriate use of a competing response, regardless of whether it was prompted or unprompted, the parent should provide praise. This may be expressed with a statement such as "*Nice job using your exercise(s),*" "*I can see you're working hard at using your exercise(s),*" or "*Way to go!*"

The clinician should model these strategies for the support person in session as the patient practices using the competing response. If the clinician notices the patient has used a competing response contingent upon the presence of a tic, or urge/earliest tic movement or sound, the clinician should stop whichever session activity is happening to praise the patient and draw attention to the achievement. If the clinician notices that the patient has had a tic and did not use the competing response, then the clinician should stop the topic of discussion momentarily to gently prompt use of the competing response. The clinician should ask the support person to help with this activity so that the clinician can assess the tone and phrasing of the support person's statements, in addition to the patient's reception of the feedback. For homework, the support person should provide prompts and praise during both planned practice of the competing response and any unplanned times in the day when noticing the patient has appropriately used a competing response or has ticced without using a competing response.

When discussing social support with the family, it is helpful for the clinician to preemptively troubleshoot any potential problems that may arise before the family leaves the session. Clinicians may consider asking the parent to specify, which prompting and praising statements he/she plans to say to the child when outside of the treatment session so as to ensure their appropriateness. It is also important to check with the patient to make sure these statements are well received.

For adults, a spouse, significant other, parent, or friend may serve as a social support person. However, the social support component may be less practical for adults depending on the individual's living situation and social environment. Furthermore, the therapeutic benefit of prompting and praising use of competing responses is less certain for adults. It is possible that for some adults, receiving prompts and praise for competing response use may place strain on their relationship with the social support person. Therefore it is important to approach the social support component with sensitivity and flexibility. For adults, social support may be more beneficial when addressed more broadly. For example, the clinician may consider how the significant other can best show support for the patient's treatment efforts generally (e.g., checking in with the patient to hear how treatment is going, or helping to make a home environment conducive to practicing skills learned in session). It would be helpful to have the identified social support person be present for this discussion, and to have the patient voice how best the significant other or family member can support him/her during HRT treatment.

The following is an example of dialog between a clinician, parent, and patient regarding a social support difficulty and how to resolve it. In this example, the family is experiencing some setbacks with the social support component as traditionally performed.

Clinician:	*How have things been going at home with the social support piece?*
Parent:	*Well...we've had some problems with that this week actually.*
Clinician:	*What's been going on?*
Parent:	*I had been reminding Tommy to complete the exercises when I would see the tics occur and he seemed to be responding well to it...*
Child [interjects]:	*It's annoying.*
Parent:	*...it was going fine at first. I would remind him to use his exercises when I noticed him having his tics and he would do the competing response. But over the weeks his younger brother and sister have begun copying me and reminding Tommy to use his exercises too. They're four years old so they don't really understand what's going on.*
Patient:	*They kept saying "remember to use your exercises", "remember to use your exercises". I don't like them making fun of me.*
Clinician:	*I'm sorry. That's really frustrating. How did you handle it?*
Patient:	*I told them to shut up.*
Clinician:	*They're really young and may not understand what's going on.*
Parent:	*They ended up arguing back and forth. I tried switching to reminding him when they were out of earshot, but by then it was too late and they were still pestering him even when I was not around. So for the past few days I haven't been saying anything when I notice the tics because I don't want to upset him.*
Clinician:	*Well we really don't want this to result in arguments. It sounds like the prompts were helpful and well-received at first. Perhaps there's a different way your mom can remind you to use your exercises. What do you think Tommy?*
Patient:	*Like how?*
Clinician:	*Maybe there's some way your mom can signal you to remind you to use your exercises so that only you know what she means, but your brother and sister don't.*

Patient:	*Oh like a secret signal.*
Clinician:	*Exactly.*
Mom:	*Yeah that could work.*
Clinician:	*What do you want your secret signal to be? You'll want it to be something that your mom is comfortable doing and that your brother and sister won't easily notice or ask about.*
Patient:	*Ummm...I don't know.*
Parent:	*What about if I subtly raise a finger like you do in session or, if I'm close, tap my pointer finger on my arm to get your attention.*
Clinician:	*That's a great idea! And how will you handle your brother and sister if they tell you to stop using your exercises again?*
Parent:	*I've already told Tommy to ignore them when they say anything like that. But he's been having some trouble doing that.*
Clinician:	*Can we agree to give what your mom is suggesting a try over the next week? Let's try harder to ignore your brother and sister if they say anything else. Let your mom handle it if they are bothering you.*
Patient:	*Okay.*
Clinician:	*Great!*

The above dialog depicts how a nonverbal prompt may be used instead of a verbal one to achieve the same purpose of reminding the patient to use their competing response contingent upon tic occurrence. Beyond sibling difficulties, there are many other situations and settings in which a nonverbal prompt could be useful, including in public situations during which others may hear—attracting unwanted attention, or in quiet settings during which providing prompts may be disruptive to others. In the same vein, providing praise in nonverbal formats (e.g., high-five, thumbs up) may also be beneficial and should be discussed as a potential option.

One conceptual issue, which may arise, is that families and patients may have difficulty reconciling guidance encouraging the minimizing of attention towards tics, with instructions to provide attention as part of social support. This may seem paradoxical. However, in social support the support person is providing a gentle reminder to use the exercise, and praising effort towards managing tics. Although the support person may feel that he/she is inadvertently drawing attention to the tics, the social support directly pertains to use of the exercises (and not tic occurrence). This is very different than telling a child to stop ticcing, or comforting a child after he/she tics. In short, while it is important to decrease attention to tics, it is generally fine to discuss tics as related to treatment when done in a respectful manner.

Social Support Overview

- Explain rationale for social support.
- Identify social support person.
- Model prompt and praise statements for support person

- For child patients, gauge appropriateness of prompt and praise statements by parent during practice session.
- For adult patients, gauge appropriateness of prompt and praise statements/assess social support needs that will encourage treatment adherence.
- Troubleshoot potential problems.
- For homework, support person should prompt and praise appropriate tic contingent competing response use during planned practice and during unplanned times, or follow alternative support plan as specified.

SELF-MONITORING

Self-monitoring refers to time spent actively attending to and tracking tic occurrence. Self-monitoring supports the building of tic and urge awareness. Self-monitoring should first be implemented as a homework assignment prior to beginning HRT for the first tic and is given as a homework assignment throughout treatment to target the next tic(s) selected for intervention in subsequent sessions. To do this, the patient and the support person should identify a time and setting when the tic is most likely to occur. This could be while watching television, eating a snack, doing homework, reading, playing video games, using the computer, etc. The patient and support person should be sure to mark down the date and activity happening during monitoring. The patient and support person should each count the number of times the tic occurs during this period. The patient and support person should each track the targeted tic independently of each other during the same time period. Prior to monitoring, the patient and support person should discuss the topography of the tic to ensure the validity of their tic counts. The amount of time spent monitoring will vary based on the frequency of the tic but may range from 15 to 60 minutes. For example, for a tic occurring once every minute on average, 15 minutes of self-monitoring may be appropriate. However, for a tic occurring every 10 minutes on average, monitoring for a longer time period, such as 1 hour may be more beneficial. Neither the social support person nor the patient should announce or gesture that tics have occurred during this period. Self-monitoring of each targeted tic or set of tics should take place a minimum of three times in a given week. The social support person should not use this time to prompt the patient to manage tics. After the monitoring period has ended, the patient and support person should share their frequency counts to see how their results compare. If the support person has a higher frequency count than the patient, this may suggest that the patient is failing to notice some tics and needs to work on building greater awareness. On the contrary, this might mean the support person misjudged a normal behavior as a tic. For this reason, it is important for the patient and support person to agree on the tic topography beforehand.

For adults who do not have a support person, this activity may be completed by recording the self-monitoring session with a video camera or cellular phone while marking down a tic count. After the self-monitoring period, the patient can watch the video recording and count the number of observed tics. The patient can compare this with the original tic count to see if it differs. See Woods et al. (2008), for example of self-monitoring forms.

Self-Monitoring Overview

- Identify time of day and setting when next tic targeted for treatment is most likely to occur.
- Establish duration of monitoring period and frequency of practice.
- Ensure patient and support person agree on the topography of the targeted tic.
- Tell patient and support person to count tics independently during set time period, and then compare and discuss discrepancies in ratings.
- Patients self-monitoring alone without a support person may record themselves on video and compare live tic frequency counts with those observed in the recording.

RELAXATION TRAINING

Relaxation training is beneficial in treatment for several reasons. First, tics may result in muscle tension or even pain; and tension or distress may be an antecedent for tic exacerbation. Second, relaxation training—specifically, diaphragmatic breathing, is used to target vocal tics, as previously mentioned. This section outlines two common relaxation techniques, which include diaphragmatic breathing and PMR to help relieve tension and stress. These techniques are outlined below. Once the clinician has trained the patient in these strategies during session, it is recommended that the patient practice them for homework. Practicing for at least three times each week for about 10 minutes each time is suggested, but this is completely flexible depending on the patient's schedule. Consequently, it is important to work with the patient to determine how many times he/she will practice each week, how long he/she will practice, and where he/she will practice. The patient may practice in whichever setting promotes relaxation (i.e., a setting free of noise and other distractions). This might be at school, home, or in a private work office for example. This will provide the patient with autonomy over their practice sessions and may boost adherence. With respect to the timing of relaxation training during the course of HRT, introduction of these skills within the first few (i.e., three to four) sessions is optimal; however, relaxation training can be implemented anytime throughout treatment to promote relaxation. And as previously stated in the description of competing response training, if vocal tics are present then it is recommended that clinicians train the patient in use of diaphragmatic breathing before teaching the competing response for vocal tics, which is controlled or diaphragmatic breathing.

Diaphragmatic Breathing

Diaphragmatic or relaxed breathing involves slow, deep and steady inhalation and exhalation and can result in lowered stress and reduced muscle tension. This type of breathing is produced by using the diaphragm; so as the patient's lungs fill with air, his/her belly region should appear to expand outwards, and as the patient exhales, his/her belly should appear to deflate. The patient's shoulders and chest should not rise as they might while engaging in shallow breathing. Following an introduction to the benefits of relaxation training, as described above, the clinician may use the following script to explain diaphragmatic breathing to the patient:

> *Let's begin with diaphragmatic or relaxed breathing. Diaphragmatic breathing involves slow, deep inhalation and exhalation. This is different than the shallow breathing most people use on a day-to-day basis during which the chest expands. Learning to manage your breathing can help reduce stress, ease stiffness in your muscles, and bring on an overall sense of calm. So let's get started. In order to do this, first place one hand on your belly and one hand on your chest. As you are breathing, you should notice the hand on your belly rise and lower as your belly expands and deflates. The hand on your chest should not move at all during this exercise. During this exercise, you'll breathe in for three to four seconds and out for about 6 seconds. The slow exhale is even more important than the inhale.*
>
> *Okay, are you ready? Let's start. I'll count out loud to help guide you. Remember your breathing should be slow. Try not to let your chest or shoulders rise. 1...2...3...4...now begin exhaling for 6 seconds. 1...2...3...4...5...6. How do you feel? Let's try it again except this time we'll keep going for a minute. Begin...1...2...3...4...and exhale...1...2...3...4...5...6.*

Progressive Muscle Relaxation

PMR involves tensing and relaxing muscle groups with the intension of training the patient to notice and ease tension within the body. Typically, PMR involves isolating different muscle groups, and alternating between squeezing them tightly and relaxing them completely. Tensing muscles tightly serves to make the subsequent relaxed state much more salient, allowing the patient to notice what it feels like to be fully relaxed. However, the purpose of PMR is also to learn to become aware of the feeling of tension within the muscles so one can remember to relax them. Individuals who carry tension in their muscles throughout the day do not typically tense them as dramatically as one would do during traditional PMR. For example, have you ever caught yourself sitting or standing with tense raised shoulders? How high were your shoulders raised when you noticed yourself doing this? They probably were not raised very high—perhaps only an inch or half-inch higher than a fully relaxed position, and perhaps not even enough to be noticeable to anyone around you. Yet, they were still tense and you may have been walking around in that position for a while without noticing. This subtle tension can lead to body aches and headaches. In order to teach the patient to learn to recognize this type of tension, a modified PMR exercise, involving subtle tensing of muscle groups, is also described. The clinician should feel free to train the patient in either or both methods depending on the patient's clinical presentation and/or the patient's preference.

Now we're going to do an exercise to help you learn to relax your muscles. It's called Progressive Muscle Relaxation or PMR. Right now, we're going to do some exercises involving tensing and relaxing different muscles. Over time if you keep using these exercises, this will help you learn to notice the difference between tense or tight feelings within your muscles and relaxed feelings. So let's begin. Hold each exercise for 10 seconds and then fully relax for 20 seconds. I'll do this with you to show you how. First, we are going to have you go back and forth between squeezing very tightly and fully relaxing with the exercises. This will help you to notice what it feels like to be relaxed. And after, we will have you move back and forth between more subtle tensing of your muscles to complete relaxing of your muscles to help you notice tension as it may occur naturally as you go about your daily activities, and learn to adjust your body to a relaxed state.

So let's begin with the tight tensing. We'll hold each movement for 10 seconds and then have you relax for 20 seconds. First, I'd like you to raise your shoulders high towards your ears. Raise them as high as you can, squeezing them tightly. Hold…hold…hold for 10 seconds. Now relax and let your body go limp. Lean back in your chair. Do you notice the difference?

Next, clench your teeth together as if you're chewing something really tough. Keep them clenched tight. And release.

Now clench your fist as if you are about to slam it down on a table. Notice what it feels like to hold your fist so tight. Squeeze it for the full 10 seconds. And now relax, open your palms and let your hands flop and feel heavy.

Now, close your eyes, and press your eyelids together tightly. Squeeze them tight the way you would if lemon juice accidentally squirted into your eyes or you were standing around cut onions. And now gently open them.

Now squeeze both your elbows into your sides. Squeeze your sides tight. And then release.

Next scrunch your toes as tight as you can as if you're trying to squeeze a pencil between your toes.

Next, straighten your legs and point your toes as if you are stretching…then release.

Next, remain seated with your feet flat on the floor and squeeze your thighs together like you're trying to pop a balloon between them. Squeeze…and relax.

Now, finally squeeze your stomach in tight as if you are trying to squeeze yourself between a tiny space between two walls. Hold…hold…hold, and then sit back in your chair and relax and breathe.

And now, we're going to have you move back and forth between subtly tensing specific muscles for 30 seconds as you might do by accident as you go about your day, and fully relaxing them for 20 seconds so you learn the difference between these physical feelings. So let's do some exercises that mirror what it might feel like when your muscles are in a tense position without you noticing. Sometimes people tense their bodies ever so slightly through the day without even noticing. They may catch themselves doing this momentarily, but later return to the tense position again without noticing. This can lead to muscle aches over time.

So let's begin with your shoulders. Raise your shoulders upwards very slightly only about an inch. And now hold this position for 30 seconds. Do you feel your shoulders beginning to become tense? Notice how this feels in your shoulders and neck. And now let your shoulders completely relax. How do you feel now? Can you tell the difference?

Now make two fists as if your fingers are wrapped around a pen…keep them closed but not too tightly…and now open your hands and let them go limp.

Now place your hands on a hard surface with your fingers slightly spread. Press the pads of your fingers onto the surface. Notice how your palm tenses…and now relax.

Next, place your feet flat on the floor. Press the very tips of your toes into the floor and slightly squeeze them. And now let your toes relax.

Next, press your teeth together gently. Hold this for 30 seconds. And release. Did you notice the difference in how your jaw felt?

Now close your eyes and press your eyelids together so you feel just the slightest pressure. Hold this for 30 seconds. Now let your eyelids fully relax.

Now squeeze or furrow your brow ever so slightly. . .then relax for 20 seconds.

Now that you have finished trying out these exercises, it's important for you to practice at home. How many times a week do you think you could practice? And where is the best place to practice where you'll feel most relaxed?

Clinicians should note, the greater subtlety of this modified tensing may draw comparisons to the act of using a competing response. As a result, parents and patients might express concern that performing competing responses may lead to muscle tension over time. However, please notify the patient that he/she would not be expected to maintain the competing response for long durations. Additionally, the patient would consciously be engaging their muscles during competing response training. This is in contrast to someone who unknowingly tenses their muscles throughout the day. The goal of this modified exercise is to train awareness of naturally occurring tension within the body.

CONCLUSION

In conclusion, HRT is an empirically-supported behavioral treatment for tics (McGuire et al., 2014). It features treatment components which have been well described in various publications over the years. The components outlined in this chapter provide a solid treatment foundation. Nonetheless, HRT should be individualized to meet the unique needs of each patient by supplementing this intervention with additional therapeutic strategies outlined in this text.

Diaphragmatic Breathing Practice

Instructions: Diaphragmatic or relaxed breathing involves slow, deep inhaling, and exhaling. This is different than the shallow breathing most people use on a day-to-day basis during which the chest expands. Learning to manage your breathing can help reduce stress, ease stiffness in your muscles, and make you feel calm.

During this exercise, you will breathe in for about 3–4 seconds and out for about 6 seconds. As you are breathing you should notice the hand on your belly rise and lower as your belly expands and deflates. The hand on your chest and your shoulders should not move up and down during this exercise.

(*Continued*)

(Continued)

Be sure to write down the number of times you will practice each week, in addition to the length of time (in minutes) you will spend practicing. Finally, also consider where you will practice. A location without distractions or noise is best. This may be in your home, school, work office, or some other location depending on your schedule.

Progressive Muscle Relaxation Practice

Instructions: PMR involves tensing and relaxing the different muscles in your body. PMR will help you to learn and notice the difference between tense or tight feelings within your muscles and relaxed feelings so you are better able to reduce tension.

Traditional Progressive Muscle Relaxation

Traditional PMR involves switching between tensing muscles tightly and relaxing them fully. Tensing muscles tightly makes the relaxed state much more noticeable allowing you to notice what it truly feels like to be fully relaxed. Practice holding each movement below for 10 seconds and relaxing for 20 seconds.

Shoulders: Raise your shoulders high towards your ears. Raise them as high as you can, squeezing them tightly as if it's freezing cold outside and you are trying to stay warm.

Jaw: Clench your teeth together as if you're chewing something really tough.

Hands: Clench your fist as if you are about to slam it down on a table.

Eyelids: Close your eyes, and press your eyelids together tightly. Squeeze them tight the way you would if lemon juice accidentally squirted into your eyes or you were standing around cut onions.

Arms: Squeeze both your elbows into your sides. Squeeze your sides tight. And then release.

Toes: Scrunch your toes as tight as you can as if you are trying to squeeze a pencil between your toes.

Legs: Straighten your legs and point your toes as if you are stretching...then release.

Thighs: Sit with your feet flat on the floor and squeeze your thighs together like you are trying to pop a balloon between your thighs.

Belly: Squeeze your belly in tight as if you are trying to squeeze yourself between a tiny space between two walls.

Modified Progressive Muscle Relaxation

Instructions: Modified PMR involves switching between subtly tensing specific muscles for 30 seconds as you might do accidentally as you go about your day, and fully relaxing them for 20 seconds so you learn the difference between these physical feelings. This exercise will help you build awareness of when your muscles may be stiff.

(*Continued*)

(Continued)

Shoulders: Raise your shoulders upwards very slightly only about an inch.

Hands: Make two fists as if your fingers are wrapped around a pen.

Fingers: Press your palms flat on a hard surface with your fingers slightly spread. Press the tips of your fingers into the hard surface.

Toes: Place your feet flat on the floor. Press the pads of your toes into the floor and slightly squeeze them.

Jaw: Press your teeth together slightly but do not clench.

Eyelids: Close your eyes and imagine you are trying to go to sleep. Slightly press your eyelids together so you feel a little bit of pressure.

Brow: Squeeze or furrow your brow ever so slightly as if you are trying to see something outside of your line of vision.

REFERENCES

Azrin, N. H., & Nunn, R. G. (1973). A method of eliminating nervous habits and tics. *Behaviour Research and Therapy*, *11*, 619–628.

Azrin, N. H., & Peterson, A. L. (1989). Reduction of an eye tic by controlled eye blinking. *Behavior Therapy*, *20*, 467–473.

Azrin, N. H., & Peterson, A. L. (1990). Treatment of Tourette syndrome by habit reversal: A waiting list control group comparison. *Behavior Therapy*, *21*, 305–318.

Blount, T. H., Raj, J. J., & Peterson, A. L. (2017). Intensive outpatient comprehensive behavioral intervention for tics: A clinical replication series. *Cognitive and Behavioral Practice*, *25*, 156–167.

Finney, J. W., Rapoff, M. A., Hall, C. L., & Christophersen, E. R. (1983). Replication and social validation of habit reversal treatment for tics. *Behavior Therapy*, *14*, 116–126.

Himle, M. B., Woods, D. W., Piacentini, J. C., & Walkup, J. T. (2006). Brief review of habit reversal training for Tourette syndrome. *Journal of Child Neurology*, *21*, 719–725.

Kennedy, T. M., Morris, A. T., Walkup, J. T., Barash, M., Gettings, J. M., Hankinson, J., … Specht, M. W. (2016). Rapid-response behavioral triage for tics (RRBTT): A 2-week clinical case series. *Clinical Practice in Pediatric Psychology*, *4*, 373–382.

Leckman, J. F., King, R. A., & Bloch, M. H. (2014). Clinical features of Tourette syndrome and tic disorders. *Journal of Obsessive-Compulsive and Related Disorders*, *3*, 372–379.

McGuire, J. F., McBride, N., Piacentini, J., Johnco, C., Lewin, A. B., Murphy, T. K., & Storch, E. A. (2016). The premonitory urge revisited: An individualized premonitory urge for tics scale. *Journal of Psychiatric Research*, *83*, 176–183.

McGuire, J. F., Piacentini, J., Brennan, E. A., Lewin, A. B., Murphy, T. K., Small, B. J., & Storch, E. A. (2014). A meta-analysis of behavior therapy for Tourette syndrome. *Journal of Psychiatric Research*, *50*, 106–112.

McGuire, J. F., Piacentini, J., Scahill, L., Woods, D. W., Villareal, R., Wilhelm., … Peterson, L. (2015). Bothersome tics in patients with chronic tic disorders: characteristics and individualized treatment response to behavior therapy. *Behaviour Research and Therapy*, *70*, 56–63.

Miltenberger, R. G., Fuqua, R. W., & McKinley, T. (1985). Habit reversal with muscle tics: Replication and component analysis. *Behavior Therapy*, *16*, 39–50.

Neal, M., & Cavanna, A. E. (2013). "Not just right experiences" in patients with Tourette syndrome: Complex motor tics or compulsions? *Psychiatry Research, 15*, 559–563.

Reese, H. E., Scahill, L., Peterson, A. L., Crowe, K., Woods, D. W., Piacentini, J., ... Wilhelm, S. (2014). The premonitory urge to tic: Measurement, characteristics, and correlates in older adolescents and adults. *Behavior Therapy, 45*, 177–186.

Sharenow, E. L., Fuqua, W., & Miltenberger, R. G. (1989). The treatment of muscle tics with dissimilar competing response practice. *Journal of Applied Behavior Analysis, 22*, 35–42.

Woods, D. W., & Miltenberger, R. G. (1996). A review of habit reversal with childhood habit disorders. *Education and Treatment of Children, 19*, 197–214.

Woods, D. W., Piacentini, J., Himle, M. B., & Chang, S. (2005). Premonitory Urge for Tics Scale (PUTS): Initial psychometric results and examination of the premonitory urge phenomenon in youths with tic disorders. *Journal of Developmental & Behavioral Pediatrics, 26*, 397–403.

Woods, D. W., Piacentini, J., Chang, S. W., Deckersbach, T., Ginsburg, G., Peterson, A. L., ... Wilhelm, S. (2008). *Managing Tourette syndrome: A behavioral intervention for children and adults: Therapist guide*. New York, NY: Oxford University Press Inc.

FURTHER READING

Conelea, C. A., & Wellen, B. C. M. (2017). Multi-media field test: Tic treatment goes tech: A review of TicHelper.com. *Cognitive and Behavioral Practice, 24*, 374–381.

Edwards, K. R., & Specht, M. (2016). A review of the literature regarding behavioral therapy for chronic tic disorders (CTDs): Where do we go from here? *Current Developmental Disorders Reports, 3*, 222–228.

Himle, M. B., Freitag, M., Walther, M., Franklin, S. A., Ely, L., & Woods, D. W. (2012). A randomized pilot trial comparing videocoference versus face-to-face delivery of behavior therapy for childhood tic disorders. *Behaviour Research and Therapy, 50*, 565–570.

Jakubovski, E., Reichert, C., Karch, A., Buddensiek, N., Breuer, D., & Müller-Vahl, K. (2016). The ONLINE-TICS study protocol: A randomized observer-blind clinical trial to demonstrate the efficacy and safety of internet-delivered behavioral treatment for adults with chronic tic disorders. *Front Psychiatry, 7*, 119.

Ricketts, E. J., Goetz, A. R., Capriotti, M. R., Bauer, C. C., Brei, N. G., Himle, M. B., ... Woods, D. W. (2016). A randomized waitlist-controlled pilot trial of voice over Internet protocol-delivered behavior therapy for youth with chronic tic disorders. *Journal of Telemedicine and Telecare, 22*, 153–162.

Scahill, L., Woods, D. W., Himle, M. B., Peterson, A. L., Wilhelm, S., Piacentini, J. C., ... Mink, J. W. (2013). Current controversies on the role of behavior therapy in Tourette syndrome. *Movement Disorders, 28*, 1179–1183.

Chapter 4

Pharmacological Management of Tic Disorders in Youth

Babar M. Saggu, MD[1], Sana Shad, MA[2], Alicia A. Barnes, DO, MPH[3] and Cathy L. Budman, MD[2,4]

[1]Department of Psychiatry, Butler Hospital, Providence, RI, United States, [2]Long Island Center for Tourette & Associated Disorders, Great Neck, NY, United States, [3]Department of Psychiatry, Saint Louis University School of Medicine, St. Louis, MO, United States, [4]Zucker School of Medicine at Hofstra-Northwell, Hempstead, NY, United States

INTRODUCTION

Tics are sudden, nonrhythmic, and repetitive abnormal movements and/or sounds that typically first emerge during early childhood. Tics are either "simple" (i.e., brief rapid movements of a single muscle group) or "complex" (i.e., involving multiple muscle groups and/or performed in an orchestrated pattern) in nature. Tics are the cardinal symptoms in a spectrum of tic disorders including: *Provisional Tic Disorder* (i.e., when motor and/or vocal tics have been present for <1 year), *Chronic Motor or Chronic Vocal Tic Disorder* (i.e., when motor or vocal tics have persistent for >1 year), and *Tourette Disorder* (i.e., when *both* motor and at least one or more vocal tics have been present during the course of the disorder, not necessarily concurrently, and tic symptoms have been active for at least 1 year or more) (American Psychiatric Association, 2013). Tics wax and wane in severity and, also change in type, location, and character. Tics may increase in response to stress or excitement, through suggestion or by demonstration, and may be elicited by certain triggers (Sanger et al., 2010). Tics are categorized as either "primary" (i.e., idiopathic) or "secondary" (i.e., due to an identifiable cause such as neurodegenerative diseases, substance abuse, pregnancy, autoimmune disorders or infections, and medications) (Donaldson, Marsden, Schneider, & Bhatia, 2012; Jankovic & Lang, 2015; Juncos, 2012; Mejia & Jankovic, 2005; Mills & Hedderly, 2014; Ropper, Samuels, & Klein, 2014). Table 4.1 presents a description of primary and secondary tics and tic disorders.

The Clinician's Guide to Treatment and Management of Youth with Tourette Syndrome and Tic Disorders.
DOI: https://doi.org/10.1016/B978-0-12-811980-8.00004-2

TABLE 4.1 Characterization of Primary and Secondary Tics and Tic Disorders

Primary Tics (American Psychiatric Association, 2013)	Secondary Tics (Donaldson et al., 2012; Jankovic & Lang, 2015; Juncos, 2012; Mejia & Jankovic, 2005; Mills & Hedderly, 2014; Ropper et al., 2014)
Provisional Tic Disorder: • One or more motor tics or vocal tics. • Duration from onset is less than 12 months. • Onset before age 18 years. • Tics are not secondary to a medical condition or substance abuse. • Does not meet criteria for persistent tic disorder or Tourette disorder. Persistent (Chronic) Motor or Vocal Tic Disorder: • One or more motor tics or vocal tics. • Duration from onset is more than 12 months. • Onset before age 18 years. • Tics are not secondary to a medical condition or substance abuse. • Does not meet criteria for Tourette disorder Tourette Disorder: • Two or more motor tics *and* at least one vocal tic, although these may not always occur at the same time. • Duration from onset is more than 12 months. • Tics are not secondary to a medical condition or substance abuse.	Neurodevelopmental Disorders: • Down's syndrome • Tuberous sclerosis • Citrullinemia • Neuroacanthocytosis • Neurodegeneration with brain iron accumulation type 1 (NBIA1) • Wilson disease • Duchenne muscular atrophy • XYY karyotype • Fragile X syndrome Cerebral Hemorrhage and Infarction Perinatal CNS Trauma Infections: • Pediatric autoimmune neuropsychiatric syndromes • Encephalitis lethargica • Sydenham's chorea • Creutzfeldt–Jakob disease • HIV CNS Tumors Drug Induced Tics: • L-Dopa • Anticholinergics • Antihistamines • Phenobarbital • Lamotrigine • Stimulant abuse • Antipsychotics

The pharmacological treatment of tics in Tourette disorder and other persistent tic disorders (collectively referred to as TD) requires their recognition and appropriate distinction from other repetitive behaviors, familiarity with the natural course of tics, and comprehensive medical evaluation including an assessment of their impact on daily functioning. Evidence-informed treatment strategies must be further individualized, taking into consideration relevant bio-psycho-social influences. When discussing tics and tic disorders, children and parents often have many questions and may be unclear how the clinician has arrived at the current diagnosis. The example below presents a common interaction regarding tics in a 9-year-old boy and sample responses to common parent questions.

Parent: *How do you know that this is a "tic" and not some other condition?*

Clinician: *The diagnosis of a tic disorder is based on the presence of characteristic symptoms that typically unfold during childhood and follow a fairly predictable course. There is no specific test or laboratory finding that confirms a diagnosis of a "tic disorder." The diagnosis of tics is made once other medical conditions are excluded.*

Parent: *My 9-year-old son has had a number of abnormal movements for the past year and a half, but never made any funny noises. That means it's not Tourette's, right?*

Clinician: *It is possible that your son may have experienced minor phonic tics that were not very conspicuous and easily unnoticed. Indeed, it's easy to overlook simple phonic tics such as soft repetitive sniffing or throat clearing. Moreover, since your son is only 9-years-old, it is still possible that he may develop phonic tics, which would meet criteria for a diagnosis of Tourette's Disorder. Also, it's important to understand that from a clinical standpoint, there may be little practical significance whether your son's diagnosis is Tourette's Disorder or persistent motor tic disorder in terms of the treatment.*

GENERAL CONSIDERATIONS

Currently, there are currently no established preventative pharmacological therapies for TD. The decision to embark on medication management of TD must be carefully weighed against the risk of known and unforeseen adverse effects. When there is sufficient evidence that daily functioning is impaired, due to: (1) disruption of academic, social or workplace performance; (2) pain, or (3) tic-associated medical and/or surgical morbidity; the potential benefits of medication treatment of tics may outweigh its potential risks. When tics do not cause significant functional impairment, conservative (i.e., nonpharmacological) interventions are preferred whenever possible (see Chapter 1: Introduction to Treatment and Management of Youth with Tourette Disorders and Tic Disorders, Chapter 2: Psychoeducation about Tic Disorders and Treatment, and Chapter 3: Habit Reversal Training).

Prior to embarking on medication management of tics, a comprehensive history focusing on the assessment of motor and/or vocal tics and their associated features, detailed assessment of cooccurring psychiatric and/or medical conditions, evaluation of impact on family, peer, and school functioning, investigation of other relevant features (e.g., neurological examination, possible laboratory and/or neuroimaging workups to rule out organic causes of secondary tics), and the use of standardized measures of TD severity remain standards of good clinical practice (Murphy, Lewin, Storch, & Stock, 2013; see Chapter 1, Introduction to Treatment and Management of Youth with Tourette Disorders and Tic Disorders, for further information on recommended assessments). This chapter presents the current evidence base for the psychopharmacological management of tics in youth, and summarizes the treatment options that are considered in context of commonly cooccurring conditions. Given general treatment guidelines, ultimately the indication for medication management and the choice of a particular therapy must be carefully assessed for each individual case, taking into consideration factors such as: tic symptom severity, functional impairment and severity of cooccurring medical and psychiatric condition, age at presentation, duration of illness, adequacy and efficacy of other treatment strategies, and tolerability of single or combined treatments. In many instances the treatment of cooccurring psychiatric conditions such as Attention Deficit Hyperactivity Disorder (ADHD), Anxiety Disorders, Mood Disorders, or Obsessive Compulsive Disorder (OCD) may take precedence, as the functional impairment caused by these cooccurring disorders may have a more significant clinical impact on overall quality of life than tic symptoms (Murphy et al., 2013). When discussing the recommendation for medication, some children and families may be hesitant. The following text continues the previous example of the 9-year-old boy with tics and serves as one approach of how to answer parents' questions and alleviate concerns.

Parent: *We are uncomfortable with using medications to treat our child's tics, but we are also worried that he is getting depressed and seems to be spending too much time alone.*

Clinician: *I can understand your reluctance to use medication to treat your child's tics. We always try to avoid using medications to treat tics unless there are really compelling reasons to do so. The benefits of using medication must always be very carefully weighed against the potential risks including both short-term and longer-term side effects. Importantly, tics are not always the main problem. You mentioned that your child seems more depressed and I'd like to explore this further. There are a number of different conditions that frequently precede, co-occur with, or develop after tics first emerge including: anxiety, obsessive compulsive thoughts and behaviors, sadness or irritability, problems with focusing, and excessive impulsivity. When unrecognized, these conditions may wreck havoc with a child's life, negatively impacting on school, relationships with peers and with family members. Depression may result from such untreated conditions, may occur on its own, and may also be the result of bullying, poor academic performance, etc. So, it's important that we examine and try to understand your child and his symptoms from a biopsychosocial standpoint, meaning that we consider all the different factors that may be relevant before we move forward with a particular treatment strategy. Even when medication management is the appropriate treatment choice, we still need to carefully assess environmental influences on symptoms and intervene accordingly.*

In general, most tic disorders have a remitting, relapsing course, with exacerbations and periods of improvement. In many instances, tics in children are mild and may not require ongoing treatment if there is minimal or no functional impairment (Black, Black, Greene, & Schlaggar, 2016). Education regarding the course of illness including anticipated changes in tic type and severity over time, the benefits and risks of treatment, and the influences of cooccurring psychiatric conditions on overall morbidity is essential (see Chapter 2, Psychoeducation about Tic Disorders and Treatment, for information about psychoeducation). Once the baseline characteristics of tic severity and functional impairment have been established, a collaborative approach towards choosing the appropriate treatment modality must be undertaken with the patient and family. The patient's age and weight, any known metabolic factors or medical comorbidity (e.g., liver, kidney, or other concurrent medical disease) and compliance optimization should always be taken into account. Adjustments in medication dosing must also take into consideration the waxing/waning nature of tics so that inadvertent escalation of medication dosage does not occur unless truly warranted. While some parents may be hesitant to initiate pharmacotherapy, other parents may want more aggressive treatment to do whatever it takes to provide their child relief (as noted in the role play below with an 13-year-old girl).

Parent: *My daughter's tics have been increasing for the past two weeks, ever since Halloween and it's already nearly Thanksgiving. I think it's time to start medication, although she doesn't even seem to be aware of her tics.*

Clinician: *It sounds like your daughter may be experiencing what is a very typical tic "waxing" period. Tics often increase during certain times of the year, and not uncommonly around the holidays, possibly due to increased excitement and stress. You mention that she doesn't seem particularly bothered by this most recent bout of increased tics. Are there any areas where you feel your daughter's tics are negatively impacting her, such as school work, relationships with friends or with family?*

Parent: *Well, to be honest, not really. She is a great student, gets straight A's, and she is also a really good soccer goalie. Everyone seems to like her including her friends, teachers, neighbors, and the soccer coach. It's just that I feel really bad when I see her ticcing. It makes me feel so upset that my child has these tics, even if it doesn't seem to bother her.*

Clinician: *I can understand how upsetting it must feel to see your daughter having these tics and how worried you must feel about the future. That's a pretty normal reaction for any parent; you'd like to make these tics go away. However, it's important to understand that tics do come and go, so we don't want to start medications unnecessarily, particularly if your daughter is going through a tic waxing period but is otherwise functioning very well in all areas.*

The choice of a particular pharmacological treatment strategy for tics requires a cautious risks/benefits analysis, including consideration of medication side effect profile, potential interactions with concomitant medications, and comorbidity (Singer, 2006). Provided below is an overview of the various pharmacological options for tic management, which is stratified on treatment strategies of common psychiatric cooccurring conditions (see Tables 4.2 and 4.3). Level 1 medications are considered "first-line" pharmacological treatments for TD based on mild side effect profiles and demonstrated efficacy for treating combined TD and ADHD symptoms. Given that subthreshold and clinically significant ADHD symptoms are common among youth with TD, such properties are highly advantageous. Moreover, Level 1 medications offer a beneficial alternative to psychostimulant medication

TABLE 4.2 Summary of Evidence-based Pharmacological Treatments for Tic Disorders

Pharmacotherapy	Summary of Evidence
Level 1	
Clonidine (Oral)	Moderate quality evidence from 2 studies of a total of 173 children, showing a medium to large effect size (Kurlan et al., 2002; Singer et al., 1995).
Clonidine (Patch)	Moderate quality evidence, from 1 study of 437 children, showing a small effect size (Du et al., 2008).
Guanfacine	Moderate quality evidence from 2 studies of a total of 58 children, showing large effect size (Cummings, Singer, Krieger, Miller, & Mahone, 2002; Scahill et al., 2001).
Level 2	
Topiramate	Low quality evidence, from 14 mixed studies of 1003 children, showing a small to moderate effect size (Donegan et al., 2015).
Atomoxetine	Moderate quality evidence, from 1 study of 145 children, showing small to moderate effect size (Allen et al., 2005).
Baclofen	Very low quality evidence, from 1 study of 10 children, showing overall improvement, but not tic severity (Singer et al., 2001).
Clonazepam	Very low quality evidence, from case reports and expert opinions (Goetz, 1992; Gonce & Barbeau, 1977; Steingard et al., 1994).
Level 3	
Haloperidol	Low quality evidence, from 1 study of 22 children, showing moderate effect size (Sallee et al., 1997; Budman, 2014).
Pimozide	Low quality evidence from 2 studies of a total of 42 children, showing moderate effect size (Sallee et al., 1997; Shapiro & Shapiro, 1984).
Risperidone	Low quality evidence, from 2 studies of a total of 45 children, showing large effect size (Gilbert, Batterson, Sethuraman, & Sallee, 2004; Scahill et al., 2003).
Olanzapine	Low quality evidence, from 1 study of 60 children, showing a moderate effect size similar to haloperidol (Ji, Li, Li, & Guo, 2005).

(*Continued*)

TABLE 4.2 (Continued)

Pharmacotherapy	Summary of Evidence
Ziprasidone	Low quality evidence, from 1 study of 27 children, showing large effect size (Sallee et al., 2000).
Aripiprazole	Low quality evidence, from 2 studies of a total of 67 children, showing a moderate effect size, similar to other antipsychotics (Liu et al., 2011; Yoo et al., 2013).

Source: Evidence is largely drawn from the following sources: Hollis, C., Pennant, M., Cuenca, J., Glazebrook, C., Kendall, T., Whittington, C., ... Stern, J. (2016). Clinical effectiveness and patient perspectives of different treatment strategies for tics in children and adolescents with Tourette syndrome: A systematic review and qualitative analysis. Health Technology Assessment, 20(4); Thenganatt, M. A., & Jankovic, J. (2016). Recent advances in understanding and managing Tourette Syndrome. F1000Research, 5 (F1000 Faculty Rev):152; Waldon, K., Hill, J., Termine, C., Balottin, U., & Cavanna, A. E. (2013). Trials of pharmacological interventions for Tourette syndrome: A systematic review. Behavioural Neurology, 26(4), 265–273; Weisman, H., Qureshi, I. A., Leckman, J. F., Scahill, L., & Bloch, M. H. (2013). Systematic review: Pharmacological treatment of tic disorders—Efficacy of antipsychotic and alpha-2 adrenergic agonist agents. *Neuroscience & Biobehavioral Reviews, 37*(6), 1162–1171; Whittington, C., Pennant, M., Kendall, T., Glazebrook, C., Trayner, P., Groom, M., ... Hollis, C. (2016). Practitioner review: Treatments for Tourette syndrome in children and young people—A systematic review. *Journal of Child Psychology and Psychiatry, 57*(9), 988–1004.

TABLE 4.3 Grading of Recommendations Assessment, Development and Evaluation (GRADE)

Quality of Evidence	Definition
High	Further research is very unlikely to change our knowledge of effects. Several high-quality studies have been conducted, with consistent results or a large multicenter trial with adequate power and design exists in some circumstances.
Moderate	More research is required and likely to change our knowledge of results. Either a single high quality study with adequate power exists, or there are several small studies with appropriate design.
Low	Further research is very likely to change our knowledge of effects. One or more studies with severe limitations exist.
Very low	Any estimate of effects is uncertain. One or more studies with very severe limitations exist, entire knowledge is based on expert opinions, some case studies exist or no significant research has been conducted.

Source: Modified from GRADE work group: Guyatt, G. H., Oxman, A. D., Vist, G. E., Kunz, R., Falck-Ytter, Y., Alonso-Coello, P., & Schünemann, H. J. (2008). GRADE: An emerging consensus on rating quality of evidence and strength of recommendations. *BMJ: British Medical Journal, 336* (7650), 924–926.

when decreased appetite, weight loss, and/or insomnia are concerns. Level 2 medications are considered "second-line" agents. While the evidence base for tic suppression is less robust than Level 1 medications, the side effect profiles of Level 2 medications are still relatively mild. Some of these agents may also be helpful for ADHD (e.g., atomoxetine), anxiety or agitation (e.g., benzodiazepines and topiramate), and may provide some degree of muscle relaxation (e.g., diazepam and baclofen). In comparison to Level 1 and Level 2 medications, Level 3 medications appear superior in terms of an evidence base and efficacy for overall tic suppression. Additionally, Level 3 agents (particularly the second generation antipsychotics, SGA) may also attenuate some psychiatric cooccurring symptoms such as anxiety, mood disorders, and aggression. However, as Level 3 medications are associated with more significant adverse effects, they are usually reserved for cases that are refractory to Levels 1 and 2 medications or for youth presenting with severe TD and/or severe cooccurring psychiatric conditions. Indeed, balancing the sometimes competing objectives of optimizing both tic suppression and tolerability is a considerable clinical challenge.

When selecting a particular medication factors such as cost and insurance coverage, ease of administration (e.g., whether the preparation is available in a liquid formulation for children who will not swallow pills, taste, whether a particular medication is available in both long and short-acting formulations), and leveraging side effects to also potentially treat cooccurring problems (e.g., taking advantage of sedating side effects to administer at night time for youth who have trouble falling asleep, using topiramate for youth with comorbid migraine, excessive sweating, or obesity) are important considerations. Simplifying medication titration and dosing schedule while providing clear information about expected therapeutic doses, duration of a particular medication trial, common and subtler medication side effects are important. Treatment compliance requires close monitoring of potential side effects and risk factors such as parental psychiatric morbidity (e.g., ADHD, depression, anxiety, etc.) that can impact on medication adherence.

LEVEL 1 MEDICATIONS

Alpha-2 Adrenergic Agonists

Alpha-2 agonists have demonstrated efficacy for the treatment of ADHD (Hirota, Schwartz, & Correll, 2014) and remain a primary treatment strategy for TD with comorbid ADHD, although the evidence supporting their efficacy for treatment of tics without comorbid ADHD is less impressive (Egolf & Coffey, 2014; Murphy et al., 2013; Murphy et al., 2017; Waldon, Hill, Termine, Balottin, & Cavanna, 2013; Weisman, Qureshi, Leckman, Scahill, & Bloch, 2013). Nonetheless, due to their relatively milder side effect profile, alpha-2 agonists (including oral preparations of regular or extended release clonidine and guanfacine, transdermal clonidine) are commonly tried before employing stronger tic medications with more serious side effects (Du et al., 2008; Egolf & Coffey, 2014; Murphy et al., 2013; Rizzo, Gulisano, Calì, & Curatolo, 2013; Weisman et al., 2013; Waldon et al., 2013). Common side effects include daytime fatigue, dry mouth and nasal mucosa, and headache. Lowered blood pressure, orthostatic hypotension and bradycardia may also occur. Baseline screening for cardiac arrhythmias and orthostatic blood pressure monitoring is recommended, especially when initiating and/or changing dosages. Although sedation is the most commonly reported side effect, excitability and changes in mood (including symptoms of hypomania or mania) have also been reported (Horrigan & Barnhill, 1999). Abruptly stopping these medications can result in rebound hypertension, and therefore discontinuation requires a gradual tapering (Kisicki, Fiske, & Lyne, 2007; Geyskes, Boer, & Dorhout Mees, 1979). These agents are usually started at a very low dose and carefully titrated over a period of weeks with regular monitoring of blood pressure, pulse, and adverse effects. Clinical responses are not expected until a therapeutic dose has been achieved and continued for several weeks (Shier, Reichenbacher, Ghuman, & Ghuman, 2013). Although local skin reactions appear common, a large study of clonidine patch showed mild efficacy in decreasing tic severity (Du et al., 2008; Zhong, Zhou, & Hu, 2007). Consider the sample case of a 9-year-old boy with TD and cooccurring ADHD.

Jeremy is a 9-year-old male with ADHD and TD. Although his symptoms had been managed without medication until last year, his ADHD symptoms are now adversely impacting his academic performance and peer relationships. He was recently kicked off his soccer team due to his disruptive behaviors, and his parents are concerned that he is no longer being invited over to his friends' homes. Jeremy has also been having more conflicts at home, particularly with his brother with whom he is sometimes excessively aggressive. Jeremy has always had difficulty falling asleep at night and his parents wonder whether this is adding to his problems with concentration in school.

Two brief trials with psychostimulants were attempted last fall, but were accompanied by excessive side effects including decreased appetite and weight loss, which concerned his parents as Jeremy is among the shorter boys in his grade. His motor tics have increased in number, frequency, and intensity in the past year, and are now very annoying to Jeremy. In particular, Jeremy reported that his head shaking/head rolling and shoulder tics and his newest abdominal tensing tic cause him distress. Jeremy's parents worry that he may be experiencing bullying at school, but Jeremy denies this is a problem.

Jeremy is not interested in "therapy" at this time, but he told his parents and his doctor that he would like to try medication for his tics; he seems even less aware of his ADHD symptoms. His clinician suggested a trial with an alpha agonist to treat his combined ADHD and tics, and reviewed general side effects and dosing schedule, emphasizing that a therapeutic dose must be achieved by titrating every 7 days and then maintained for approximately 4–6 weeks before efficacy can be assessed. Jeremy's parents initially express concern that a blood pressure medication may cause him to faint at school. The clinician reassures that Jeremy's dose will be gradually increased and that his blood pressure can be monitored by the school nurse as needed and will be checked at each subsequent office visit. The clinician performs pre-medication ratings of TD and ADHD symptoms, then reviews the different options including both short- and long-acting preparations, noting that guanfacine appears to be less sedating than clonidine, and longer-acting preparations are more easily administered and tolerated than short-acting preparations.

Initially Jeremy is prescribed clonidine ER, but since his insurance company will only cover guanfacine ER, his clinician opts to start this medication at 1.0 mg at bedtime, increasing after 7 days if tolerated to 2.0 mg once daily at bedtime and requests Jeremy to return for a follow-up visit after he has been maintained on this dose for about 2–4 weeks, with telephone feedback by his parents in the interim.

At the next follow-up visit, Jeremy is tolerating the 2.0 mg dose for the past 3 weeks very well with no reported side effects, but only minimal improvement. His clinician suggests increasing the dose to 3.0 mg daily with follow-up in one month and encourages Jeremy's parents to call with any concerns during the interim. At the follow-up visit, his parents report that he is sleeping better and seems to be less disruptive in class. His tics have decreased somewhat in intensity and number, although it is not clear whether this is from his medication or due to a waning period. His clinician advises that Jeremy stay on this same dose, return for follow-up in one month, and also provides a rating scale for his teacher to complete on a weekly basis so that at next visit improvements in Jeremy's ADHD symptoms can be better assessed.

LEVEL 2 MEDICATIONS

Topiramate

Topiramate is a broad spectrum antiepileptic (i.e., anti-seizure) medicine that can be a useful option for the treatment of tics, especially in patients with comorbid obesity, insomnia, or migraine headaches. Due to its sedating effects, topiramate is typically administered at bedtime. A relatively minimal weight loss may be associated with its use (Ferraro & Di Trapani, 2008; Kuo & Jimenez-Shahed, 2010; Yang, Zhang, Zeng, Huang, & Liu, 2013). Other common side effects of topiramate include: cognitive problems (such as word-finding difficulties and impaired attention), taste changes, anxiety, and anorexia (Donegan, Dixon, Hemming, Tudur-Smith, & Marson, 2015). Some patients may respond to a lower dosage of topiramate, while others may require higher doses (Jankovic, Jimenez-Shahed, & Brown, 2010). While there are several small, low quality trials of topiramate that showed a small-to-moderate effect size in meta-analysis (Donegan et al., 2015), a double-blind placebo controlled study of topiramate showed a moderate-to-large effect size (Jankovic et al., 2010). Similar to alpha agonists, improvement in tics may not occur until treatment has been sustained for a few weeks (Cavanna & Nani, 2013).

Baclofen

Baclofen is a skeletal muscle relaxant that has some evidence supporting its use for the treatment of TD, which comes from a single placebo controlled trial. While this single trial demonstrated that baclofen decreased overall TD-related impairment, it did not produce significant improvement in motor or vocal tic related scores (Singer, Wendlandt, Krieger, & Giuliano, 2001; Pringsheim et al., 2012; Whittington et al., 2016). However, compared with stronger Level 3 medications, baclofen is considered to have a relatively mild side effect profile and because it is a muscle relaxant, it is sometimes used clinically for treating dystonia (Greene & Fahn, 1992). Due to its sedating effects, it is recommended that baclofen dosing is initiated at bedtime with daytime doses added only as needed, and at the lowest effective dose to minimize excessive daytime sedation. Additional possible side effects include confusion, hypotonia, and the risk for abuse, tolerance, and withdrawal (Novartis Pharmaceuticals Canada Inc., 2013; Reeves, Ladner, Perry, Burke, & Laizer, 2015).

Botulinium Toxin

Onabotulinumtoxin A (formerly known as "botulinium toxin type A") is administered via injections that are often required to be repeated every few months. Onabotulinumtoxin A is considered in cases where typical oral therapy and/or behavioral therapy are ineffective for managing a particularly disruptive and focal tic. Onabotulinumtoxin A injection directly into the affected muscle(s) acts to weaken the specific muscle(s) that produces the tic. While a significant decrease in simple motor tics and in premonitory urges was found in one placebo-controlled crossover study (Marras, Andrews, Sime, & Lang, 2001), the overall improvement in impairment is usually modest (Egolf & Coffey, 2014; Ferraro & Di Trapani, 2008; Jankovic, 1994; Marras et al., 2001; Porta, Maggioni, Ottaviani, & Schindler, 2004). Patients who have complex tics involving multiple muscle groups are generally not suitable for this particular therapy. Referral to a movement disorders specialist with expertise in the administration of onabotulinumtoxin A is required, and in cases of vocal tics, additional specialists and hospitalization are usually necessary. Common side effects are site specific, but may include dystonia or weakness of the muscle groups injected which can lead to paresis or paralysis of the muscle, pain and/or bruising (Hallett et al., 2013). Consider the following example of a patient who might benefit from onabotulinumtoxin A.

Patient:	*Doctor, I am very self-conscious about my eye blinking tic. I tried behavior therapy and medications, but nothing seems to help this particular tic and I will be going on college interviews soon. Are there any other specific treatments for this tic?*
Clinician:	*You may want to consider getting a consultation for "Botox." This treatment is particularly helpful for eye blinking tics, which are often very automatic. A small amount of Botulinum toxin is injected into the muscle and weakens it so that it won't contract so vigorously and generally treatments are given every three months. Uncommonly some develop an allergic reaction to this but for many, it can be a highly effective treatment for eye blinking tics.*

Atomoxetine

Atomoxetine, a selective norepinephrine reuptake inhibitor with little affinity for serotonergic receptors, is a nonstimulant medication used for the treatment of ADHD (Bymaster et al., 2002). Atomoxetine has been shown to be effective for treating ADHD in youth with TD and appears to reduce both ADHD symptoms and tic severity (Kratochvil et al., 2011). Therapeutic dosage is calculated based on weight and is usually titrated over a period of weeks. Similar to alpha agonists, clinical benefits in terms of reduction of ADHD symptoms and decreased tic severity will not occur for some time. Common side effects associated with atomoxetine include: nausea, headache, stomachache, irritability, and behavioral activation in some patients (Allen et al., 2005; Bloch, Panza, Landeros-Weisenberger, & Leckman, 2009; Cortese et al., 2015).

Benzodiazepines

Clonazepam is a benzodiazepine that some consider clinically helpful for the treatment of TD (Gonce & Barbeau, 1977). There are some reports suggesting its efficacy for reducing tic severity is superior to that of short-acting oral clonidine; however, others suggest it has only a moderate benefit for reducing tic severity at best and only when it is used as an adjuvant treatment strategy (Goetz, 1992; Steingard, Goldberg, Lee, & DeMaso, 1994). The use of clonazepam or other benzodiazepines for treatment of youth with TD can be complicated by common side effects such as sedation, disinhibition (Commander, Green, & Pendergast, 1991), and the risk for abuse, dependence, and drug diversion (Coffey, 2009). While there are no systematic studies of either shorter- or longer-term clonazepam use for TD, there may be a role for its use in the acute treatment of severe anxiety disorders cooccurring with TD, as a reduction in anxiety (which is a common trigger for tic exacerbation) may secondarily decrease tic severity in adolescents and adults (Eddy, Rickards, & Cavanna, 2011). Consider the example case of a 16-year-old male patient with both TD and cooccurring anxiety.

Mitchell is a 16-year-old male with Tourette's Disorder, mild obsessive symptoms, and generalized anxiety. Most of the time, he manages his tics and anxiety well without medications. However, during particularly stressful periods such as finals or when attending large family gatherings, he finds his anxiety symptoms often spiral "out of control" and are associated with an increase in tics.

Mitchell's clinician suggests using clonazepam on an "as needed basis" to manage occasions anticipated to worsen anxiety symptoms, and taking clonazepam more regularly during predictable time-limited periods of stress. Mitchell and his parents like this treatment option, as it avoids having to take ongoing medication. After a two-week trial of 0.25–0.5 mg 2–3 times daily during finals, Mitchell returns for follow-up and happily reports that he could focus on his studies and exams due to decreased anxiety with decreased intensity and disruption of tics. His dose of clonazepam is tapered and discontinued without any rebound in tic or anxiety symptoms.

LEVEL 3 MEDICATIONS

Dopamine-2 Receptor Antagonists

Second Generation Antipsychotics

Aripiprazole is a partial D2 receptor agonist and also a partial agonist for serotonin (5-HT) 2A and 2C receptors, as well as D3 receptors, with some affinity for histamine and alpha-adrenergic receptors (Shapiro et al., 2003). Aripiprazole acts as a D2 receptor antagonist at higher doses, which may account in part for its efficacy in reducing tic severity and also for possible adverse effects shared with the first-generation antipsychotics (FGA) such as acute dystonic reactions, akathisia, and parkinsonism (Budman, 2014). Apart from haloperidol and pimozide, aripiprazole is the only other agent approved by the United States' Food and Drug Administration (FDA) for the indication of treating TD. Indeed, there is considerable clinical and empirical evidence supporting its efficacy for reducing tic severity in adults and children (Budman et al., 2008; Ghanizadeh, Tordjman, & Jaafari, 2015; Ho, Chiu, Tseng, & Huang, 2014; Lyon et al., 2009; Murphy et al., 2009; Yoo et al., 2013).

There is also evidence supporting the efficacy of the SGA risperidone and to a lesser extent for ziprasidone, with even less or little evidence for other agents in this category such as olanzapine, quetiapine, and/or paliperidone (Budman, 2014; Sallee et al., 2000; Scahill, Leckman, Schultz, Katsovich, & Peterson, 2003; Yamamuro, Makinodan, Ota, Iida, & Kishimoto, 2014). Although the SGAs are considered to have comparable tic suppressing efficacy with a generally reduced risk for extrapyramidal side effects such as parkinsonism and acute dystonias when compared with FGAs (Budman, 2014), these agents are associated with significant weight gain and risk for developing metabolic syndrome; youth treated with SGAs appear to be at even higher risk for developing such complications (Ames et al., 2016; Correll & Kane, 2007; De Hert, Dobbelaere, Sheridan, Cohen, & Correll, 2011; Roerig, Steffen, & Mitchell, 2011). Since olanzapine is associated with particularly high risk for weight gain with metabolic syndrome, despite some evidence supporting its usefulness for treatment of tics, it should only be considered in very limited cases (McCracken, Suddath, Chang, Thakur, & Piacentini, 2008; Onofrj, Paci, D'Andreamatteo, & Toma, 2000).

The consequences of long-term use of these agents in TD are not well established. Routine monitoring at appropriate intervals should be undertaken for measures of weight, height, waist circumference, BMI, serum glucose and lipid levels, adhering to published guidelines, and the lowest-most effective dose should be used, especially for younger patients (Ames et al., 2016; Pringsheim, Panagiotopoulos, Davidson, Ho, & for the CAMESA guideline group, 2011). There is some evidence supporting the use of SGAs for addressing comorbid conditions such as tic-associated OCD, especially when the symptoms are severe or refractory to standard treatments (Budman, 2014; Waldon et al., 2013). It is important to keep in mind that all D2 receptor antagonists, whether first- or second-generation agents, can cause a variety of movement disorders as side effects. In some instances, it may be difficult to distinguish medication-induced movement disorders from tics. Hence, baseline symptom severity rating scales for TD (such as the Yale Global Tic Severity Scale; Leckman et al., 1989) and for monitoring treatment-emergent abnormal involuntary movements (such as the Abnormal Involuntary Movement Scale; Lane, Glazer, Hansen, Berman, & Kramer, 1985) should be routinely used by an experienced clinician and administered at baseline and follow-up visits. Consider the following discussion between a parent and clinician regarding the initiation of a SGA.

Parent: *My 14-year-old has seen quite a few different doctors, has tried a number of medications and also behavior therapy. However, his tics have been so severe for the past several months that he is in nearly constant pain from head, neck, and shoulder twitching and a repetitive kicking movement that interrupts him while walking. He finds it nearly impossible to get his words out now due to his loud grunting, and cannot use his computer mouse without banging on it repeatedly. We are scared and don't know what to do, does he need surgery?*

Clinician: *I see that he has not yet been tried on a stronger tic medication such as aripiprazole or risperidone. These medications often have greater side effects than the ones he has already tried, but are also more effective in treating such moderate-severe tics. Aripiprazole is less likely to cause problems with breast enlargement or severe weight gain and is FDA approved for treating Tourette's Disorder. We can start at a very low dose, even as little as 1–2 mg at bedtime and gradually increase the dose each week until your son achieves some degree of relief. Most youth with TD experience improvement with doses in the range of 5–15 mg daily; we will aim for the lowest dose that effectively decreases his tics without causing unacceptable untoward side effects. We will review common side effects now and stay in close contact should any concerns arise. It will also be necessary to schedule regular follow-up visits each month and periodic blood tests so that we can monitor progress, changes in weight, and other possible side effects.*

First Generation Antipsychotics

FGAs are potent blockers of dopamine-2 (D2) receptors (Meltzer, Matsubara, & Lee, 1989; Scahill et al., 2006). Until very recently in the United States the only medications with FDA approval for treatment of tics were the FGAs haloperidol and pimozide (Mogwitz, Buse, Ehrlich, & Roessner, 2013; Sallee, Nesbitt, Jackson, Sine, & Sethuraman, 1997). Fluphenazine is another FGA with a higher affinity for D2 receptors, which is preferred by some experts due to its reportedly relatively better tolerability compared to haloperidol or pimozide (Singer, 2006; Wijemanne, Wu, & Jankovic, 2014). While the FGAs are associated with stronger efficacy for reducing tic severity than Levels 1 and 2 medications, many patients find their side effects intolerable and require discontinuation. Use of these agents may be contraindicated or cautioned in the presence of certain medical conditions (e.g., liver disease, cardiovascular disease, leukopenia, and neutropenia) and in combination with other prescribed and over-the-counter medications (e.g., CNS depressants and anticholinergics). Adverse side effects include: acute dystonia, Parkinsonism, akathisia, tardive dyskinesia, neuroleptic malignant syndrome, cognitive dulling, dysphoria, hyperprolactinemia, excessive sedation, cardiac arrhythmias, lowered seizure threshold, and weight gain (Arana, 2000). Due to the current availability of other tic medications with less severe side effects, these agents are now generally reserved only for patients who do not respond to first or second line treatments. Baseline and regular screening for abnormal involuntary movements along with other laboratory testing is required prior to initiation and during ongoing treatment (Kenney, Kuo, & Jimenez-Shahed, 2008). The risks of serious side effects such as the prolongation of the cardiac QTc interval (which can lead to deadly arrhythmias) is associated with this class of medications, and is of particular concern when using pimozide since some patients metabolize this medicine more slowly. Prior to initiating treatment, specific genotyping to assess a patient's metabolizer status and a baseline

EKG are required to identify those at significantly greater risk for higher serum drug concentrations of pimozide and associated problems (Preskorn, 2012; Pringsheim & Marras, 2009). EKGs should be repeated at regular intervals and with increase in dose.

Vesicular Monoamine Transporter Inhibitors

Tetrabenazine is among a class of agents called vesicular monoamine transporter-2 (VMAT2) inhibitors that impede the presynaptic release of monoamine neurotransmitters such as dopamine, serotonin, norepinephrine, epinephrine, and histamine (Guay, 2010). Due to its ability to deplete the presynaptic release of dopamine, tetrabenazine is used for the treatment of severe hyperkinetic movement disorders such as Huntington's disease and tardive dyskinesia (Kenney & Jankovic, 2006). There is evidence suggesting that many patients with TD experience mild-to-marked improvement in tics when treated with tetrabenazine in comparison to conventional neuroleptics, although there has not been a large double-blind placebo trial (Fasano & Bentivoglio, 2009). However, tetrabenazine has been associated with a number of intolerable side effects including, hypotension, akathisia, Parkinsonism, insomnia, depressive symptoms, and suicidal ideation which has limited its use (Kenney & Jankovic, 2006; Fasano & Bentivoglio, 2009; Porta et al., 2008). Tetrabenazine's efficacy and reduced tolerability have prompted the further investigation and the development of more selective inhibitors of VMAT2 such as deutrabenazine and valbenazine, which may show similar efficacy with improved tolerability for the treatment of certain movement disorders including TD (Huntington Study Group et al., 2016; Jankovic et al., 2016; Neurocrine Biosciences, 2016; Thenganatt & Jankovic, 2016).

NOVEL AGENTS AND EXPERIMENTAL THERAPIES

Cannabinoids

A number of case reports, and at least two small randomized placebo-controlled trials suggest that tic severity is improved by tetrahydrocannabinol (THC) (Hasan et al., 2010; Kluger, Triolo, Jones, & Jankovic, 2015; Müller-Vahl et al., 2003; Müller-Vahl et al., 2002; Müller-Vahl, 2013). While a Cochrane systematic review concluded that there is not sufficient evidence at this time demonstrating the efficacy of cannabinoids for treatment of TD, it was suggested that THC may have some role in the treatment of otherwise refractory cases (Curtis, Clarke, & Rickards, 2009). Commonly reported side effects associated with cannabinoids include: fatigue, dizziness, dry mouth, anxiety, depersonalization, and panic attacks (Jacobus, Squeglia, Sorg, Nguyen-Louie, & Tapert, 2014; Müller-Vahl, 2013). Cannabinoid receptors are found throughout the brain and are instrumental in neurotransmission across the neural systems (Jacobus & Tapert, 2014). Several neuroimaging studies have found that adolescent marijuana users are more susceptible to neurocognitive impairments (i.e., deficits in learning, memory, attention, and other executive functioning) compared to adult users. Although many studies suggest the more subtle cognitive impairments are likely to resolve after an extended period of abstinence, early onset marijuana users may in fact continue to see persistent deficits in executive functioning (Jacobus & Tapert, 2014; Schweinsburg, Brown, & Tapert, 2008). Of note, a neuroimaging study comparing adolescent marijuana users to nonusers found changes in the amygdala in female users was associated with an increase in reported depression and anxiety symptoms (Jacobus & Tapert, 2014). Hence, given the insufficient evidence at this time to support the efficacy of cannabinoids for tic management, its use in youth (who may be more susceptible to increased risks for neurocognitive and affective effects as well as psychosis) is not recommended. As this question may be raised in treatment, the following text serves as one approach on how to answer parents and/or patients questions regarding the use of THC for tics.

Parent: *I read online that marijuana might help my child's tics. Is this true?*

Clinician: *Unfortunately, we do not have enough evidence to say whether THC, the active ingredient in marijuana, would decrease tics and for this reason, medical marijuana currently does not have an approved indication for treatment of TD in nearly all states. There are also many different cannabinoid products advertised on the internet that promise all sorts of possible benefits, but presently there is insufficient scientific evidence demonstrating efficacy and safety for treating tics. In light of evidence associating marijuana use with increased risks for psychosis, mood disorders, and cognitive problems in youth, plus the current lack of compelling evidence supporting marijuana's safety and efficacy for treatment of tics, it is not recommended at this time. Let's review the medications that you have tried previously and see what options that are evidence-based can be considered.*

AZD5213

A novel histamine-3 receptor inverse agonist, AZD5213 is currently being studied for the treatment of TD (AstraZeneca, 2013). Based on a genetic linkage study implicating inherited disturbances of histamine metabolism identified in an unusual cohort of familial cases of TD, this agent is being investigated due to its effects on histamine release (Ercan-Sencicek et al., 2010). The most common adverse effects reported thus far are headaches, activation, insomnia, and dizziness (Jucaite et al., 2013).

Ecopipam

Ecopipam is a dopamine-1 (D1) receptor antagonist that has shown possible benefits for reducing tics in an open-label study of adults with TD. Ecopipam appears to be generally well tolerated with sedation as its most commonly reported side effect; less commonly reported adverse effects include: fatigue, insomnia, anxiety, headaches, and muscle twitching (Gilbert, Budman, Singer, Kurlan, & Chipkin, 2014). A placebo-controlled clinical trial is currently underway for children and adolescents with TD (Gilbert et al., 2014).

Miscellaneous Pharmacological Agents

While the following agents appear to be used for treatment of TD by some clinicians, the evidence base for these agents is either entirely lacking or has been shown to be negative. Therefore, the use of these medications specifically to treat tics is not generally recommended. These medications include the following: levetiracetam (Smith-Hicks, Bridges, Paynter, & Singer, 2007), valproic acid (Yang, Zhang, Lin, & Guo, 2015), N-acetylcysteine and of omega-3 fatty acids (Bloch et al., 2016; Gabbay et al., 2012), pramipexole (Kurlan et al., 2012), pergolide (Gilbert, Sethuraman, Sine, Peters, & Sallee, 2000; Gilbert et al., 2003), selegiline (Feigin et al., 1996), ondansetron (Nicolson, Craven-Thuss, Smith, McKinlay, & Castellanos, 2005; Toren, Weizman, Ratner, Cohen, & Laor, 2005), mecamylamine (Silver et al., 2001), and nicotine patch (Howson et al., 2004).

COMBINED TREATMENT OF TICS AND COOCCURRING PSYCHIATRIC DISORDERS

In many cases, the clinician may opt to pharmacologically target tic symptoms by using medications that are more typically used to treat anxiety and other psychiatric conditions. However, whether such strategies offer meaningful benefits remains unclear. For example, in a very small clinical study, treatment with the serotonin reuptake inhibitor (SRI) fluoxetine demonstrated a slight improvement of tic severity, with no reported changes in obsessive compulsive symptoms (Kurlan, Como, Deeley, McDermott, & McDermott, 1993). Additionally, the tricyclic antidepressant desipramine, which can be used to treat anxiety, depression, and ADHD, was examined in a clinical study that treated children with ADHD comorbid with tics and showed a statistically significant reduction of both ADHD and tic symptoms (Müller-Vahl, 2013). However, concerns about desipramine's common and more serious side effects, as well as its toxicity in overdose, make it less appealing for widespread use (Müller-Vahl, 2013).

As close to 90% of patients with TD are also affected by symptoms of cooccurring ADHD and/or OCD (Wright, Rickards, & Cavanna, 2012), clinical concerns about how treating psychiatric comorbidity affects tic severity are highly pertinent. Such high rates of psychiatric comorbidity highlight the complexity of treating TD and emphasize the importance of accurately accessing the primary contributions to clinical presentation and functional morbidity. While the treatment of other and of multiple psychiatric disorders and tics is extremely important, such discussion is beyond the scope of this chapter. Therefore, this chapter will only briefly describe how evaluation and management strategies for TD should be approached whenever cooccurring ADHD or OCD symptoms are also significantly interfering with overall functioning. It is in such circumstances that appropriately recognizing and prioritizing primary, secondary, and additional treatment objectives is most critical.

Treatment of TD With Comorbid ADHD

The evaluation of ADHD symptoms in patients with TD should be comprehensive and follow standardized parameters and well-established guidelines (e.g., clinical assessment and use of ADHD rating scales, e.g., Vanderbilt or Conner's) (Pliszka & The AACAP Work Group on Quality Issues, 2007). Severe tics can interfere with attention and concentration, while the anxiety related to tics and premonitory urges can be very distracting and may also present as fidgetiness (Robertson, 2000). The alpha-2 agonists, clonidine and guanfacine, are the recommended first line pharmacological treatments for combined ADHD and tics (Connor, Fletcher, & Swanson, 1999). Systematic reviews and large scale meta-analyses have not found psychostimulant medications to worsen tic severity (Cohen et al., 2015). Although individual cases of tic exacerbation may still occur, psychostimulants such as long and short acting formulations of methylphenidate, amphetamine, dexmethylphenidate, and mixed amphetamine salts remain an effective strategy with good effect sizes for ADHD symptom management and may be used as first line agents for ADHD symptoms (Cohen et al., 2015; Pringsheim & Steeves, 2011). Additionally, there is empirical support from a large multicenter randomized placebo controlled trial that the combination of an alpha agonist with a psychostimulant is highly effective to treating both ADHD and tics (Tourette's Syndrome Study Group, 2002). Meanwhile, atomoxetine is an effective nonstimulant prescribed for the treatment of ADHD that has been shown to be helpful for combined ADHD and tics (Allen et al., 2005). Given the fact that cooccurring ADHD is a major source of morbidity in youth with TD, its evaluation and prompt treatment is extremely important (Bloch et al., 2009). Consider the case of a patient with ADHD and a history of TD, and how the clinician addresses possible parental concerns when discussing psychostimulant use.

Parent: *Ben is a 7-year-old boy who has moderately severe ADHD, and an older brother who has been diagnosed with Tourette's Disorder. Ben is very fidgety and having significant problems focusing in class. He is disruptive not only at school, but also at home and at his afterschool religious class. Ben's pediatrician has recommended a trial with a psychostimulant to treat his ADHD, but since Ben has experienced a few minor and transient motor tics such as repetitive blinking and facial twitches in the past, Ben's mother is very concerned that treating his ADHD with stimulants may "bring out his tics."*

Clinician: *It's important to recognize that psychostimulants are considered frontline medications for treating ADHD, and have an established history of safety and evidence-based efficacy. Doctors used to avoid using psychostimulants in children with tics due to reports that these medications worsened tics. However, there is an abundance of compelling data that clearly demonstrates treating children who have tics and ADHD with psychostimulants does not lead to worsening of tics. So the overwhelming majority of children with ADHD, who are at risk for tics or who already have tics, can safely and effectively be treated with psychostimulants. That said, like trying any other medication, your son could experience intolerable side effects with psychostimulants and if so, a different medication option can be considered. It's important to remember too, that your son already has tics and we know that given the natural history of tic disorders, these may increase or worsen even without any medication intervention.*

Treatment of TD With Comorbid OCD

The phenomenology and presentation of obsessive compulsive symptoms in youth with TD also requires careful assessment, since complex tics may manifest with repetitive behaviors that may be confused with and misdiagnosed as compulsive symptoms. Not infrequently, certain repetitive behaviors in youth with TD have both urge-like and compulsion-like qualities, prompting some investigators to characterize such symptoms as "impulsions" (Worbe et al., 2010). CBT is considered first-line treatment for pediatric OCD (McGuire et al., 2015). Furthermore, it has been demonstrated in many well-controlled clinical trials and by meta-analyses that tic-related OCD does not respond as well to typical OCD medication management (Ginsburg, Kingery, Drake, & Grados, 2008). When considering treatment, adding CBT with pharmacotherapy for tic-related OCD, the SRIs have been well studied in pediatric OCD and are reported to be relatively effective and safe (The Pediatric OCD Treatment Study (POTS) Team, 2004). While no individual differences exist between various SRIs in terms of efficacy, choosing an agent based on relative side effect profile and ease of dosing strategy is worthwhile (Soomro, Altman, Rajagopal, & Oakley Browne, 2008).

CONCLUSIONS

Medication management of TD in youth is rarely successful in isolation, and generally needs to be viewed as an optional component of an overall integrated medical, psychological, and social treatment approach. Once initiated, the need for ongoing medication management of tics requires regular review, especially since tic symptoms tend to improve over time for the majority of individuals. Vigilance to detect untoward adverse medication effects or interactions, and ongoing assessment of medication benefits vs risks is extremely important. Medication management of psychiatric cooccurring disorders may often take precedence over the medication management of tics.

KEY POINTS

1. Tic disorders that interfere with functioning may be treated with pharmacological agents, in appropriately selected patients, after careful baseline assessment of tic severity, comorbidity and overall psychosocial functioning.
2. Comorbid conditions such as ADHD or OCD should help guide treatment strategies and the most distressing symptoms should be a priority of treatment.
3. Relative side effect profiles of various agents should be considered in choosing the initial or second level treatment strategy.
4. Appropriate medication side effect monitoring strategies should be used for all patients on pharmacological therapies.
5. Periodic reevaluation of the medication treatment plan should occur, as tic disorder symptoms evolve, with exacerbations and remissions in the natural course of illness and in most cases improve over time.

DISCLOSURES

1. Dr. Saggu does not have any financial or other conflicts of interest to disclose.
2. Dr. Barnes does not have any financial or other conflicts of interest to disclose.
3. Ms. Shad does not have any financial or other conflicts of interest to disclose.
4. Dr. Budman receives support for clinical research from: Psyadon Pharmaceuticals, Assurex/TEVA Pharmaceuticals, Synchroneuron Pharmaceuticals, Neurocrine Pharmaceuticals, is a consultant for Bracket, and is a speaker for the Tourette Association of America—Center for Disease Control Partnership.

REFERENCES

Allen, A. J., Kurlan, R. M., Gilbert, D. L., Coffey, B. J., Linder, S. L., Lewis, D. W., ... Spencer, T. J. (2005). Atomoxetine treatment in children and adolescents with ADHD and comorbid tic disorders. *Neurology*, *65*(12), 1941–1949.

American Psychiatric Association. (2013). *Diagnostic and statistical manual of mental disorders* (5th ed.). Arlington, VA: American Psychiatric Publishing.

Ames, D., Carr-Lopez, S. M., Gutierrez, M. A., Pierre, J. M., Rosen, J. A., Shakib, S., & Yudofsky, L. M. (2016). Detecting and managing adverse effects of antipsychotic medications: Current state of play. *Psychiatric Clinics of North America*, *39*(2), 275–311.

Arana, G. W. (2000). An overview of side effects caused by typical antipsychotics. *The Journal of Clinical Psychiatry*, *61*(Suppl. 8), 5–11.

AstraZeneca. (2013). *A 6-month, multicenter, randomized, safety, tolerability, pharmacokinetic, and preliminary efficacy study of AZD5213 in adolescents with Tourette's disorder*. [Online] Available from https://clinicaltrials.gov/ct2/show/NCT01904773 Accessed 30.03.16.

Black, K. J., Black, E. R., Greene, D. J., & Schlaggar, B. L. (2016). Provisional Tic disorder: What to tell parents when their child first starts ticking. *F1000Research, 5*, 696.

Bloch, M. H., Panza, K. E., Landeros-Weisenberger, A., & Leckman, J. F. (2009). Meta-analysis: Treatment of attention-deficit/hyperactivity disorder in children with comorbid Tic disorders. *Journal of the American Academy of Child and Adolescent Psychiatry, 48* (9), 884–893.

Bloch, M. H., Panza, K. E., Yaffa, A., Alvarenga, P. G., Jakubovski, E., Mulqueen, J. M., ... Leckman, J. F. (2016). N-acetylcysteine in the treatment of pediatric Tourette syndrome: Randomized, double-blind, placebo-controlled add-on trial. *Journal of Child and Adolescent Psychopharmacology, 26*(4), 327–334.

Budman, C., Coffey, B. J., Shechter, R., Schrock, M., Wieland, N., Spirgel, A., & Simon, E. (2008). Aripiprazole in children and adolescents with Tourette disorder with and without explosive outbursts. *Journal of Child and Adolescent Psychopharmacology, 18*(5), 509–515.

Budman, C. L. (2014). The role of atypical antipsychotics for treatment of Tourette's syndrome: An overview. *Drugs, 74*(11), 1177–1193.

Bymaster, F. P., Katner, J. S., Nelson, D. L., Hemrick-Luecke, S. K., Threlkeld, P. G., Heiligenstein, J. H., ... Perry, K. W. (2002). Atomoxetine increases extracellular levels of norepinephrine and dopamine in prefrontal cortex of rat: A potential mechanism for efficacy in attention deficit/hyperactivity disorder. *Neuropsychopharmacology, 27*(5), 699–711.

Cavanna, A. E., & Nani, A. (2013). Chapter 12. Antiepileptic drugs and Tourette syndrome. In D. Martino, & A. E. Cavanna (Eds.), *International review of neurobiology* (Vol. 112, pp. 373–389). London, UK: Academic Press.

Coffey, B. J. (2009). Anxiolytics for children and adolescents: Traditional and new drugs. *Journal of Child and Adolescent Psychopharmacology, 1*(1), 57–83.

Cohen, S. C., Mulqueen, J. M., Ferracioli-Oda, E., Stuckelman, Z. D., Coughlin, C. G., Leckman, J. F., & Bloch, M. H. (2015). Meta-analysis: Risk of tics associated with psychostimulant use in randomized, placebo-controlled trials. *Journal of the American Academy of Child & Adolescent Psychiatry, 54*(9), 728–736.

Commander, M., Green, S. H., & Pendergast, M. (1991). Behavioral disturbances in children treated with clonazepam. *Developmental Medicine and Child Neurology, 33*(4), 362–363.

Connor, D. F., Fletcher, K. E., & Swanson, J. M. (1999). A meta-analysis of clonidine for symptoms of attention-deficit hyperactivity disorder. *Journal of the American Academy of Child & Adolescent Psychiatry, 38*(12), 1551–1559.

Correll, C. U., & Kane, J. M. (2007). One-year incidence rates of tardive dyskinesia in children and adolescents treated with second-generation antipsychotics: A systematic review. *Journal of Child and Adolescent Psychopharmacology, 17*(5), 647–655.

Cortese, S., Panei, P., Arcieri, R., Germinario, E. A., Capuano, A., Margari, L., ... Curatolo, P. (2015). Safety of methylphenidate and atomoxetine in children with attention-deficit/hyperactivity disorder (ADHD): Data from the italian national ADHD registry. *CNS Drugs, 29* (10), 865–877.

Cummings, D. D., Singer, H. S., Krieger, M., Miller, T. L., & Mahone, E. M. (2002). Neuropsychiatric effects of guanfacine in children with mild Tourette syndrome: A pilot study. *Clinical Neuropharmacology, 25*(6), 325–332.

Curtis, A., Clarke, C. E., & Rickards, H. E. (2009). Cannabinoids for Tourette's syndrome. *Cochrane Database of Systematic Reviews, 4*, CD006565.

De Hert, M., Dobbelaere, M., Sheridan, E. M., Cohen, D., & Correll, C. U. (2011). Metabolic and endocrine adverse effects of second-generation antipsychotics in children and adolescents: A systematic review of randomized, placebo controlled trials and guidelines for clinical practice. *European Psychiatry*, *26*(3), 144–158.

Donaldson, I., Marsden, C. D., Schneider, S. A., & Bhatia, K. P. (2012). Section 6. Tics. In I. Donaldson, C. D. Marsden, S. A. Schneider, & K. P. Bhatia (Eds.), *Marsden's book of movement disorders*. Oxford, UK: Oxford University Press.

Donegan, S., Dixon, P., Hemming, K., Tudur-Smith, C., & Marson, A. (2015). A systematic review of placebo-controlled trials of topiramate: How useful is a multiple-indications review for evaluating the adverse events of an antiepileptic drug? *Epilepsia*, *56*(12), 1910–1920.

Du, Y. S., Li, H. F., Vance, A., Zhong, Y. Q., Jiao, F. Y., Wang, H. M., ... Wu, J. B. (2008). Randomized double-blind multicentre placebo-controlled clinical trial of the clonidine adhesive patch for the treatment of tic disorders. *Australian and New Zealand Journal of Psychiatry*, *42*(9), 807–813.

Eddy, C. M., Rickards, H. E., & Cavanna, A. E. (2011). Treatment strategies for tics in Tourette syndrome. *Therapeutic Advances in Neurological Disorders*, *4*(1), 25–45.

Egolf, A., & Coffey, B. J. (2014). Current pharmacotherapeutic approaches for the treatment of Tourette syndrome. *Drugs of Today*, *50*(2), 159–179.

Ercan-Sencicek, A. G., Stillman, A. A., Ghosh, A. K., Bilguvar, K., O'Roak, B. J., Mason, C. E., ... State, M. W. (2010). L-Histidine decarboxylase and Tourette's syndrome. *The New England Journal of Medicine*, *362*(20), 1901–1908.

Fasano, A., & Bentivoglio, A. R. (2009). Tetrabenazine. *Expert Opinion on Pharmacotherapy*, *10*(17), 2883–2896.

Feigin, A., Kurlan, R., McDermott, M. P., Beach, J., Dimitsopulos, T., Brower, C. A., & Jankovic, J. (1996). A controlled trial of deprenyl in children with Tourette's syndrome and attention deficit hyperactivity disorder. *Neurology*, *46*(4), 965–968.

Ferraro, D., & Di Trapani, G. (2008). Topiramate in the prevention of pediatric migraine: Literature review. *The Journal of Headache and Pain*, *9*(3), 147–150.

Gabbay, V., Babb, J. S., Klein, R. G., Panzer, A. M., Katz, Y., Alonso, C. M., ... Coffey, B. J. (2012). A double-blind, placebo-controlled trial of omega-3 fatty acids in Tourette's disorder. *Pediatrics*, *129*(6), e1493–e1500.

Geyskes, G. G., Boer, P., & Dorhout Mees, E. J. (1979). Clonidine withdrawal. Mechanism and frequency of rebound hypertension. *British Journal of Clinical Pharmacology*, *7*(1), 55–62.

Ghanizadeh, A., Tordjman, S., & Jaafari, N. (2015). Aripiprazole for treating irritability in children & adolescents with autism: A systematic review. *The Indian Journal of Medical Research*, *142*(3), 269–275.

Gilbert, D. L., Batterson, J. R., Sethuraman, G., & Sallee, F. R. (2004). Tic reduction with risperidone versus pimozide in a randomized, double-blind, crossover trial. *Journal of the American Academy of Child & Adolescent Psychiatry*, *43*(2), 206–214.

Gilbert, D. L., Budman, C. L., Singer, H. S., Kurlan, R., & Chipkin, R. E. (2014). A D1 receptor antagonist, ecopipam, for treatment of tics in Tourette syndrome. *Clinical Neuropharmacology*, *37*(1), 26–30.

Gilbert, D. L., Dure, L., Sethuraman, G., Raab, D., Lane, J., & Sallee, F. R. (2003). Tic reduction with pergolide in a randomized controlled trial in children. *Neurology*, *60*(4), 606–611.

Gilbert, D. L., Sethuraman, G., Sine, L., Peters, S., & Sallee, F. R. (2000). Tourette's syndrome improvement with pergolide in a randomized, double-blind, crossover trial. *Neurology*, *54*(6), 1310–1315.

Ginsburg, G. S., Kingery, J. N., Drake, K. L., & Grados, M. A. (2008). Predictors of treatment response in pediatric obsessive-compulsive disorder. *Journal of the American Academy of Child & Adolescent Psychiatry*, *47*(8), 868–878.

Goetz, C. G. (1992). Clonidine and clonazepam in Tourette syndrome. *Advances in Neurology*, *58*, 245–251.

Gonce, M., & Barbeau, A. (1977). Seven cases of Gilles de la tourette's syndrome: Partial relief with clonazepam: A pilot study. *Canadian Journal of Neurological Sciences*, *4*(4), 279–283.

Greene, P. E., & Fahn, S. (1992). Baclofen in the treatment of idiopathic dystonia in children. *Movement Disorders*, *7*(1), 48–52.

Guay, D. R. P. (2010). Tetrabenazine, a monoamine-depleting drug used in the treatment of hyperkinetic movement disorders. *The American Journal of Geriatric Pharmacotherapy*, *8* (4), 331–373.

Guyatt, G. H., Oxman, A. D., Vist, G. E., Kunz, R., Falck-Ytter, Y., Alonso-Coello, P., & Schünemann, H. J. (2008). GRADE: An emerging consensus on rating quality of evidence and strength of recommendations. *BMJ: British Medical Journal*, *336*(7650), 924–926.

Hallett, M., Albanese, A., Dressler, D., Segal, K. R., Simpson, D. M., Truong, D., & Jankovic, J. (2013). Evidence-based review and assessment of botulinum neurotoxin for the treatment of movement disorders. *Toxicon*, *67*(1), 94–114.

Hasan, A., Rothenberger, A., Münchau, A., Wobrock, T., Falkai, P., & Roessner, V. (2010). Oral delta 9-tetrahydrocannabinol improved refractory Gilles de la Tourette syndrome in an adolescent by increasing intracortical inhibition: A case report. *Journal of Clinical Pharmacology*, *30*(2), 190–192.

Hirota, T., Schwartz, S., & Correll, C. U. (2014). Alpha-2 agonists for attention-deficit/hyperactivity disorder in youth: A systematic review and meta-analysis of monotherapy and add-on trials to stimulant therapy. *Journal of the American Academy of Child and Adolescent Psychiatry*, *53*(2), 153–173.

Ho, C. S., Chiu, N. C., Tseng, C. F., & Huang, Y. L. (2014). Clinical effectiveness of aripiprazole in short-term treatment of tic disorder in children and adolescents: A naturalistic study. *Pediatrics & Neonatology*, *55*(1), 48–52.

Hollis, C., Pennant, M., Cuenca, J., Glazebrook, C., Kendall, T., Whittington, C., ... Stern, J. (2016). Clinical effectiveness and patient perspectives of different treatment strategies for tics in children and adolescents with Tourette syndrome: A systematic review and qualitative analysis. *Health Technology Assessment*, *20*(4).

Horrigan, J. P., & Barnhill, L. J. (1999). Guanfacine and secondary mania in children. *Journal of Affective Disorders*, *54*(3), 309–314.

Howson, A. L., Batth, S., Ilivitsky, V., Boisjoli, A., Jaworski, M., Mahoney, C., & Knott, V. J. (2004). Clinical and attentional effects of acute nicotine treatment in Tourette's syndrome. *European Psychiatry*, *19*(2), 102–112.

Huntington Study Group., Frank, S., Testa, C. M., Stamler, D., Kayson, E., Davis, C., ... Christopher, E. (2016). Effect of deutetrabenazine on chorea among patients with huntington disease: A randomized clinical trial. *JAMA*, *316*(1), 40–50.

Jacobus, J., Squeglia, L. M., Sorg, S. F., Nguyen-Louie, T. T., & Tapert, S. F. (2014). Cortical thickness and neurocognition in adolescent marijuana and alcohol users following 28 days of monitored abstinence. *Journal of Studies on Alcohol and Drugs*, *75*(5), 729–743.

Jacobus, J., & Tapert, S. F. (2014). Effects of cannabis on the adolescent brain. *Current Pharmaceutical Design*, *20*(13), 2186–2193.

Jankovic, J. (1994). Botulinum toxin in the treatment of dystonic tics. *Movement Disorders*, *9* (3), 347–349.

Jankovic, J., Jimenez-Shahed, J., & Brown, L. W. (2010). A randomised, double-blind, placebo-controlled study of topiramate in the treatment of Tourette syndrome. *Journal of Neurology, Neurosurgery & Psychiatry*, *81*(1), 70–73.

Jankovic, J., Jimenez-Shahed, J., Budman, C., Coffey, B., Murphy, T. K., Shprecher, D., & Stamler, D. (2016). A pilot study of SD-809 (deutetrabenazine) in tics associated with Tourette syndrome. *Movement Disorders*, *31*(Suppl. 2), [abstract].

Jankovic, J., & Lang, A. E. (2015). Diagnosis and assessment of parkinson disease and other movement disorders. In R. B. Daroff, J. Jankovic, J. C. Mazziotta, & S. L. Pomeroy (Eds.), *Neurology in clinical practice* (7th ed.). Philadelphia, PA: Elsevier.

Ji, W. D., Li, Y., Li, N., & Guo, B. Y. (2005). Olanzapine for treatment of Tourette syndrome: A double-blind randomized controlled trial. *Chinese Journal of Clinical Rehabilitation*, *9*, 66–68.

Jucaite, A., Takano, A., Boström, E., Jostell, K. G., Stenkrona, P., Halldin, C., … Nyberg, S. (2013). AZD5213: A novel histamine H3 receptor antagonist permitting high daytime and low nocturnal H3 receptor occupancy, a PET study in human subjects. *International Journal of Neuropsychopharmacology*, *16*(6), 1231–1239.

Juncos, J. L. (2012). Chapter 39. Tourette syndrome and related disorders. In R. L. Watts, D. G. Standaert, & J. A. Obeso (Eds.), *Movement disorders* (3rd ed.). New York, NY: McGraw-Hill Education.

Kenney, C., & Jankovic, J. (2006). Tetrabenazine in the treatment of hyperkinetic movement disorders. *Expert Review of Neurotherapeutics*, *6*(1), 7–17.

Kenney, C., Kuo, S. H., & Jimenez-Shahed, J. (2008). Tourette's syndrome. *American Family Physician*, *77*(5), 651–658.

Kisicki, J. C., Fiske, K., & Lyne, A. (2007). Phase I, double-blind, randomized, placebo-controlled, dose-escalation study of the effects on blood pressure of abrupt cessation versus taper down of guanfacine extended-release tablets in adults aged 19 to 24 years. *Clinical Therapeutics*, *29*(9), 1967–1979.

Kluger, B., Triolo, P., Jones, W., & Jankovic, J. (2015). The therapeutic potential of cannabinoids for movement disorders. *Movement Disorders: Official Journal of the Movement Disorder Society*, *30*(3), 313–327.

Kratochvil, C. J., Vaughan, B. S., Stoner, J. A., Daughton, J. M., Lubberstedt, B. D., Murray, D. W., … March, J. S. (2011). A Double-blind, placebo-controlled study of atomoxetine in young children with ADHD. *Pediatrics*, *127*(4), e862–e868.

Kuo, S. H., & Jimenez-Shahed, J. (2010). Topiramate in treatment of Tourette syndrome. *Clinical Neuropharmacology*, *33*(1), 32–34.

Kurlan, R., Como, P. G., Deeley, C., McDermott, M., & McDermott, M. P. (1993). A pilot controlled study of fluoxetine for obsessive-compulsive symptoms in children with Tourette's syndrome. *Clinical Neuropharmacology*, *16*(2), 167–172.

Kurlan, R., Crespi, G., Coffey, B., Mueller-Vahl, K., Koval, S., Wunderlich, G., & Pramipexole for TS Trial Investigators. (2012). A multicenter randomized placebo-controlled clinical trial of pramipexole for Tourette's syndrome. *Movement Disorders*, *27*(6), 775–778.

Kurlan, R., Goetz, C. G., McDermott, M. P., Plumb, S., Singer, H., Dure, L., … Greiner, A. (2002). Treatment of ADHD in children with tics: A randomized controlled trial. *Neurology*, *58*(4), 527–536.

Lane, R. D., Glazer, W. M., Hansen, T. E., Berman, W. H., & Kramer, S. I. (1985). Assessment of tardive dyskinesia using the abnormal involuntary movement scale. *Journal of Nervous & Mental Disease*, *173*(6), 353–577.

Leckman, J. F., Riddle, M. A., Hardin, M. T., Ort, S. I., Swartz, K. L., Stevenson, J., & Cohen, D. J. (1989). The yale global tic severity scale: Initial testing of a clinician-rated scale of tic severity. *Journal of the American Academy of Child & Adolescent Psychiatry*, *28*(4), 566–573.

Liu, Z. S., Chen, Y. H., Zhong, Y. Q., Zou, L. P., Wang, H., Sun, D., ... Liao, J. X. (2011). A multicenter controlled study on aripiprazole treatment for children with Tourette syndrome in China. *Zhonghua er ke za zhi*, *49*(8), 572–576.

Lyon, G. J., Samar, S., Jummani, R., Hirsch, S., Spirgel, A., Goldman, R., & Coffey, B. J. (2009). Aripiprazole in children and adolescents with Tourette's disorder: An open-label safety and tolerability study. *Journal of Child and Adolescent Psychopharmacology*, *19*(6), 623–633.

Marras, C., Andrews, D., Sime, E., & Lang, A. E. (2001). Botulinum toxin for simple motor tics: A randomized, double-blind, controlled clinical trial. *Neurology*, *56*(5), 605–610.

McCracken, J. T., Suddath, R., Chang, S., Thakur, S., & Piacentini, J. (2008). Effectiveness and tolerability of open label olanzapine in children and adolescents with Tourette syndrome. *Journal of Child and Adolescent Psychopharmacology*, *18*(5), 501–508.

McGuire, J. F., Piacentini, J., Lewin, A. B., Brennan, E. A., Murphy, T. K., & Storch, E. A. (2015). A meta-analysis of cognitive behavior therapy and medication for child obsessive-compulsive disorder: Moderators of treatment efficacy, response, and remission. *Depression and Anxiety*, *32*(8), 580–593.

Mejia, N. I., & Jankovic, J. (2005). Secondary tics and tourettism. *Revista Brasileira de Psiquiatria*, *27*(1), 11–17.

Meltzer, H. Y., Matsubara, S., & Lee, J. C. (1989). Classification of typical and atypical antipsychotic drugs on the basis of dopamine D-1, D-2 and serotonin2 pKi values. *Journal of Pharmacology and Experimental Therapeutics*, *251*(1), 238–246.

Mills, S., & Hedderly, T. (2014). A guide to childhood motor stereotypies, tic disorders and the Tourette spectrum for the primary care practitioner. *The Ulster Medical Journal*, *83*(1), 22–30.

Mogwitz, S., Buse, J., Ehrlich, S., & Roessner, V. (2013). Chapter 10. Clinical pharmacology of dopamine-modulating agents in Tourette's syndrome. In D. Martino, & A. E. Cavanna (Eds.), *International review of neurobiology* (Vol. 112, pp. 281–349). London, UK: Academic Press.

Müller-Vahl, K. R. (2013). Treatment of Tourette syndrome with cannabinoids. *Behavioural Neurology*, *27*, 119–124.

Müller-Vahl, K. R., Schneider, U., Koblenz, A., Jöbges, M., Kolbe, H., Daldrup, T., & Emrich, H. M. (2002). Treatment of Tourette's syndrome with delta 9-tetrahydrocannabinol (THC): A randomized crossover trial. *Pharmacopsychiatry*, *35*(2), 57–61.

Müller-Vahl, K. R., Schneider, U., Prevedel, H., Theloe, K., Kolbe, H., Daldrup, T., & Emrich, H. M. (2003). Delta 9-tetrahydrocannabinol (THC) is effective in the treatment of tics in Tourette syndrome: A 6-week randomized trial. *Journal of Clinical Psychiatry*, *64*(4), 459–465.

Murphy, T. K., Fernandez, T. V., Coffey, B. J., Rahman, O., Gavaletz, A., Hanks, C. E., & Scahill, L. (2017). Extended-release guanfacine does not show a large effect on tic severity in children with chronic Tic disorders. *Journal of Child and Adolescent Psychopharmacology*, *27*(9), 762–770.

Murphy, T. K., Lewin, A. B., Storch, E. A., & Stock, S. (2013). Practice parameter for the assessment and treatment of children and adolescents with tic disorders. *Journal of the American Academy of Child & Adolescent Psychiatry*, *52*(12), 1341–1359.

Murphy, T. K., Mutch, J., Reid, J. M., Edge, Paula, Storch, E. A., Bengston, M., & Yang, M. (2009). Open Label Aripiprazole in the treatment of youth with Tic disorders. *Journal of Child and Adolescent Psychopharmacology, 19*(4), 441–447.

Neurocrine Biosciences. (2016). *A randomized, double-blind, placebo-controlled study to assess the safety and efficacy of NBI-98854 in adult subjects with Tourette syndrome.* [Online] Available from https://clinicaltrials.gov/ct2/show/NCT02581865 Accessed 30.09.16.

Nicolson, R., Craven-Thuss, B., Smith, J., McKinlay, B. D., & Castellanos, F. X. (2005). A randomized, double-blind, placebo-controlled trial of metoclopramide for the treatment of Tourette's disorder. *Journal of the American Academy of Child & Adolescent Psychiatry, 44* (7), 640–646.

Novartis Pharmaceuticals Canada Inc. (2013). *Lioresal (baclofen) [product monograph].* Dorval, Quebec: Novartis Pharmaceuticals Canada Inc.

Onofrj, M., Paci, C., D'Andreamatteo, G., & Toma, L. (2000). Olanzapine in severe Gilles de la Tourette syndrome: A 52-week double-blind cross-over study vs. low-dose pimozide. *Journal of Neurology, 247*(6), 443–446.

Pliszka, S., & The AACAP Work Group on Quality Issues. (2007). Practice parameter for the assessment and treatment of children and adolescents with attention-deficit/hyperactivity disorder. *Journal of the American Academy of Child & Adolescent Psychiatry, 46*(7), 894–921.

Porta, M., Maggioni, G., Ottaviani, F., & Schindler, A. (2004). Treatment of phonic tics in patients with Tourette's syndrome using botulinum toxin type A. *Neurological Sciences., 24* (6), 420–423.

Porta, M., Sassi, M., Cavallazzi, M., Fornari, M., Brambilla, A., & Servello, D. (2008). Tourette's syndrome and role of tetrabenazine: Review and personal experience. *Clinical Drug Investigation, 28*(7), 443–459.

Preskorn, S. H. (2012). Changes in the product label for pimozide illustrate both the promises and the challenges of personalized medicine. *Journal of Clinical Psychiatry, 73*(9), 1191–1193.

Pringsheim, T., Doja, A., Gorman, D., McKinlay, D., Day, L., Billinghurst, L., … Sandor, P. (2012). Canadian Guidelines for the evidence-based treatment of tic disorders: Pharmacotherapy. *The Canadian Journal of Psychiatry, 57*(3), 133–143.

Pringsheim, T., & Marras, C. (2009). Pimozide for tics in Tourette's syndrome. *Cochrane Database of Systematic Reviews, 15*(2), CD006996.

Pringsheim, T., Panagiotopoulos, C., Davidson, J., Ho, J., & for the CAMESA Guideline Group. (2011). Evidence-based recommendations for monitoring safety of second generation antipsychotics in children and youth. *Journal of the Canadian Academy of Child and Adolescent Psychiatry, 20*(3), 218–233.

Pringsheim, T., & Steeves, T. (2011). Pharmacological treatment for attention deficit hyperactivity disorder (ADHD) in children with comorbid tic disorders. *Cochrane Database of Systematic Reviews, 4*, CD007990.

Reeves, R. R., Ladner, M. E., Perry, C. L., Burke, R. S., & Laizer, J. T. (2015). CME: Abuse of medications that theoretically are without abuse potential. *Southern Medical Journal, 108* (3), 151–157.

Rizzo, R., Gulisano, M., Calì, P. V., & Curatolo, P. (2013). Tourette syndrome and comorbid ADHD: Current pharmacological treatment options. *European Journal of Paediatric Neurology, 17*(5), 421–428.

Robertson, M. M. (2000). Tourette syndrome, associated conditions and the complexities of treatment. *Brain, 123*(3), 425–462.

Roerig, J. L., Steffen, K. J., & Mitchell, J. E. (2011). Atypical antipsychotic-induced weight gain: Insights into mechanisms of action. *CNS Drugs*, *25*(12), 1035–1059.

Ropper, A. H., Samuels, M. A., & Klein, J. P. (2014). Chapter 6. Tremor, myoclonus, focal dystonias, and tics. In A. H. Ropper, M. A. Samuels, & J. P. Klein (Eds.), *Adams & Victor's principles of neurology* (10th ed.). New York, NY: McGraw-Hill Education.

Sallee, F. R., Kurlan, R., Goetz, C. G., Singer, H., Scahill, L., Law, G., ... Chappell, P. B. (2000). Ziprasidone treatment of children and adolescents with Tourette's syndrome: A pilot study. *Journal of the American Academy of Child & Adolescent Psychiatry*, *39*(3), 292–299.

Sallee, F. R., Nesbitt, L., Jackson, C., Sine, L., & Sethuraman, G. (1997). Relative efficacy of haloperidol and pimozide in children and adolescents with Tourette's disorder. *American Journal of Psychiatry*, *154*(8), 1057–1062.

Sanger, T. D., Chen, D., Fehlings, D. L., Hallett, M., Lang, A. E., Mink, J. W., ... Valero-Cuevas, F. (2010). Definition and classification of hyperkinetic movements in childhood. *Movement Disorders: Official Journal of the Movement Disorder Society*, *25*(11), 1538–1549.

Scahill, L., Chappell, P. B., Kim, Y. S., Schultz, R. T., Katsovich, L., Shepherd, E., ... Leckman, J. F. (2001). A placebo-controlled study of guanfacine in the treatment of children with tic disorders and attention deficit hyperactivity disorder. *American Journal of Psychiatry*, *158*(7), 1067–1074.

Scahill, L., Erenberg, G., Berlin, C. M., Budman, C., Coffey, B. J., Jankovic, J., ... Walkup, J. (2006). Contemporary assessment and pharmacotherapy of Tourette syndrome. *NeuroRx*, *3* (2), 192–206.

Scahill, L., Leckman, J. F., Schultz, R. T., Katsovich, L., & Peterson, B. S. (2003). A placebo-controlled trial of risperidone in Tourette syndrome. *Neurology*, *60*(7), 1130–1135.

Schweinsburg, A. D., Brown, S. A., & Tapert, S. F. (2008). The influence of Marijuana use on neurocognitive functioning in adolescents. *Current Drug Abuse Review*, *1*(1), 99–111.

Shapiro, A. K., & Shapiro, E. (1984). Controlled study of pimozide vs. placebo in Tourette's syndrome. *Journal of the American Academy of Child & Adolescent Psychiatry*, *23*(2), 161–173.

Shapiro, D. A., Renock, S., Arrington, E., Chiodo, L. A., Liu, L. X., Sibley, D. R., ... Mailman, R. (2003). Aripiprazole, a novel atypical antipsychotic drug with a unique and robust pharmacology. *Neuropsychopharmacology*, *28*, 1400–1411.

Shier, A. C., Reichenbacher, T., Ghuman, H. S., & Ghuman, J. K. (2013). Pharmacological treatment of attention deficit hyperactivity disorder in children and adolescents: Clinical strategies. *Journal of Central Nervous System Disease*, *5*, 1–17.

Silver, A. A., Shytle, R. D., Sheehan, K. H., Sheehan, D. V., Ramos, A., & Sanberg, P. R. (2001). Multicenter, double-blind, placebo-controlled study of mecamylamine monotherapy for Tourette's disorder. *Journal of the American Academy of Child & Adolescent Psychiatry*, *40*(9), 1103–1110.

Singer, H. S. (2006). Tourette syndrome and its associated neurobehavioral problems. In K. F. Swaiman, S. Ashwal, & D. M. Ferriero (Eds.), *Pediatric neurology. Principles and practice* (4th ed.). Philadelphia, PA: Elsevier.

Singer, H. S., Brown, J., Quaskey, S., Rosenberg, L. A., Mellits, E. D., & Denckla, M. B. (1995). The Treatment of attention-deficit hyperactivity disorder in Tourette's syndrome: A double-blind placebo-controlled study with clonidine and desipramine. *Pediatrics*, *95*(1), 74–81.

Singer, H. S., Wendlandt, J., Krieger, M., & Giuliano, J. (2001). Baclofen treatment in Tourette syndrome: A double-blind, placebo-controlled, crossover trial. *Neurology*, *56*(5), 599–604.

Smith-Hicks, C. L., Bridges, D. D., Paynter, N. P., & Singer, H. S. (2007). A double blind randomized placebo control trial of levetiracetam in tourette syndrome. *Movement Disorders*, *22*(12), 1764–1770.

Soomro, G. M., Altman, D. G., Rajagopal, S., & Oakley Browne, M. (2008). Selective serotonin re-uptake inhibitors (SSRIs) versus placebo for obsessive compulsive disorder (OCD). *Cochrane Database of Systematic Reviews*, *1*, CD001765.

Steingard, R. J., Goldberg, M., Lee, D., & DeMaso, D. R. (1994). Adjunctive clonazepam treatment of Tic symptoms in children with comorbid tic disorders and ADHD. *Journal of the American Academy of Child & Adolescent Psychiatry*, *33*(3), 394–399.

The Pediatric OCD Treatment Study (POTS) Team. (2004). Cognitive-behavior therapy, sertraline, and their combination for children and adolescents with obsessive-compulsive disorder: The pediatric OCD treatment study (POTS) randomized controlled trial. *JAMA*, *292*(16), 1969–1976.

Thenganatt, M. A., & Jankovic, J. (2016). Recent advances in understanding and managing Tourette Syndrome. *F1000Research*, *5*. (F1000 Faculty Rev):152.

Toren, P., Weizman, A., Ratner, S., Cohen, D., & Laor, N. (2005). Ondansetron treatment in Tourette's disorder: A 3-week, randomized, double-blind, placebo-controlled study. *Journal of Clinical Psychiatry*, *66*(4), 499–503.

Tourette's Syndrome Study Group. (2002). Treatment of ADHD in children with tics: A randomized controlled trial. *Neurology*, *58*(4), 527–536.

Waldon, K., Hill, J., Termine, C., Balottin, U., & Cavanna, A. E. (2013). Trials of pharmacological interventions for Tourette syndrome: A systematic review. *Behavioural Neurology*, *26* (4), 265–273.

Weisman, H., Qureshi, I. A., Leckman, J. F., Scahill, L., & Bloch, M. H. (2013). Systematic review: Pharmacological treatment of tic disorders—Efficacy of antipsychotic and alpha-2 adrenergic agonist agents. *Neuroscience & Biobehavioral Reviews*, *37*(6), 1162–1171.

Whittington, C., Pennant, M., Kendall, T., Glazebrook, C., Trayner, P., Groom, M., ... Hollis, C. (2016). Practitioner review: Treatments for Tourette syndrome in children and young people—A systematic review. *Journal of Child Psychology and Psychiatry*, *57*(9), 988–1004.

Wijemanne, S., Wu, L. J. C., & Jankovic, J. (2014). Long-term efficacy and safety of fluphenazine in patients with Tourette syndrome. *Movement Disorders.*, *29*(1), 126–130.

Worbe, Y., Mallet, L., Golmard, J. L., Béhar, C., Durif, F., Jalenques, I., ... Hartmann, A. (2010). Repetitive behaviours in patients with Gilles de la Tourette syndrome: Tics, compulsions, or both? *PLoS One*, *5*(9), e12959.

Wright, A., Rickards, H., & Cavanna, A. E. (2012). Impulse-control disorders in Gilles de la Tourette syndrome. *The Journal of Neuropsychiatry and Clinical Neurosciences*, *24*(1), 16–27.

Yamamuro, K., Makinodan, M., Ota, T., Iida, J., & Kishimoto, T. (2014). Paliperidone extended release for the treatment of pediatric and adolescent patients with Tourette's disorder. *Annals of General Psychiatry*, *13*, 13.

Yang, C. S., Zhang, L. L., Lin, Y. Z., & Guo, Q. (2015). Sodium valproate for the treatment of Tourette's syndrome in children: A systematic review and meta-analysis. *Psychiatry Research*, *226*(2), 411–417.

Yang, C. S., Zhang, L. L., Zeng, L. N., Huang, L., & Liu, Y. T. (2013). Topiramate for Tourette's syndrome in children: A meta-analysis. *Pediatric Neurology*, *49*(5), 344–350.

Yoo, H. K., Joung, Y. S., Lee, J. S., Song, D. H., Lee, Y. S., Kim, J. W., ... Cho, S. C. (2013). A multicenter, randomized, double-blind, placebo-controlled study of aripiprazole in children and adolescents with Tourette's disorder. *Journal of Clinical Psychiatry*, *74*(8), e772–e780.

Zhong, Y. Q., Zhou, W. Z., & Hu, W. G. (2007). Randomized double-blind controlled study on treatment of tic disorders in children with transcutaneous patch of clonidine. *Zhonghua er ke za zhi*, *45*(10), 785–787.

FURTHER READING

Awaad, Y., Michon, A. M., & Minarik, S. (2005). Use of levetiracetam to treat tics in children and adolescents with Tourette syndrome. *Movement Disorders*, *20*(6), 714–718.

Bloch, M. H., Landeros-Weisenberger, A., Kelmendi, B., Coric, V., Bracken, M. B., & Leckman, J. F. (2006). A systematic review: Antipsychotic augmentation with treatment refractory obsessive-compulsive disorder. *Molecular Psychiatry*, *11*(7), 622–632.

Fernández-Jaén, A., Fernández-Mayoralas, D. M., Muñoz-Jareño, N., & Calleja-Pérez, B. (2009). An open-label, prospective study of levetiracetam in children and adolescents with Tourette syndrome. *European Journal of Paediatric Neurology*, *13*(6), 541–545.

Hedderick, E. F., Morris, C. M., & Singer, H. S. (2009). Double-blind, crossover study of clonidine and levetiracetam in Tourette syndrome. *Pediatric Neurology*, *40*(6), 420–425.

McDougle, C. J., Goodman, W. K., Leckman, J. F., Lee, N. C., Heninger, G. R., & Price, L. H. (2004). Haloperidol addition in fluvoxamine-refractory obsessive-compulsive disorder: A double-blind, placebo-controlled study in patients with and without tics. *Archives of General Psychiatry*, *51*(4), 302–308.

Varigonda, A. L., Jakubovski, E., & Bloch, M. H. (2016). Systematic review and meta-analysis: Early treatment responses of selective serotonin reuptake inhibitors and clomipramine in pediatric obsessive-compulsive disorder. *Journal of the American Academy of Child & Adolescent Psychiatry*, *55*(10), 851–859, e2.

Chapter 5

Cognitive Restructuring About Tics

Flint M. Espil, PhD[1] and David C. Houghton, MS[2]
[1]Department of Psychiatry and Behavioral Sciences, Stanford University School of Medicine, Stanford, CA, United States, [2]Department of Psychology, Texas A&M University, College Station, TX, United States

COGNITIVE RESTRUCTURING ABOUT TICS

One challenge that can present itself during treatment of persistent tic disorders (PTDs, including Tourette's disorder) is that affected children and adolescents (hereafter referred to collectively as "youth") sometimes have negative beliefs about themselves and their tics. Tics are often experienced as annoying and embarrassing, and they can get in the way of life activities. Moreover, even with the best treatments, tics rarely remit completely, and PTDs tend to persist through adolescence (Bloch & Leckman, 2009), a period when bullying is most common (Nansel et al., 2001). As such, it is understandable that youth with PTDs might feel tempted to avoid activities and develop poor self-esteem. These negative thought patterns may disrupt or impair individuals' ability to function across social, academic, or occupational domains, and lead to reduced quality of life.

Accordingly, clinicians should be attentive to how youth understand their tics and how tics affect their identity and behavior. If youth present with negative thought patterns regarding their tics or other problems, then therapeutic techniques derived from traditional cognitive-behavioral approaches, namely cognitive restructuring (CR), may help clients overcome negative patterns and reengage in their lives. In the following chapter, we will review research on maladaptive thought patterns in PTDs and present a cognitive-behavioral model of maladaptive cognition in PTDs. We will also review the evidence supporting CR and discuss how to assess for and treat maladaptive cognitions in PTDs.

The Clinician's Guide to Treatment and Management of Youth with Tourette Syndrome and Tic Disorders.
DOI: https://doi.org/10.1016/B978-0-12-811980-8.00005-4

Negative Impact of Chronic Tic Disorders

In order to understand the experience of children with PTDs, it is important to acknowledge that tics are often stigmatizing. Several studies indicate youth with tics are viewed more negatively by peers compared to those without tics (Boudjouk, Woods, Miltenberger, & Long, 2000; Friedrich, Morgan, & Devine, 1996; Stokes, Bawden, Camfield, Backman, & Dooley, 1991). Like children with other medical and psychological disabilities (Miller, 1984; Van Cleave & Davis, 2006), youth with PTDs also experience high rates of peer victimization (Storch et al., 2007b; Zinner, Conelea, Glew, Woods, & Budman, 2012). Conelea et al. (2011) found that 75% of youth with PTDs reported being treated differently because of their tics, 20.6% had been asked to leave a school setting, 20% had been discriminated against or treated rudely by a business, and 13.5% had been asked to leave a public space. The impact of social maltreatment appears to be significant, as the level of peer victimization positively correlates with tic severity, loneliness, anxiety, internalizing and externalizing symptoms, and reduced quality of life (Storch et al., 2007b; Zinner et al., 2012). Further, research on peer victimization across child and adolescent populations shows that bullying is associated with negative consequences, such as psychosomatic problems, poor academic achievement, and increased suicide risk (Gini & Polizzi, 2013; Glew, Fan, & Katon, 2005; Klomek, Sourander, & Gould, 2010; Kumpulainen, Räsänen, & Henttonen, 1999).

In addition to the negative emotional consequences of peer victimization, youth with PTDs also report difficulties interacting with others. Tics that are severe or noticeable enough to cause physical pain or embarrassment can interfere with various activities (e.g., academics, social life, private leisure and vacations, home life) and result in a tendency to avoid such events (Bawden, Stokes, Camfield, Camfield, & Salisbury, 1998; Conelea et al., 2011; Shady, Fulton, & Champion, 1988; Storch et al., 2007a). These impacts appear to be significant, as evidence suggests that tic-related impairment and activity restriction is associated with lower quality of life and poorer emotional functioning (Conelea, Busch, Catanzaro, & Budman, 2014). Accordingly, many parents of youth with PTDs report (a) that tics lead to the development of emotional disorders, (b) that tics have exacerbated emotional problems in themselves and their spouse, and (c) that they have sought professional help in dealing with reactions to their child's tics (Conelea et al., 2011). Symptoms of depression, anxiety, and stress are also higher in PTDs than in the general population (Conelea et al., 2011), and youth with PTDs have poor self-concept (Hanks, McGuire, Lewin, Storch, & Murphy, 2015). In fact, youth with TDs have higher rates of suicidal ideation and suicidal behavior than community youths (Storch et al., 2015).

Given the significant emotional consequences and life impairment associated with tics, it is perhaps unsurprising that many youth seeking treatment for PTDs are eager to get rid of their tics. However, there are several problems with the notion of eliminating all tics. First, although it is sometimes the case that youth respond well to interventions and see drastic reductions in tic frequency and severity, tics often fail to remit completely (Jeon et al., 2013). Because of the chronicity of tic disorders during childhood and adolescence, clinicians should advise affected youth and their parents that the aim of treatment is to manage, not eliminate, all tics (Woods et al., 2008). Accordingly, youth usually need to cope with ongoing tic-related issues, such as dealing with occasional tics or accepting that new tics may come and go over time. Second, while some tics are clearly impairing, in that they can cause pain or embarrassment (e.g., a shrieking vocal tic), occur too frequently (e.g., every few seconds), or get in the way of valued activities (e.g., a hand-shaking tic that makes writing difficult), many tics are not inherently associated with negative consequences. For instance, tics that are low intensity and infrequent may rarely cause interference and impairment, or be noticed by others (e.g., mild eye blinking tic or mild sniffing tic). When youth express a desire to get rid of all of their tics, a thorough assessment may indicate that not all of their tics are truly problematic, with some mild and transient tics not causing significant problems. In such cases, youth may believe that all of their tics are "bad," based on negative reactions to their problematic tics. This brings us to the third consideration: some youth with PTDs develop negative attitudes about their tics and themselves, meaning that they believe they cannot do certain activities, cannot fit in socially, or have less value than others because of tics.

The cases in which youth have negative attitudes or behavior patterns related to tics are the subject of the current chapter. Accordingly, the aim of cognitive interventions for PTDs is to help affected youth reengage with valued life activities and develop a more positive view of themselves and their tics. This is particularly important because evidence suggests that negative psychosocial experiences can have a significant impact on quality of life, and tics themselves. For example, psychosocial distress over a 2-year period in youth with PTDs predicts future depressive symptoms and tic severity (Lin et al., 2007), and stress and anxiety tend to exacerbate tic severity (Conelea & Woods, 2008; Himle et al., 2014). In the following section, we will present a cognitive-behavioral model of how youth with PTDs develop negative beliefs about themselves and their tics.

A Cognitive-Behavioral Model of Cognition, Affect, and Behavior in Persistent Tic Disorders

A central tenet of cognitive-behavioral approaches to psychopathology is that thoughts, feelings, and behaviors are related. For instance, when one has negative beliefs about themselves and the world, they tend to feel anxious and withdraw from normal activities. This reduction in valued behavior leaves fewer opportunities for reinforcement; thus decreasing positive effect, which in turn engenders further negative attributions about one's circumstances. These negative thoughts in turn lead to increased negative affect and behavior, which further strengthen negative thought patterns. Cognitive-behavioral theory holds that this reciprocal, interactive relationship represents a negative feedback loop that reinforces and maintains depression and anxiety (see Fig. 5.1).

In PTDs, the negative feedback loop can start with others' negative reactions to tics and develop into a pernicious cycle of depressive thoughts, feelings, and behaviors. When tics first develop (generally between ages 4–6; Bloch & Leckman, 2009), they typically involve simple motor tics, such as eye blinking or nose movements. These first tics are likely experienced as benign and receive few negative reactions; the child and others may not even notice initial tics. As such, tics in their early stages are spurious behaviors that have neutral valence, but as tics increase in number and severity into early adolescence (Bloch & Leckman, 2009), they often begin to elicit negative reactions. People may ask, "*Why do you keep making that strange face?*" or "*Are you making a noise under your breath?*" Unfortunately, as parents and others begin noticing tics, they may ask the youth to stop, which is typically impossible, if not extremely difficult. As negative reactions to tics continue, youth usually become more aware of their tics, which begin to acquire an increasingly negative valence. Whenever a tic occurs, or youth sense that a tic is about to occur, they simultaneously anticipate negative feedback or other unwelcome attention. Youth may even experience

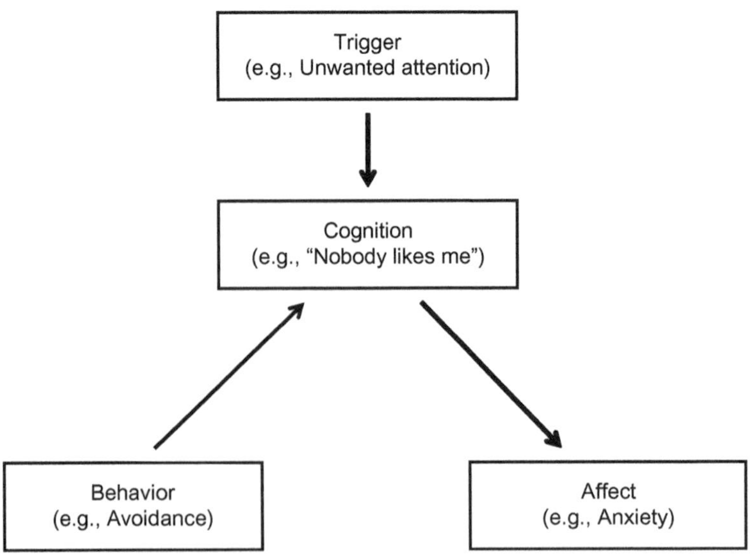

FIGURE 5.1 Cognitive-behavioral model.

frustration in trying repeatedly to suppress their tics without success. Eventually, youth may develop anxiety around social situations and cultivate negative thoughts about themselves and their tics. Negative thoughts and congruent affect may then lead to avoidance of valued life activities, which then precipitates other negative outcomes, such as fewer opportunities to make friends and failure to engage in activities that provide reinforcement and skill-building (i.e., extracurricular organizations and sports).

When youth with PTDs develop these negative beliefs and feelings, their clinical presentation becomes remarkably similar to those with depressive and anxiety disorders. In these instances, the presence of negative beliefs about themselves and the tendency to avoid pleasurable activities overlap with those found in depression, and the feelings related to social rejection, maltreatment from others, and low self-efficacy commonly present in anxiety disorders. It is thus reasonable to borrow from psychotherapeutic techniques that work with depressive and anxiogenic thinking for use in youth with PTDs. In the section below, we describe a technique often used in CBT, CR, and the evidence supporting its efficacy.

Cognitive Restructuring: Description and Efficacy

CR is based on the notion that maladaptive thought patterns contribute to psychopathology, and that a clinician can point out the inaccuracies in these beliefs to help the client develop more positive and adaptive views of themselves and the world. The roots of CR go back to Albert Ellis' Rational Emotive Behavior Therapy (REBT; Ellis, 1973). Ellis believed that psychopathology was caused by irrational beliefs that were objectively wrong. For instance, social phobia would be conceptualized as being caused by the irrational belief that one is not liked by others. Using REBT, the clinician would challenge such beliefs on an intellectual level, pointing out logical fallacies and the lack of evidence for certain assumptions that one uses to support irrational beliefs. Furthermore, Ellis believed that, on some level, negative beliefs did not have to dictate behavior. When working with a client with social phobia, Ellis might have stated something like, "*Who cares if people do not like you? So what? You cannot win over everyone. You should just live your life and stop caring about what other people think so much.*" With clients who believe they are intellectually deficient, he might have said, "*So what if you're stupid? Big deal!*" Ellis also supported the use of behavioral experiments designed to disprove negative beliefs, and would ask clients to engage in activities aimed at disconfirming their irrationality through corrective learning experiences. Evidence indicates that REBT is effective for a variety of conditions (Gonzalez et al., 2004; Lyons & Woods, 1991), but some have argued that the REBT approach to CR can be too brash and condescending (Johnson, Ridley, & Nielsen, 2000).

Modern treatment approaches, such as cognitive therapy, include a modified version of CR. Instead of viewing negative thoughts as irrational, contemporary thinkers proposed that depressed and anxious individuals develop overly negative belief systems that do not accurately reflect positive qualities and facilitate healthy behaviors. CR borrows from humanistic psychotherapy, in that all clients are regarded positively and the clinician helps promote positive thinking so that the client can feel less depressed, more self-efficacious, and engaged in valued life activities (Meichenbaum & Cameron, 1974). Beck's cognitive model of depression and anxiety described affected individuals as having negative core beliefs about themselves, the future, and the world (Beck, 1979). Negative core beliefs are reflected in automatic thoughts and distortions of reality. For instance, one might have the core belief that he or she is worthless, leading the individual to have automatic thoughts, such as "I do everything wrong" or "Everyone hates me." Furthermore, this individual might misinterpret messages from others, such as misconstruing constructive criticism from a teacher at school to mean that they have failed miserably and will probably fail the course, which then reinforces automatic thoughts and core beliefs about worthlessness.

When implemented correctly, CR is a powerful intervention that has shown efficacy in a variety of conditions. Although an exhaustive review of the literature is outside the scope of the present chapter, there is a positive evidence for the use of CR in social phobia (Mattick, Peters, & Clarke, 1989; Taylor, 1996), test anxiety (Goldfried, Linehan, & Smith, 1978), generalized anxiety disorder (Woodward & Jones, 1980), stuttering (Murphy, Yaruss, & Quesal, 2007), and even schizophrenia (Bouchard, Vallières, Roy, & Maziade, 1996). Moreover, meta-analyses of cognitive behavior therapy, which usually contains CR, have found positive results in anxiety disorders, depression, somatoform disorders, bulimia, anger control, and general stress (Butler, Chapman, Forman, & Beck, 2005; Hofmann, Asnaani, Vonk, Sawyer, & Fang, 2012).

Few studies have examined the role of CR for individual with PTDs. This may stem from the fact that several researchers have argued that psychoeducation alone can have powerful effects at dispelling negative beliefs about tics (Woods et al., 2008; Zinner et al., 2012). Indeed, youth and parents can be relieved to learn that tics have a definite neurobiological origin, that medications are not the only treatment approach, and that many individuals with tics, including a number of well-known and highly successful people, live fulfilling lives. However, the effects of psychoeducation on negative beliefs about tics and oneself have never been empirically tested. Two studies tested a cognitive-behavioral treatment package, called Living With Tics (LWT), which includes psychoeducation, CR, problem solving, parent training, overcoming tic-related avoidance, and improving self-esteem. Results of the initial pilot study of LWT on eight youth with PTDs found promising results (Storch et al., 2012), and a recent randomized controlled trial found significant improvements in tic-related impairment and quality of life for those who received LWT when compared to a wait-list control (McGuire et al., 2015). Additionally, the intervention was well tolerated by both youth and parents. A second study tested a group-based intervention that included cognitive-behavioral techniques for identifying negative automatic thoughts and generating alternative, more adaptive thoughts (Murphy & Heyman, 2007). Qualitative results of this pilot study indicated that it was well attended and viewed favorably by participants, but no quantitative data were obtained. The intervention also consisted of many other components, making it difficult to determine if CR was effective. Finally, a third study tested a modified version of anger control training that included CR for youth with Tourette's Disorder and comorbid disruptive behavior (Sukhodolsky et al., 2009). Although the intervention was effective at reducing disruptive behavior, treatment was not directly aimed at negative tic-related cognitions.

In sum, there is a positive preliminary evidence for CR in youth with PTDs, and although more research should be conducted, we believe there is sufficient evidence for the use of CR in youth with PTDs who experience negative attitudes/thoughts, maladaptive behavioral patterns, and comorbid mood problems (e.g., depression and anxiety) related to their tics. In the following sections, we will elucidate this process using a "how-to" approach.

Applying Cognitive Restructuring to Persistent Tic Disorders

As most clinicians interested in treating individuals with PTDs will likely have at least some previous exposure to the process of cognitive therapy, cognitive models of psychopathology, and the technique of CR, the goal of the following section is not to train clinicians to be experts in cognitive therapy, but to instead provide guidelines for its use within the context of treating PTDs. In this context, CR can be implemented to help clients challenge distorted cognitions related to tics and associated problems in order to minimize the impact these constructs have on mood, self-esteem, quality of life, and overall functioning. Clinical judgment on the part of the clinician should be used to decide if and when CR may be helpful as an adjunctive technique in addition to treating tics themselves, and whether the problem areas being targeted through restructuring should take a central role (see Chapter 1: Introduction to Treatment and Management of Youth With Tourette Disorders and Tic Disorders for further discussion on selection and prioritization of therapeutic techniques). For example, if a clinician learns that a client has become severely depressed during the course of treating tics, it may be prudent to shift both the focus and techniques in therapy to the depressive symptomology.

The basic approach to CR involves identifying the role of negative thinking in underlying beliefs and negative emotions. When pointing out automatic thoughts, clinicians should highlight the role of such thoughts within the cognitive model, specifically mentioning the interplay among thoughts, emotions, and behavior. Clinicians should then work together with clients to identify and challenge negative thoughts through a process commonly referred to as "collaborative empiricism," which means that the clinician and client come to a mutual decision about what is really happening to the client and why he or she feels as they do. To assess the types and frequencies of negative thoughts, clinicians may employ strategies, such as thought records, Socratic questioning, the "downward arrow" technique, and others depending on the type of cognitive therapy (e.g., Cognitive-Behavioral Therapy, Rational Emotive Therapy, etc.). More generally, clinicians should ask clients "*what is going through your mind right now*" when they notice a shift in effect during sessions. Retrospectively, clinicians can also ask clients to describe difficult situations that have occurred previously and then inquire about the thoughts experienced during those situations. Regardless of the specific technique, assessing for negative thoughts within the course of treating PTDs may occur more formally, if there is reason to suspect other psychopathology, or informally as clients bring up stressful situations at home, school, or other contexts. For example, clients may report higher levels of ticcing during stressful school exams and subsequently reveal thoughts of being an underachiever, or worry about being a disappointment to their parents. Individuals with tics might also have negative thoughts surrounding the long-term consequences of ticcing, such as the inability to acquire a romantic partner, make friends during college, or get a job. During such occasions, clinicians can use CR to evaluate potentially negative beliefs—which may also be contributing to higher levels of stress, mood symptoms, and subsequent ticcing.

When using CR, clinicians should make efforts to tailor the techniques to the developmental and cognitive abilities of the client. Younger children may not be able to understand higher levels of abstract thinking or attend to their thoughts with the same level of attention as older adolescents and adults. Although some tailoring may be necessary, research indicates that developmentally appropriate cognitive interventions can be effective for younger clients (Grave & Blissett, 2004; Ishikawa, Okajima, Matsuoka, & Sakano, 2007). For example, when working with children as young as 6–8 years old, techniques examining irrational thoughts might use more concrete picture or story-based approaches. Children might express their negative thinking in terms of a "thought monster," with the goal of CR being recognition of the thought monster's influence and learning to fight back. In addition to providing an overview of the cognitive, or cognitive-behavioral model, it can also be helpful to provide clients examples of common types of negative thoughts, or cognitive errors, people often make. These can include probability overestimation, catastrophizing (jumping to conclusions), all-or-none thinking, fortune telling, mind reading, overgeneralization, disqualifying the positive, over-using "should" statements, and several others. A brief list of these errors, including definitions and examples, can be found in Table 5.1.

After identifying automatic thoughts, the role of the clinician is to use Socratic questioning, or questions that stimulate curiosity and inquisitiveness, to help gradually reveal dysfunctional thought patterns and behaviors. Examples of Socratic questions might include "*What is the evidence for this thought?*," "*Is there an alternative explanation?*," and "*What is the worst that could happen?*," with the overall goal of evaluating and challenging

TABLE 5.1 Cognitive Errors

Cognitive Error	Definition	Example
Probability overestimation, or jumping to conclusions	Greatly inflating the likelihood of a negative outcome.	"If I tic in class then others will laugh at me"
Catastrophizing/ fortune telling	Predicting negative future outcomes.	"My tics will never get any better, even if I participate in therapy"
		"I'll never make friends because of my tics"
All-or-nothing thinking	Viewing a situation as only two possible outcomes or categories.	"My tics will either go away completely or get a lot worse"
		"If I cannot control my tics, I won't go in certain places"
Mind reading	Believing one knows what others are thinking.	"My teacher thinks my tics are annoying"
Overgeneralization	Making broad, negative conclusions that go well beyond a given situation.	"My tics made it harder for me to concentrate during my math test. I'll never be able to pass any of my classes"
Personalization	Thinking others are behaving negatively because of one's own actions.	"The other kids at school do not invite me to sit with them in the cafeteria because of my tics"
Oversimplifying	Focusing on one negative aspect of a given situation, to the exclusion of the broader context	"Everyone just sees me as the kid with tics"
Over-using "should" statements	Blaming oneself for any perceived failures	"I should be able to control my tics, and be like other kids"

such thoughts in order to reduce their effects on emotion and behavior. Socratic questioning is a methodical process that is designed to identify inconsistencies and logical flaws, and it should appear that the clinician is asking specific questions in order to better understand the situation. It should not feel condescending to the client. In fact, the client should ideally come to the realization, on their own, that their interpretation of an event is not completely accurate. The clinician should avoid telling the client outright that they are wrong, as this tends to create resistance and doubt, and the client is unlikely to change his or her perspective based on a clinician's reassurance alone. As this process advances, the clinician digs deeper into negative self-statements by connecting them to core beliefs (i.e., the downward arrow technique). Ideally, as maladaptive belief system slowly unravels, the client becomes more willing to entertain new ways of thinking and try new behaviors. Once the client has achieved some flexibility in their thinking, behavioral experiments can be employed to test belief systems in the real world. For instance, if youth with PTDs believe they are worthless and cannot make friends due to their tics, clinicians might ask them to start an innocuous conversation with a peer and test what happens. Ideally, the child has a positive experience, or at least finds it to be less aversive than anticipated. This corrective experience facilitates a further unraveling of the maladaptive belief system. Given parents' involvement in tic disorder treatment, it may also be helpful to enlist their support when implementing cognitive strategies. For example, parents can help youth follow through with thought record homework, identify negative thoughts when youth are struggling emotionally, model healthy thought patterns and interpretations, and use challenging techniques when appropriate to help youth engage in treatment more generally. Clinical judgment should be exercised on the part of the clinician to ensure the appropriateness of involving parents in CR sessions.

Troubleshooting Problems and Barriers

Several challenges can arise during the process of CR. First, youths' "negative" views of their world may accurately reflect their experiences. For instance, parents may not feel that their child is being bullied, but the child reveals that his or her schoolmates make derogatory comments without teachers and parents noticing. Youth who claim to be socially isolated may indeed have few friends and a history of negative interactions with peers. As such, it is unwise to challenge beliefs unless there is a significant reason to suspect that they are not accurate. Moreover, in such cases, clinicians can utilize problem-solving techniques, social skills interventions, and other approaches to ameliorate problematic environments (see Chapter 6: Improving Self-Esteem for Youth with Tourette Syndrome and Tic Disorders, Chapter 7: Talking about Tics with Peers and Coping in Social Interactions, Chapter 8: Tourette's in The Classroom: Support and Guidance on Education Issues for Clinicians, Chapter 9: Overcoming Tic-Related Avoidance, and Chapter10: Problem-Solving Strategies to Overcome Common Challenges Associated with Tourette Syndrome). Youth may also become uncomfortable discussing negative thoughts or beliefs, outright refuse to engage in restructuring, or possess low insight into their dysfunctional cognitions about tics and other problems. If youth become noticeably distressed or verbalize discomfort while discussing negative beliefs, clinicians may try revisiting the cognitive model and use the present moment as evidence of the relationship between thoughts and emotions. Specifically, clinicians can point out how in-session discomfort is related to clients' thoughts and beliefs about specific problem areas. Additionally, it is often helpful to introduce the cognitive model and the effects of negative thoughts by initially using examples unrelated to youth's thoughts/fears/beliefs in order to ensure understanding, and then subsequently apply the model to actual experiences.

If youth refuse to engage in CR or any of the associated strategies, clinicians should evaluate this behavior within the context of the child's behavior more generally. Does the child have a history of oppositional or defiant behavior, or does this refusal serve another function entirely? Discussions with both youth and parents may bring insight into their behavior. Additionally, motivational techniques (e.g., Miller & Rollnick, 2012) may be helpful to increase engagement in both CR as well as therapy more generally.

If youth present with dysfunctional cognitions about tics and also possess poor insight into the nature of these thoughts, then CR can be especially challenging. In such situations, clinicians should take care to break concepts down into much smaller components, spend more time on each concept, and ensure understanding from youth before moving onto the next component of CR. In such cases, it may also be helpful to have youth engage in behavioral experiments to test their beliefs. For example, youth who believe nobody will want to talk to them if they start ticcing could engage in brief exposures with their clinician to test his hypothesis. Additionally, youth with PTDs might learn vicariously by watching documentaries or other educational media about other youth with PTDs who live meaningful lives (e.g., "I have Tourette's, but Tourette's doesn't have me," Kent, 2005).

CASE EXAMPLES

The following case examples demonstrate the process of identifying and challenging maladaptive thoughts. Each illustrates a part of the CR process, including strategies to introduce the cognitive model, identify negative thinking patterns, and challenge negative thoughts. The clinicians also use developmentally appropriate concepts and language as well as examples from clients' history, and also praise effort within session. In the first example, the clinician introduces the idea of CR and addresses a common error, probability overestimation. Given that PTDs are more prevalent in males, we use male-gendered pronouns when referring to each client in these case examples.

Clinician: *Your parents mentioned that you don't want to enroll in basketball this year, even though it's your favorite sport. Would you mind sharing with me why you decided to change your mind?*
Child: *I don't know. I guess I'm afraid that others will notice my tics while I'm playing.*
Clinician: *I see. Well thank you for being honest with me about your reasons. I know we've just begun monitoring your tics, but do you know if they usually happen while you are playing?*
Child: *They don't happen when I'm on the court, but sometimes I tic while sitting on the bench.*
Clinician: *I'm impressed by the fact that you're able to pick up on when your tics are happening. A lot of kids struggle with knowing when and where their tics occur. We can certainly work on helping you manage your tics while you are on the bench, but I want to talk a little bit about your thoughts more generally. Do you know what a crystal ball is?*
Child: *I think so. It's the thing people use to make predictions about the future.*
Clinician: *That's right. Fortune tellers claim they can predict individuals' futures using crystal balls, palm reading, and other devices. Although there isn't any evidence to suggest these methods work, we as human beings tend to have all kinds of thoughts about what may happen to us in the future. What are some predictions you might make about your day tomorrow? For example, what will happen after you wake up?*
Child: *I'll get out of bed, take a shower, and have breakfast.*
Clinician: *Sounds pretty straightforward. And what's likely to happen at school?*
Child: *I'll go to class and take a test in Math.*
Clinician: *And how do you think you'll do on that test?*
Child: *I think I'll do pretty well. Math is my favorite subject and it's pretty easy.*
Clinician: *Good! That's an example of when we predict good things that might happen to us, like doing well on a test. What are some examples of bad predictions people might make about school?*
Child: *That we might fail a test?*
Clinician: *Also correct! Have you ever predicted you wouldn't do well on a test?*
Child: *Yeah, especially in English class.*
Clinician: *Right, people make predictions all the time about how they might perform on tests, interact with other kids their age, or whether their teachers will like them. These are all common, but not necessarily as likely to happen. For example, will you always do well or always do poorly on tests?*
Child: *No, it depends on how much I study.*
Clinician: *Right, the more you study, the more likely you are to do well on a test. And what if you don't study?*
Child: *I guess I wouldn't do very well.*
Clinician: *Correct! Different outcomes are more or less likely to occur depending on a variety of circumstances. We usually refer to the likelihood of events as the "probability" of something happening. For example, what is the likelihood, or probability, that you win the lottery or get struck by lightning tomorrow?*
Child: *Pretty low.*

Clinician: *Correct. And what is the probability that you eat lunch?*
Child: *A lot higher. I usually eat lunch every day.*
Clinician: *Exactly. Some events are more probable and some are less probable. Unfortunately, sometimes people get stuck in making only bad or negative predictions about what might happen to them, regardless of probability. Why do you think it would be bad for someone to always predict that bad things will happen to them, regardless of probability?*
Child: *I do not know. Bad?*
Clinician: *Let's try using an example. Let's pretend you have a friend who loves to ride his bicycle, it's his favorite thing in the world. Now what if he stopped riding his bicycle because he constantly worried that he would be hit by a car?*
Child: *I think he would be pretty sad.*
Clinician: *Right, he would probably feel both worried about being struck by a car and also pretty sad that he couldn't do his activity. How do you think he would feel if he was constantly predicting that all of his activities would go badly?*
Child: *He would feel really bad.*
Clinician: *So always predicting bad things will happen leads us to always feeling down, unhappy, and worried. Does this mean we should never worry about outcomes?*
Child: *I do not think so.*
Clinician: *When can worrying about outcomes be helpful?*
Child: *When you worry about Math tests!*
Clinician: *Good! The point is not to avoid worrying always, but to make sure our worry is realistic. If you haven't studied it makes sense to be a little worried and then go study! In some ways, worry can be motivating, but in other ways it can stop us from doing things we enjoy—especially when we always predict something bad will happen. How likely is it that your friend be injured by a car while riding his bike?*
Child: *Well it could happen.*
Clinician: *True, it is possible, but how probable is it? You ride your bike around regularly and yet here you are, safe and sound and in one piece. It doesn't stop you, does it?*
Child: *Nope.*
Clinician: *Exactly. And so your friend has become stuck making scary predictions that are not very probable. As such he feels terrible and has stopped riding his bike. What would you tell him to do?*
Child: *I would tell him to get back on his bike.*
Clinician: *So would I. Now do you remember why we started talking about thoughts, predictions, and outcomes in the first place?*
Child: *Yeah, I think I know where you are going with this.*
Clinician: *You mentioned not wanting to play your favorite sport, basketball, this year because you were worried about others noticing your tics. How likely is it that others will notice your tics while you're out on the court?*
Child: *Not very likely. They sometimes happen while on the bench, but not out on the court.*
Clinician: *Exactly. Do you think you might be stuck in predicting that things will definitely go badly?*
Child: *I think you might be right.*
Clinician: *Maybe I am and maybe I'm not, but I want you to start paying attention to situations where you tend to make more negative predictions about what will happen to you and how that influences your behavior. Your parents mentioned basketball season isn't for another month, so we can continue this*

	discussion as we develop strategies to help manage your tics while on the bench well before the season starts. You can decide then whether or not you want to play. Does that sound ok to you?
Child:	*Yeah, that sounds good.*

The clinician was able to introduce probability overestimation and also demonstrate the relationship among thoughts, emotions, and behavior. An appropriate goal for the next session would be to review the events of the past week with a particular emphasis on situations in which the child was feeling down or worried (in relation to tics and otherwise), and also revisit the child's thoughts on participating in the activity. A logical next step might be for the clinician to introduce thought records to help the child identify when negative thoughts about tics and related symptoms are occurring, and how they are related to his mood.

In this second example, the child and clinician have been using a behavioral treatment for managing tics, habit reversal training, to develop competing responses to block the child's various tics. Although the child has been having some success, he is worried that his newly developed competing response will be noticeable when using it in the classroom. The following is an example of how clinicians might employ cognitive techniques to identify maladaptive thoughts and help youth challenge them on issues that arise within the session.

Child:	*I am afraid that everyone will see me using my exercise.*
Clinician:	*And why would it be bad if others see you using your exercises?*
Child:	*If they saw me doing them, it would be embarrassing.*
Clinician:	*Ok, so it would be embarrassing for you if others saw you using your exercises. I know we came up with treatment strategies you could use that are not very noticeable, but let's pretend others did notice them. What would be so bad about being embarrassed?*
Child:	*I would feel terrible.*
Clinician:	*I agree with you in that feeling embarrassed does not feel very good at all. Remember when we talked about that "urge" to tic and how it is uncomfortable?*
Child:	*Yeah.*
Clinician:	*And when we first introduced using exercises to block your tics you were worried that the urge would get worse and worse and never go away, right?*
Child:	*Yeah, I was pretty scared.*
Clinician:	*But what happened to that urge?*
Child:	*It went away eventually.*
Clinician:	*Right, so that uncomfortable feeling went away. I wonder if that terrible feeling of being embarrassed might also go away, and if you think you might be able to handle it just as well as you did with your urges to tic?*
Child:	*It wouldn't feel good, but I could probably handle it.*
Clinician:	*I agree with you. We've talked about other situations where you have also been successful handling uncomfortable situations, including overcoming your worry about coming to therapy.*
Child:	*That's true. It actually was not as bad as I thought it would be.*

Clinician: *You've really come a long way and put in a lot of hard work. Good for you! Sometimes we assume the worst when we are feeling nervous or anxious about the future, but things turn out a lot better than we expect. This type of thinking is called catastrophizing, and everybody does it to some extent.*

From here, the clinician could expand on how catastrophizing is a common thinking error with several negative consequences, using both general as well as specific examples from the child's experiences. The clinician also pointed out the child's past successes and praised effort within session.

The third and final case example illustrates more extensive use of CR techniques. In this scenario, negative thoughts have come up in a previous session. To begin the process of CR, the client was instructed to use a thought record over the previous week.

Clinician: *Over the past week I had you monitor your thoughts and write down the scary ones in your thought record. How did it go?*

Child: *It was tough at first, but became easier the more I did it.*

Clinician: *Nice job following through and completing the work. What did you learn from it?*

Child: *That I have a lot of these thoughts!*

Clinician: *Well let's discuss some of those thoughts. Is there one in particular that you noticed having several times throughout the week?*

Child: *Yeah, I kept thinking that I'll never fit in with normal people.*

Clinician: *What do you mean by "normal people?"*

Child: *People who don't have tics like I do.*

Clinician: *Yeah. This is something that lots of people with tics deal with over their lives. As we've discussed, in some ways the tics make it harder for you to do some things. How were you feeling when you were thinking you would never fit in?*

Child: *I was feeling terrible.*

Clinician: *Ok, and what were the specific sensations you were experiencing in your body? Did you remember to write them down?*

Child: *Yeah. I felt sick to my stomach and my heart was beating pretty fast.*

Clinician: *Ok, so you were feeling sick and probably a little nervous or worried. This is consistent with what we discussed about the connection between negative thoughts and their connection to physical sensations in your body. Were these sensations consistently present throughout the week when you had this thought?*

Child: *Pretty consistent, yeah.*

Clinician: *So in a way these symptoms are warning signs that you may be having negative or worrisome thoughts. Do you remember what you did in these situations?*

Child: *I tried not to think about it.*

Clinician: *And was that helpful?*

Child: *No, not at all, actually. I think it made things worse.*

Clinician: *Funny how that works, isn't it? The more we try not to think of something the harder it becomes! This brings us to the next step in changing our negative thoughts—replacing them with alternative, healthier thoughts. So let's pretend you're having the thought of not fitting in again. What would be some alternative, more positive thoughts you might have?*

Child: *Hmmm...maybe that I actually do fit in?*

Clinician: *Ok, and what evidence do you have that you actually do fit in?*
Child: *I don't know. I guess that, maybe, I have friends?*
Clinician: *Sure. What else?*
Child: *I get along pretty well with classmates and teachers.*
Clinician: *Good. And what about your relationship with your judo team?*
Child: *I get along well with them. I've known those guys for several years now.*
Clinician: *So you get along well with classmates and teachers, have several friends, and also a close relationship with your teammates. Thinking about all of this evidence, how are you feeling now?*
Child: *(laughs) Much better, actually.*
Clinician: *Again, your thoughts and feelings are moving in the same direction. Replacing your negative thoughts with more positive thoughts improves your feelings. As I mentioned earlier, it is common for people with tics to think they may not fit in, but when you break things down you actually fit in very well. You can't stop yourself from having your thoughts, but what can you do the next time you think you do not fit in?*
Child: *I guess I can tell myself that I actually do fit in. It just happens so quickly sometimes I forget.*
Clinician: *This is also very common. We have these thought so quickly and automatically that we do not stop to evaluate them. This is why I had you monitor and record both your thoughts and associated feelings over the past week. The more you do this the better you will come at "catching" them as they occur and then implementing the next step, challenging them with alternative thoughts!*
Child: *That makes sense. But I have so many thoughts I'm not sure I'll be able to challenge them all.*
Clinician: *I'm glad you mentioned this. It make sense given you are new to the whole process. I want you to think about this the same way you approached our work on developing strategies to manage your tics. Were those easy when we started?*
Child: *No way. It was pretty hard!*
Clinician: *It was a lot of work initially, yes. Did things change at all?*
Child: *Yeah, it got a lot easier as we went along.*
Clinician: *Precisely. Think of monitoring and challenging your thoughts the same way. It's a skill like any other and the more you practice, the easier it becomes. You have already accomplished a lot by noticing them and writing them down and should be very proud of yourself. This is the merely the next step.*

CONCLUSION

In this chapter, we first discussed the distress and impairment commonly experienced by youth with PTDs, and how such experiences may lead to patterns of negative thinking. Second, we introduced the cognitive-behavioral model and how thoughts, feelings, and behavior may all interact to negatively influence the lives of youth with PTDs. Third, we provided an overview of cognitive therapies and associated techniques, with specific emphasis on CR and how it can be used to help youth with PTDs. Although CR is not designed to directly reduce tic frequency and severity, it can be a valuable tool for addressing comorbid problems and distress in youth with PTDs, and in doing so, enhance the functioning and quality of life in these individuals.

REFERENCES

Bawden, H. N., Stokes, A., Camfield, C. S., Camfield, P. R., & Salisbury, S. (1998). Peer relationship problems in children with Tourette's disorder or diabetes mellitus. *Journal of Child Psychology and Psychiatry, 39*(5), 663–668.

Beck, A. T. (1979). *Cognitive therapy of depression*. Guilford Press.

Bloch, M. H., & Leckman, J. F. (2009). Clinical course of Tourette syndrome. *Journal of Psychosomatic Research, 67*(6), 497–501.

Bouchard, S., Vallières, A., Roy, M. A., & Maziade, M. (1996). Cognitive restructuring in the treatment of psychotic symptoms in schizophrenia: a critical analysis. *Behavior Therapy, 27* (2), 257–277.

Boudjouk, P. J., Woods, D. W., Miltenberger, R. G., & Long, E. S. (2000). Negative peer evaluation in adolescents: effects of tic disorders and trichotillomania. *Child & Family Behavior Therapy, 22*(17), 17–28.

Conelea, C. A., Busch, A. M., Catanzaro, M. A., & Budman, C. L. (2014). Tic-related activity restriction as a predictor of emotional functioning and quality of life. *Comprehensive Psychiatry, 55*(1), 123–129.

Conelea, C. A., & Woods, D. W. (2008). The influence of contextual factors on tic expression in Tourette's syndrome: a review. *Journal of Psychosomatic Research, 65*(5), 487–496.

Conelea, C. A., Woods, D. W., Zinner, S. H., Budman, C., Murphy, T., Scahill, L. D., et al. (2011). Exploring the impact of chronic tic disorders on youth: Results from the Tourette syndrome impact survey. *Child Psychiatry and Human Development, 42*(2), 219–242.

Ellis, A. (1973). *Humanistic psychotherapy: A rational-emotive approach*. Three Rivers Press.

Friedrich, S., Morgan, S. B., & Devine, C. (1996). Children's attitudes and behavioral intentions toward a peer with Tourette syndrome. *Journal of Pediatric Psychology, 21*(3), 307–319.

Gini, G., & Pozzoli, T. (2013). Bullied children and psychosomatic problems: A meta-analysis. *Pediatrics, 132*(4), 720–729.

Glew, G. M., Fan, M. Y., & Katon, W. (2005). Bullying, psychosocial adjustment, and academic performance in elementary school. *Archives of Pediatrics & Adolescent Medicine, 159*(11), 1026–1031.

Goldfried, M. R., Linehan, M. M., & Smith, J. L. (1978). Reduction of test anxiety through cognitive restructuring. *Journal of Consulting and Clinical Psychology, 46*(1), 32–39.

Gonzalez, J. E., Nelson, J. R., Gutkin, T. B., Saunders, A., Galloway, A., & Shwery, C. S. (2004). Rational emotive therapy with children and adolescents: A meta-analysis. *Journal of Emotional and Behavioral Disorders, 12*(4), 222–235.

Grave, J., & Blissett, J. (2004). Is cognitive behavior therapy developmentally appropriate for young children? A critical review of the evidence. *Clinical Psychology Review, 24*(4), 399–420.

Hanks, C. E., McGuire, J. F., Lewin, A. B., Storch, E. A., & Murphy, T. K. (2015). Clinical correlates and mediators of self-concept in youth with chronic tic disorders. *Child Psychiatry & Human Development, 47*(1), 64–74.

Himle, M. B., Capriotti, M. R., Hayes, L. P., Ramanujam, K., Scahill, L., Sukhodolsky, D., ... Piacentini, J. (2014). Variables associated with tic exacerbation in children with chronic tic disorders. *Behavior Modification, 38*(2), 163–183.

Hofmann, S. G., Asnaani, A., Vonk, I. J. J., Sawyer, A. T., & Fang, A. (2012). The efficacy of cognitive behavioral therapy: A review of meta-analyses. *Cognitive Therapy and Research, 36*, 427–440.

Ishikawa, S. I., Okajima, I., Matsuoka, H., & Sakano, Y. (2007). Cognitive behavioural therapy for anxiety disorders in children and adolescents: A meta-analysis. *Child and Adolescent Mental Health, 12*(4), 164–172.

Jeon, S., Walkup, J. T., Woods, D. W., Peterson, A., Piacentini, J., Wilhelm, S., . . . Scahill, L. (2013). Detecting a clinically meaningful change in tic severity in Tourette syndrome: A comparison of three methods. *Contemporary Clinical Trials, 36*(2), 414–420.

Johnson, W. B., Ridley, C. R., & Nielsen, S. L. (2000). Religiously sensitive rational emotive behavior therapy: Elegant solutions and ethical risks. *Professional Psychology: Research and Practice, 31*(1), 14–20.

Kent, E.G. (2005). I have Tourettes's but Tourette's doesn't have me. *Estados Unidos: USA-TV-PG.*

Klomek, A. B., Sourander, A., & Gould, M. (2010). The association of suicide and bullying in childhood to young adulthood: A review of cross-sectional and longitudinal research findings. *Canadian Journal of Psychiatry, 55*(5), 282–288.

Kumpulainen, K., Räsänen, E., & Henttonen, I. (1999). Children involved in bullying: psychological disturbance and the persistence of the involvement. *Child Abuse & Neglect, 23*(12), 1253–1262.

Lin, H., Katsovich, L., Ghebremichael, M., Findley, D. B., Grantz, H., Lombroso, P. J., et al. (2007). Psychosocial stress predicts future symptom severities in children and adolescents with Tourette syndrome and/or obsessive-compulsive disorder. *Journal of Child Psychology and Psychiatry, 48*(2), 157–166.

Lyons, L. C., & Woods, P. J. (1991). The efficacy of rational-emotive therapy: A quantitative review of the outcome research. *Clinical Psychology Review, 11*(4), 357–369.

Mattick, R. P., Peters, L., & Clarke, J. C. (1989). Exposure and cognitive restructuring for social phobia: A controlled study. *Behavior therapy, 20*(1), 3–23.

McGuire, J. F., Arnold, E., Park, J. E., Nadeau, J. M., Lewin, A. B., Murphy, T. K., & Storch, E. A. (2015). Living with tics: Reduced impairment and improved quality of life for youth with chronic tic disorders. *Psychiatry Research, 225*(3), 571–579.

Meichenbaum, D., & Cameron, R. (1974). The clinical potential of modifying what clients say to themselves. *Psychotherapy: Theory, Research & Practice, 11*(2), 103–117.

Miller, M. (1984). Social acceptability characteristics of learning disabled students. *Journal of Learning Disabilities, 17*(10), 619–621.

Miller, W. R., & Rollnick, S. (2012). *Motivational interviewing: Helping people change.* Guilford Press.

Murphy, T., & Heyman, I. (2007). Group work in young people with Tourette syndrome. *Child and Adolescent Mental Health, 12*(1), 46–48.

Murphy, W. P., Yaruss, J. S., & Quesal, R. W. (2007). Enhancing treatment for school-age children who stutter: I. Reducing negative reactions through desensitization and cognitive restructuring. *Journal of Fluency Disorders, 32*(2), 121–138.

Nansel, T. R., Overpeck, M., Pilla, R. S., Ruan, W. J., Simons-Morton, B., & Scheidt, P. (2001). Bullying behaviors among US youth: Prevalence and association with psychosocial adjustment. *Journal of the American Medical Association, 285*(16), 2094–2100.

Shady, G. A., Fulton, W. A., & Champion, L. M. (1988). Tourette syndrome and educational problems in Canada. *Neuroscience & Biobehavioral Reviews, 12*(3–4), 263–265.

Stokes, A., Bawden, H. N., Camfield, P. R., Backman, J. E., & Dooley, J. M. (1991). Peer problems in Tourette's disorder. *Pediatrics, 87*(6), 936–942.

Storch, E. A., Hanks, C. E., Mink, J. W., McGuire, J. F., Adams, H. R., Augustine, E. F., et al. (2015). Suicidal thoughts and behaviors in children and adolescents with chronic tic disorders. *Depression and Anxiety*, *32*(10), 744–753.

Storch, E. A., Lack, C. W., Simons, L. E., Goodman, W. K., Murphy, T. K., & Geffken, G. R. (2007a). A measure of functional impairment in youth with Tourette's syndrome. *Journal of Pediatric Psychology*, *32*(8), 950–959.

Storch, E. A., Morgan, J. E., Caporino, N. E., Brauer, L., Lewin, A. B., Piacentini, J., & Murphy, T. K. (2012). Psychosocial treatment to improve resilience and reduce impairment in youth with tics: An intervention case series of eight youth. *Journal of Cognitive Psychotherapy*, *26*(1), 57–70.

Storch, E. A., Murphy, T. K., Chase, R. M., Keeley, M., Goodman, W. K., Murray, M., & Geffken, G. R. (2007b). Peer victimization in youth with Tourette's syndrome and chronic tic disorder: relations with tic severity and internalizing symptoms. *Journal of Psychopathology and Behavioral Assessment*, *29*(4), 211–219.

Sukhodolsky, D. G., Vitulano, L. A., Carroll, D. H., McGuire, J. F., Leckman, J. F., & Scahill, L. (2009). Randomized trial of anger control training for adolescents with Tourette's syndrome and disruptive behavior. *Journal of the American Academy of Child & Adolescent Psychiatry*, *48*(4), 413–421.

Taylor, S. (1996). Meta-analysis of cognitive-behavioral treatments for social phobia. *Journal of Behavior Therapy and Experimental Psychiatry*, *27*(1), 1–9.

Van Cleave, J., & Davis, M. M. (2006). Bullying and peer victimization among children with special health care needs. *Pediatrics*, *118*(4), e1212–e1219.

Woods, D. W., Piacentini, J. C., Chang, S. W., Deckersbach, T., Ginsburg, G. S., Peterson, A. L., ... Wilhelm, S. (2008). *Managing Tourette syndrome: A behavioral intervention for children and adults*. Oxford University Press.

Woodward, R., & Jones, R. B. (1980). Cognitive restructuring treatment: A controlled trial with anxious patients. *Behaviour Research and Therapy*, *18*(5), 401–407.

Zinner, S. H., Conelea, C. A., Glew, G. M., Woods, D. W., & Budman, C. L. (2012). Peer victimization in youth with Tourette syndrome and other chronic tic disorders. *Child Psychiatry and Human Development*, *43*(1), 124–136.

Chapter 6

Improving Self-Esteem for Youth With Tourette Syndrome and Tic Disorders

Meghan C. Schreck[1] and Christine A. Conelea[2]
[1]McLean Hospital, Harvard University Medical School, Belmont, MA, United States,
[2]University of Minnesota, Minneapolis, MN, United States

LOW SELF-ESTEEM IN YOUTH WITH TICS

Many youth with tic disorders have low self-esteem and report feeling abnormal and different because of their tics (Conelea et al., 2011; Hanks, Mcguire, Lewin, Storch, & Murphy, 2016; Hesapçıoğlu, Tural, & Kandil, 2014). These youth may experience discrimination, peer victimization, and impairment in family, social, and academic functioning (Cavanna et al., 2013; Conelea et al., 2011; Zinner, Conelea, Glew, Woods, & Budman, 2012). In some cases, functional impairment and low self-worth experienced as a result of having tics can be more distressing than the tics themselves. Additionally, there is a high comorbidity rate between tic disorders and other psychiatric conditions associated with low self-esteem and lower quality of life (i.e., attention-deficit hyperactivity disorder (ADHD), obsessive–compulsive disorder (OCD), anxiety and depressive disorders, and developmental delays; CDC, 2009; Guillon, Crocq, & Bailey, 2003; Hanks et al., 2016). Moreover, youth with tic disorders and co-occurring psychiatric conditions, such as OCD and ADHD, have lower self-concept compared to those with tic disorders alone (Hanks et al., 2016).

The existing gold-standard behavioral treatments for tics, such as habit reversal training and comprehensive behavioral intervention for tics (CBIT), do not directly target self-esteem (Murphy, Lewin, Storch, & Stock, 2013; Piacentini et al., 2010; Woods et al., 2011). Rather, the psychosocial sequelae associated with tics, including low self-esteem, are presumed to improve secondary to reduction in tic severity. Few interventions directly target self-esteem in youth with tics. A guide for practitioners treating individuals with Tourette syndrome and tic disorders recommends targeting low

The Clinician's Guide to Treatment and Management of Youth with Tourette Syndrome and Tic Disorders.
DOI: https://doi.org/10.1016/B978-0-12-811980-8.00006-6

self-esteem by increasing perceived control of one's environment, success in meaningful activities, and independent functioning; however, it does not offer examples of *how* to implement these strategies (Woods, Piacentini, & Walkup, 2007). More recently, research has focused on the efficacy of an intervention, "Living With Tics," aimed at promoting coping and resiliency in youth with tic disorders (McGuire et al., 2015; Storch et al., 2012). The treatment package includes a module dedicated to treating low self-esteem. Results showed improved self-concept and quality of life in youth with tic disorders.

The current chapter provides an overview of the construct of self-esteem and interventions for low self-esteem as well a guide for assessing and treating low self-esteem in youth with tic disorders. First, we define self-esteem. We then outline a cognitive–behavioral conceptualization of low self-esteem and provide examples of how perceived and actual limitations of tics can influence the development and maintenance of low self-esteem. Next, we briefly discuss the treatment literature for low self-esteem in youth and define four cognitive mechanisms of low self-esteem. Finally, we outline several cognitive and behavioral strategies clinicians can use to treat tic-related low self-esteem.

DEFINITION OF SELF-ESTEEM

Self-esteem is defined as the degree to which an individual positively evaluates themselves, which often includes comparing the self to others (Harter, 1999). Individuals may evaluate themselves differently in different domains, and the influence each domain has on self-esteem depends on how important that domain is to the individual (Harter, 1986, 1999). For example, an individual may positively evaluate their academic functioning, but negatively evaluate their physical appearance. If the individual values academic performance more than physical appearance, high self-esteem may be maintained. Meanwhile, low self-esteem is thought to develop when an individual perceives themselves to be unsuccessful or incompetent in a valued area of life. Characteristics of low self-esteem include self-critical beliefs and distorted self-evaluations. Self-esteem is best understood as a cognitive or schematic representation of the self that is influenced by previous life events and behaviors (Fennell et al., 1997). As such, Beck's (1979) cognitive model provides a foundation for understanding the development and maintenance of low self-esteem.

COGNITIVE–BEHAVIORAL CONCEPTUALIZATION OF SELF-ESTEEM

Based on Beck's (1979) cognitive model, Fennell et al. (1997) proposed a conceptualization of low self-esteem, which suggests that individuals develop a global negative schema of the self or "bottom line" based on previous life events. The bottom line is made up of negative core beliefs about the self and becomes fundamental to how the individual views and experiences the world. In youth with tics, experiences of discrimination and victimization by peers and/or punishment from parents or teachers (as a result of having tics) may influence an individual's perception of themselves. Additionally, actual limitations of tics may also influence one's bottom line. For example, severe motor tics can interfere with desired actions, such as an individual's ability to eat meals, brush teeth, and get dressed, or disruptive or inappropriate vocalizations can lead to practical or social limitations (Conelea, Busch, Catanzaro, & Budman, 2014). These perceived and real-life obstacles may contribute to bottom-line beliefs, such as "I am weird," "I am different," or "I am broken."

In an effort to cope with these negative foundational beliefs about the self, the individual creates rules to live by (Fennell et al., 1997). Beck (1979) described these "rules of living" as "dysfunctional conditional assumptions," which commonly relate to acceptance, control, and achievement, and tend to be excessive and rigid in their content and/or application. For children with tics, these rules might include, "I am a failure if I cannot manage my tics" or "If I tic, people won't like and accept me," or "If I have tics, I can't succeed in school or my sports teams." Striving to live by these extreme and concrete rules can lead to disappointment and a perceived sense of failure. The perception that these rules *could be* or *may have been* broken can elicit anxious thinking (e.g., "What if I tic in front of others?" or "If I tic, people *will* tease me and *might* think I am weird"), whereas the belief that the rules *are* or *have been* broken can lead to depressive thinking (e.g., "I *am* different/weird because of my tics" or "No one likes me because of my tics"). Negative automatic thoughts elicited from the threat or perception of broken rules can lead to distressing emotions (i.e., anxiety, depression). These thoughts and feelings are then reinforced by maladaptive behaviors, including avoidance, reassurance seeking, and social isolation. In youth with tics, these maintaining behaviors may include avoiding social situations where tics occur or refusing to go to school due to tic-related academic impairment.

Shirk, Burwell, and Harter (2003) outlined four cognitive pathogenic mechanisms of low self-esteem that can guide assessment and inform the selection of treatment strategies for youth with low self-esteem. These mechanisms include (1) unrealistic self-standards, (2) inaccurate self-evaluations, (3) undifferentiated self-structure, and (4) inauthentic or false self.

Unrealistic self-standards are defined as dysfunctional attitudes that involve unattainable expectations for the self, such as rigid beliefs about performance (i.e., perfectionism) and social acceptance. In youth with tic disorders, unrealistic self-standards might include thoughts such as, "If I show any tics, I am a complete failure" or "Forgetting to use my competing response is just as bad as not using it at all," or "I cannot tic if I want to be accepted by my peers."

Inaccurate self-evaluations arise when youth misappraise their true abilities. Youth with tic-related inaccurate self-evaluations might believe, "I can't play basketball because of my tics" or "I can never have a relationship with someone because of my tics," or "I'll never be able to manage my tics."

Undifferentiated self-structure is a function of self-complexity. Self-complexity is defined as (1) the number of and (2) distinction between different aspects of the self. Research has shown that self-esteem is influenced by the importance given to each self-aspect (Harter, 1999). With few self-aspects and limited differentiation, positive or negative feedback in a given self-aspect can color an individual's global self-esteem (Linville & Higgins, 1985). For example, if a youth with tics identifies only a few aspects of self-definition with little differentiation, functional impairment from tics in any one of these domains will negatively influence their self-esteem.

Finally, *inauthentic or false self* is defined as the suppression or hiding of one's true thoughts, feelings, and behaviors. This avoidance may stem from hopelessness about pleasing others and is imbedded within a sociocultural context (Harter, Marold, Whitesell, & Cobbs, 1996). For example, stigma of Tourette syndrome and tic disorders may impose a societal pressure on youth to hide their tics or hide their status as someone with a tic disorder.

TREATMENT FOR LOW SELF-ESTEEM

Treatments for low self-esteem have included cognitive–behavioral strategies with a primary focus on changing negative cognitions about the self. Broadly, change in low self-esteem is targeted *directly* through restructuring negative cognitions and reinforcing positive beliefs about the self, and *indirectly* through reducing maladaptive behaviors, which are thought to maintain negative self-beliefs. Engaging in adaptive behaviors is thought to provide corrective information or new experiences for the individual to draw upon when evaluating themselves (Jacobson et al., 1996).

Examples of intervention strategies for low self-esteem include (1) identifying and changing pervasive, maladaptive cognitions and behaviors and (2) reinforcing positive self-beliefs and behavioral strengths of the individual (Fennell et al., 1997; Shirk et al., 2003). Shirk and colleagues summarized research showing that assertiveness training, attribution restructuring, and social reinforcement of positive self-referent statements were effective in improving low self-esteem. These authors also indicated that multicomponent treatment packages for depressive symptoms, which included both behavioral and cognitive strategies, improve low self-esteem in adolescents. Given that self-esteem is a cognitive construct, most of the strategies used to treat low self-esteem are also cognitive in nature (i.e., cognitive restructuring, identification of positive self-beliefs).

GUIDE FOR IMPROVING SELF-ESTEEM IN YOUTH WITH TIC DISORDERS

In the remainder of the chapter, we outline a guide for assessing and treating low self-esteem in youth with tic disorders. This guide draws on the literature cited earlier and from our own clinical experience treating youth with tic disorders and/or low self-esteem. It includes strategies to normalize tics and challenge self-beliefs related to the limitations of tics. The intent of these techniques is to help youth identify positive attributes and personal strengths and values, and to engage in value-consistent activities that build upon these strengths. In addition, strategies for youth to practice assertiveness for communicating their tic-related needs in different areas of functioning will also be outlined.

It is important to note that the strategies described in this chapter have not been specifically tested in the context of treating low self-esteem in youth with tics. Additionally, many treatment studies of self-esteem in youth used multicomponent interventions (McGuire et al., 2015), meaning that the efficacy of any one strategy in improving self-esteem is unclear. Clinicians using these strategies are encouraged to monitor the benefit of interventions targeting self-esteem in individual patients with evidence-based assessments. Tools that have been widely used to assess global and domain-specific self-esteem in children and adolescents are the Children's Depression Inventory-2 Self Report Form (CDI-2 SF; Kovacs, 2011), Self Perception Profiles for Children (SPPC; Harter, 1985), and Self Perception Profiles for Adolescents (SPPA; Harter, 1988). Self-esteem is a vast and complex construct, and additional strategies for improving self-esteem can be found in other chapters in this text. For example, although this chapter provides examples for how youth can challenge and restructure negative beliefs about the self, this strategy is more fully covered in Chapter 5, Cognitive Restructuring About Tics. In addition, social and academic functioning are two important domains of self-esteem in youth. Additional strategies for improving these areas of functioning can be found in Chapter 7, Talking About Tics With Peers and Coping in Social Interactions, and Chapter 8, Tourette's in the Classroom: Support and Guidance on Education Issues for Clinicians.

EVALUATING SELF-ESTEEM AND TIC-SPECIFIC SELF-ESTEEM

Before implementing treatment strategies for low self-esteem in youth with tic disorders, it is important to conduct an assessment of global and domain-specific low self-esteem. As mentioned earlier, the CDI-2 SF and SPPC for children or SPPA for adolescents are evidence-based assessments that may help to identify low self-esteem. However, these measures are not tic-specific. Therefore, utilizing the domain-specific aspects of self-esteem delineated by Harter (1985, 1988), we provide examples of questions to assess tic-related global and domain-specific self-esteem. Although children with tic disorders may experience low self-esteem that is unrelated to tics, this chapter focuses on improving self-esteem that is influenced by the experience of having tics.

Define and Assess Global Self-Esteem

When defining and assessing global self-esteem, a clinician might begin by saying the following: "*All people have self-esteem. Self-esteem is how much people think positively about themselves or how good they feel about themselves. Sometimes when people feel different than others, they can start to feel bad about themselves, which affects their self-esteem. For example, some children with tics feel bad about having tics and being unable to control them. Do you ever feel this way?*"

Define and Assess Domain-Specific Self-Esteem

When defining and assessing domain-specific self-esteem, a clinician might say the following: "*Your self-esteem is made up of many different parts. For example, the way you think about yourself as a friend might be different than how you think about yourself as a student or an athlete. And, how good you think you are at math might be different than how good you think you are at spelling. The way you think about yourself might change depending on how important each area is to you.*

Some people feel bad about how tics make them look. Other people think that tics make them have less friends. I'm going to ask you questions about whether having tics ever makes you feel bad about yourself in different parts of your life. By learning more about how having tics affects different parts of who you are, we can develop ways for you to feel better about yourself.

The following questions are adapted from Harter's Self Perception Profiles (1985, 1988) and can aid in the identification of domain-specific negative beliefs about the self and functional impairment as a consequence of having tics. These questions are intended as assessment starting points for evaluating possible low self-esteem in each domain, and clinicians are encouraged to follow these questions with focused open-ended questions to elicit more specific negative beliefs. While the strategies from the current chapter can be used to treat low self-esteem in different areas of functioning (e.g., social, family, academic), we also reference additional chapters that provide treatment strategies for domain-specific tic-related functional impairment.

Self-Esteem Domain	Tic-Specific Questions	Additional Chapter
Children and Adolescents		
Academic	Do you believe you are not good at school or not as good as you could be, because of your tics? Do your tics get in the way of you doing well on your classwork or homework? Do you *avoid* completing homework or going to class because of your tics?[a]	Chapter 8, Tourette's in the Classroom: Support and Guidance on Education Issues for Clinicians
Social	Do you think people don't like you because of your tics? Do you worry about what other people think of you, because of your tics? Do you believe you have fewer friends, because of your tics? Do you *avoid* social situations because of your tics?[a]	Chapter 7, Talking About Tics With Peers and Coping in Social Interactions
Physical appearance	Are you unhappy with the way you look because of your tics? Do you believe your tics are unattractive?	
Athletic and extracurricular abilities	Do your tics hold you back from playing sports or other extracurricular activities? Do you believe you are not good at (activity) or not as good as you could be, because of your tics? Do you *avoid* (activity) because of your tics?[a]	
Behavior	Do your tics make you feel abnormal, weird, or different? Do you get in trouble at school or at home because of your tics? *If yes:* How does that make you feel about yourself at school and/or at home?	Chapters 11, Brief Trans-diagnostic Parent Training: A Strengths-Based, Parent-Centered Treatment for Youth With Tourette Syndrome, and 12, Assessing and Treating Emotion Dysregulation and Anger Management
Adolescents		
Close friendships	Do you believe you won't develop close friendships because of your tics? Do your tics prevent you from developing close friendships? Do your tics make it hard for you to have a best friend?	Chapter 7, Talking About Tics With Peers and Coping in Social Interactions

(*Continued*)

(Continued)

Self-Esteem Domain	Tic-Specific Questions	Additional Chapter
Romantic appeal	Do you believe that no one will want to date you because of your tics?	
Do you *avoid* going on dates because of your tics?[a]	Do your tics make you feel unloveable?	
Job competence	Do your tics prevent you from getting a job, or do you worry tics will make it hard to get a job when you want one? Do you believe you are not good at your job or not as good as you could be at your job, because of your tics? Do you *avoid* work/applying for a job because of your tics?[a]	

[a] *Tic-related avoidance may impact more than one domain of functioning. Strategies to overcome and elicit tic-related avoided activities and minimize family accommodation of tic-related avoidance are provided in Chapters 9, Managing Avoidance and Accommodation of Tics and Related Behaviors, and 14, Family Issues Associated With Tics.*

NORMALIZING AND REDUCING STIGMA OF TIC DISORDERS

Psychoeducation

Providing education about the prevalence, course, and treatment of tic disorders may help to normalize the experience of having tics and instill hope and self-efficacy for managing tics. We recommend reviewing Chapter 2 for relevant psychoeducation about tic disorders.

Sharing in the Experience

Increasing the patient's awareness of other youth who have tic disorders, including highly famous and successful people with tic disorders (e.g., US National Team goalkeeper, Tim Howard), may help to validate the experience of having tics, foster social acceptance, and reduce stigma. Discussing stories and showing videos of youth talking about their experiences with tic disorders may help the youth understand that they are *not alone*, that tics are a *part* of who they are but *do not define* who they are, and that they can live a successful and fulfilling life *with* tics. Stories and videos of youth with Tourette syndrome and tic disorders can be found at the Tourette Association of America (TAA) (Living with Tourette syndrome, n.d.).

Advocating for Youth With Tics

Participating in advocacy to reduce stigma related to tic disorders may also help to improve self-esteem and self-efficacy in youth with tic disorders. The TAA's *Youth Ambassador Program* is a program for youth with or without tics who want to spread tolerance and understand Tourette syndrome and tic disorders (Living with Tourette syndrome, n.d.). These youth work with their community, elected officials, and schools to talk about and advocate for youth with tics.

Teens can also participate in TAA's *social media* campaigns to raise awareness, acceptance, and knowledge of Tourette syndrome and tic disorders (Living with Tourette syndrome, n.d.). Two digital advocacy campaigns hosted by TAA are the #tiChallenge and #Rally4Tourette. The #tiChallenge campaign asks individuals to create an "I Challenge" video encouraging others to be more accepting, tolerant, compassionate, and informed about tic disorders. The #Rally4Tourette campaign encourages individuals to meet with a member of Congress to rally for legislation that impacts individuals with tic disorders. Social media is a platform for constituents to connect with Congress and the TAA provides instructions for how to most effectively use #Rally4Tourette in different social media outlets (i.e., Twitter, Facebook, Instagram). Additionally, in partnership with the CDC, the TAA hosts #TouretteChat, a monthly Twitter Chat, that promotes awareness through providing education on various topics related to Tourette syndrome and tic disorders.

COGNITIVE RESTRUCTURING

Treatments for low self-esteem have largely focused on identifying and restructuring negative beliefs about the self. According to the cognitive model, the way an individual thinks about a situation influences the way the individual feels and behaves. The automatic thoughts that arise when interpreting a situation are thought to be influenced by how a person perceives the self, the future, or the world. As previously stated in this chapter, self-esteem is a cognitive construct made up of evaluative beliefs about the self. As such, low self-esteem is largely made up of negative schemas, dysfunctional attitudes, and automatic thoughts about the self. Therefore, in using cognitive restructuring to treat low self-esteem specifically, we recommend assessing and treating the four previously mentioned cognitive mechanisms involved in negative beliefs about the self: (1) unrealistic self-standards, (2) inaccurate self-evaluations, (3) undifferentiated self-structure, and (4) inauthentic or false self. We recommend using the techniques outlined in Chapter 5, Cognitive Restructuring About Tics, to identify and restructure cognitions about the self. If the clinician notices a pattern of cognitive distortions that are self-focused, we recommend additional strategies outlined in this chapter to improve low self-esteem. Additionally, tic-related thoughts and schemas about the future and the world may also influence self-esteem. For example, youth with tics may have future-oriented thoughts like, "*I will never be able to hold a job because of my tics*" or global cognitions, such as "*The world is an unfair place for people with tics.*" These thoughts can also be treated with cognitive restructuring.

BUILDING A POSITIVE SELF-SCHEMA

In addition to restructuring inaccurate and unhelpful self-evaluations, it is also important to uncover and reinforce positive beliefs about the self, identify what is important to the patient, and engage in activities that are consistent with the patient's values. In the following exercises, youth with tics will be instructed to "catch the positives" about themselves and work toward building a more diverse and complex sense of self. Additionally, assisting youth in identifying and clarifying their values will facilitate setting treatment goals that are congruent with what is most important to them.

Before introducing activities that can help youth with tics look for positive qualities in themselves, use the following metaphor and/or experiential activity to communicate how thoughts and feelings can influence the way we experience situations.

Sunglasses Metaphor

When we are feeling sad, it is like wearing sunglasses with blue lenses—everything you see is through a blue filter. The same thing can happen when you feel sad—you might start to see things more negatively and miss the positives in life. We are going to practice taking these sunglasses off and seeing things as they really are. This way, we don't miss all the positives about ourselves and our lives. By recognizing the positives, you will start to feel better about yourself and your future (Stark et al., 2008).

Bead in Shoe Exercise

Materials: Candy, Small beads

Before you eat this piece of candy, I want you to put these beads in your shoes. Now, I want you to start eating your candy while walking around the room with the beads in your shoes. What do you notice? Can you feel the beads in your shoes? Are they uncomfortable? Is it harder for you to enjoy the candy with the beads in your shoes? Sometimes it can be difficult to notice the positives when your mind is on something that is bothering you. Practicing paying attention to the positives can help you to notice and enjoy the positives even when something uncomfortable happens. For the next minute, every time you notice the feeling of the beads, I want you to come back to paying attention to the taste of the candy. It's okay to notice and think about the beads, but keep coming back to the candy and practice describing what you like about it (Stark et al., 2008).

Catch the Positives Journal

The Catch the Positives Journal is a way for youth with tics to practice shifting their attention from negative to positive information about themselves (Stark et al., 2008). Through keeping track of positive internal and external experiences, youth can build evidence that supports adaptive alternative beliefs about the self. In addition, self-monitoring can help increase the youth's pleasant activities, coping skills, and problem-solving. The journal is an ongoing activity that youth complete daily and review weekly in session. Provide youth with a notebook and a series of prompts they can use to identify positive behaviors, thoughts, and feelings. On the first page of the notebook, write down prompts that the youth can reference each day. Youth can choose to answer any one of or all of the prompts every day or they can come up with a different prompt to answer. Encourage the youth to record any positive event they choose. They can also record thoughts and feelings associated with the positive event. Examples of prompts include:

- Name one nice thing someone did for me.
- Name one compliment someone gave me.
- Name one nice thing I said to someone else.
- Name one fun activity I did with a friend.
- Name one nice thing I did for someone else.
- Name one thing or person I am grateful for.

After the youth gains practice catching positives in their life, it can be helpful to individualize the journal. Based on recordings from the journal as well as findings from their domain-specific self-esteem assessment, it is important to help the youth focus on identifying positive experiences in vulnerable areas of their life. For example, if the youth omits positive events related to school and has identified negative beliefs about the self in this domain, encourage the youth to record positive experiences related to effort and performance in school over the next week. By individualizing the Catch the Positives Journal, clinicians can help youth expand their sense of self and identify areas of self-definition that the youth finds most important.

Positive Self-Map

The positive self–map is an activity to build a more positive self-schema (Stark et al., 2008). The self-map is a drawing consisting of a large circle in the middle and a series of smaller circles surrounding it. Each small circle has a line connecting it to the large circle. The large circle represents the whole person and the outer circles represent different roles and characteristics of the youth. The smaller circles represent different aspects of self-definition. Toward building a more positive and expansive sense of self, youth are instructed to fill in each small circle with relevant strengths about themselves. Some circles can be labeled in advance with domains that many youth use to define themselves (e.g., friend, family member, student, etc.) Blank circles should be filled in with unique areas that are important to the individual. The importance of each area and the number of strengths within each area will vary from person to person.

It is also important to solicit examples of the youth's positive qualities and strengths from parents and teachers. In addition to helping the youth recognize their own positive qualities, such an exercise can help to increase parent/teacher awareness of the youth's strengths, which may be particularly beneficial in situations where parents/teachers are overfocused on tics. In this way, instruct a parent and/or teacher to complete the same Catching the Positives Journal and positive self-map for the youth, share their positive beliefs and descriptions with the youth, and incorporate them into the self-map. Parents can also be encouraged to "catch the positives" on a more regular basis in the form of ongoing verbal praise and differential attention (i.e., increased attention directed toward activities that pull for the youth's strengths, less attention to tic-related challenges or barriers).

The Catch the Positives Journal can be used in conjunction with the positive self-map to monitor evidence that supports the components of self-definition identified on the self-map. The journal can be especially helpful in finding evidence for breaking down global positive self-statements into finer, more specific components to help broaden the youth's self-definition. For example, if the youth writes, "I am a good friend" on their self-map, ask the youth to identify and track in their journal, "*What behaviors or characteristics make you a good friend?*" "I am a good listener" and "I am loyal" are specific behaviors and qualities of a good friend. In addition, encouraging youth to document detailed evidence within domains of greater personal importance will also aid in improving self-esteem. For example, if the youth bases much of their self-worth on their academic performance, it is important to help the individual broaden what it means to be successful in this domain. To this end, the youth would be instructed to monitor in their journal their participation in class, effort on homework and tests, and pleasure from learning. Emphasizing the importance of effort, in addition to performance, is a critical message to deliver to youth developing their sense of self (Mueller & Dweck, 1998).

During this exercise, youth may uncover areas about themselves that they would like to improve or build upon. In this case, the self-map can be used to identify and set attainable goals in service of self-improvement. In order to do this, create an action list of problems to solve and realistic goals to achieve, and develop a specific behavioral plan to cope with or solve problems and achieve goals (Stark et al., 2008).

ASSERTIVENESS TRAINING

Given that many youth with tics experience actual limitations and discrimination/peer victimization due to tics (Conelea et al., 2011; Zinner et al., 2012), it is important that they learn to how to effectively communicate their needs and advocate for their rights. First, it is important for youth to understand what it means to be assertive and how it is different from being passive, aggressive, and passive–aggressive. Define each communication style for the youth and elicit examples of behaviors for each style (Mangini, 1986; McKay, Wood, & Brantley, 2007).

Communication Style	Tic-Related Example
Passive: communicating in a way that treats others' needs as more important than your own	Poking fun at self for having tics. Not communicating tic-related needs to a peer or teacher. Apologizing for having tics.
Aggressive: communicating in a way that treats your needs as more important than others' needs	Insulting others, yelling (e.g., "Stop making fun of my tics, loser!")
Passive–aggressive: communicating in indirect, subtle, and unclear ways, and denying personal responsibility for your actions	Rolling eyes at a peer who teases you because of your tics. Sighing in class when a teacher asks you to complete a task that is difficult due to your tics.
Assertiveness: communicating in a way that treats your own needs and others' needs as equally important	Expressing feelings, wants, and needs directly and honestly. "Please do not make fun of my tics." "I need extra time on tests, because of my tics." "I know my tic can sound annoying. I want you to know that I can't help doing it."

Next, identify situations where assertiveness may be particularly relevant and important. Example situations include addressing teasing from peers, difficulty competing school or homework assignments, or telling someone that they have a tic disorder. After identifying these situations, use role-playing to help the youth practice using assertiveness to communicate their needs. In addition, printing and sharing an "I have TS card" from the TAA website may be useful. These cards help youth explain the effects of TS and tic disorders. Specific strategies for how to communicate tic-related needs in important areas of daily functioning can be found in additional chapters within this text.

COMPLEX ISSUES

Reduction Versus Acceptance

The goals of symptom reduction and self-acceptance can be a delicate balance, especially in the context of treating tic disorders. Tics are very unlikely to completely remit with treatment (Woods et al., 2011), even for youth who are fully compliant with behavioral strategies and/or medication regimens. This probable outcome can pose difficulties for youth who enter treatment with low self-esteem or contribute to reduction in self-esteem over the course of treatment.

At the start of treatment, clinicians should assess for the presence of unrealistic expectations or desires for tic reduction, as well as for self-beliefs that are heavily tied to tic reduction, such as, "I am flawed unless my tics go away." When the initial treatment rationale is presented, it is important to be forthcoming about the fact that complete tic remission is not expected. Rather, treatment aims should be described as improving tic management, reducing functional impairment, improving quality of life, *and* improving the child and family's willingness to accept that some degree of ticcing is expected and does not necessarily mean that the child cannot lead a fulfilling and valued life. Drawing parallels to other medical conditions that can be managed but not cured (e.g., diabetes, asthma) may also help set realistic expectations and normalize the experience of having a tic disorder. Doing the self-map activity early in treatment may help to more concretely identify treatment targets that differ from tic reduction and illustrate to the child that tics are merely one component of who they are as a person.

Later in treatment, clinicians should be alert to youth frustration or discouragement in reaction to a lack of real or perceived progress in reducing tics, as this situation may adversely impact self-esteem (e.g., "I can't reduce my tics, so I'm a failure."). In addition to using the aforementioned strategies to boost self-esteem, clinicians might consider drawing on acceptance-based cognitive–behavioral therapies or techniques for youth (Coyne, McHugh, & Martinez, 2011). These strategies can help shift the focus of treatment from tic reduction toward values-based activity engagement (e.g., engaging in valued life activities even if tics still occur).

Actual Versus Perceived Limitations of Tics

Many of the strategies for improving low self-esteem involve restructuring inaccuracies in thinking about the self or the future. While some thoughts truly are logically inaccurate, some thoughts may reflect actual or realistic limitations caused by tics. For example, motor tics can interfere with one's ability to complete physical tasks, such as eating, writing, dressing, reading, or driving. Vocal tics can disrupt one's speech or be loud or inappropriate (i.e., coprolalia), making it difficult to do age-typical activities like go to the movies or stay in class during tests. These actual limitations can have an adverse impact on self-esteem. In these situations, it is important to emphasize the utility or helpfulness, as opposed to the accuracy, of negative thinking and to set realistic, attainable behavioral goals. Modification of activities to fit the actual limitations of tics may also be helpful in providing youth with positive reinforcement and opportunities to develop confidence and mastery (e.g., watching movies at home with friends instead of going to a theater; Conelea et al., 2014).

Low Motivation or Insight

Some children with low self-esteem may also have poor insight into the skewed nature of their negative evaluations of the self. These youth may have a difficult time recognizing errors in their thinking and identifying strengths in values. As a result, they may have less motivation to engage in behavioral treatment for tics as well as strategies to improve low self-esteem. In this case, recognizing and guiding the patient's readiness for change using evidence-based motivational interviewing principles is indicated (Miller & Rollnick, 2002; Prochaska, DiClemente, & Norcross, 1992). Uncovering the ways in which the youth's behaviors, thinking patterns, and, possibly, tics are getting in the way of living a meaningful life will be important in deriving motivation to change.

Family Context

The family context may contribute to self-esteem problems in youth with tics. Family conflict between caregivers or between patient and caregiver may negatively impact the youth's self-esteem. Excessive or negative focus on the youth's tics by family members may also adversely impact self-esteem, as could a parent's own beliefs about having a child with tics. For example, caregivers might overfocus on tics, find it challenging to identify strengths of their child, overestimate the role of tics in their child's identity, fear for their child's success and happiness because of tics, and/or accommodate tic-related avoidance. A functional assessment of the impact of the youth's tics on the family should be used to inform the selection of treatment strategies for managing common family problems related to tics. See Chapter 14, Family Issues Associated With Tics, for assessment and treatment strategies.

SUMMARY

Many youth with tic disorders have low self-esteem, yet the existing gold-standard treatment for tics (i.e., CBIT, habit reversal training) does not directly target low-self-worth and negative beliefs about the self due to having tics. The current chapter tailored evidence-based assessments and cognitive–behavioral interventions for individuals with low self-esteem for the treatment of youth tic disorders. Strategies include restructuring tic-specific cognitive distortions related to low self-esteem, including (1) unrealistic self-standards, (2) inaccurate self-evaluations, (3) undifferentiated self-structure, and (4) inauthentic or false self. Additionally, this chapter included skills for building and enhancing a positive self-schema by reinforcing both positive self-beliefs and behavioral strengths of the individual, as well as expanding one's sense of self, which includes, but is not limited to, having tics. Finally, we reviewed complex issues that may come up in the treatment of low self-esteem among youth with tic disorders, including the dialectic between tic reduction and tic acceptance, perceived versus actual limitations due to tics, low motivation or insight into one's low self-esteem, and the role of family context in the maintenance and treatment of low self-esteem in youth with tic disorders.

REFERENCES

Beck, A. T. (1979). *Cognitive therapy and the emotional disorders (Meridian book)*. New York: New American Library.

Cavanna, A. E., Luoni, C., Selvini, C., Blangiardo, R., Eddy, C. M., Silvestri, P. R., . . . Termine, C. (2013). Disease-specific quality of life in young patients with Tourette syndrome. *Pediatric Neurology*, *48*(2), 111–114. <https://doi.org/10.1016/j.pediatrneurol.2012.10.006>.

Centers for Disease Control and Prevention. (2009). Prevalence of diagnosed Tourette syndrome in persons aged 6–17 years—United States, 2007. *MMWR Morbidity and Mortality Weekly*, *58*(21).

Conelea, C., Busch, A., Catanzaro, M., & Budman, C. (2014). Tic related activity restriction as a predictor of emotional functioning and quality of life. *Comprehensive Psychiatry*, *55*(1), 1–12. <https://doi.org/10.1016/j.comppsych.2013.06.009>.

Conelea, C., Woods, D. W., Zinner, S. H., Budman, C., Murphy, T., Scahill, L. D., . . . Walkup, J. (2011). Exploring the impact of chronic tic disorders on youth: Results from the Tourette syndrome impact survey. *Child Psychiatry and Human Development*, *42*(2), 219–242. <https://doi.org/10.1007/s10578-010-0211-4>.

Coyne, L. W., McHugh, L., & Martinez, E. R. (2011). Acceptance and commitment therapy (ACT): Advances and applications with children, adolescents, and families. *Child and Adolescent Psychiatric Clinics of North America*, *20*, 379–399. Available from https://doi.org/10.1016/j.chc.2011.01.010.

Fennell, M. J. V., Abramson, L. Y., Seligman, M. E., Teasdale, J. D., Brown, G. W., Bifulco, A., . . . van den Broek, P. (1997). Low self-esteem: A cognitive perspective. *Behavioural and Cognitive Psychotherapy*, *25*(1), 1. <https://doi.org/10.1017/S1352465800015368>.

Guillon, M. S., Crocq, M., & Bailey, P. E. (2003). The relationship between self-esteem and psychiatric disorders in adolescents. *European Psychiatry*, *18*, 59–62.

Hanks, C. E., Mcguire, J. F., Lewin, A. B., Storch, E. A., & Murphy, T. K. (2016). Clinical correlates and mediators of self-concept in youth with chronic tic disorders. *Child Psychiatry and Human Development*, *47*(1), 64–74. Available from https://doi.org/10.1007/s10578-015-0544-0.

Harter, S. (1985). *Manual for the self-perception profile for children*. Denver, CO: University of Denver.

Harter, S. (1986). Processes underlying the construction, maintenance, and enhancement of self-concept in children. In J. Suls, & A. Greenwald (Eds.), *Psychological perspectives on the self* (pp. 137–181). Hillsdale, NJ: Erlbaum.

Harter, S. (1988). *Manual for the self-perception profile for adolescents*. Denver, CO: University of Denver.

Harter, S. (1999). *The construction of the self: A developmental perspective*. New York: Guilford Press.

Harter, S., Marold, D., Whitesell, N., & Cobbs, G. (1996). A model of the effects of perceived parent and peer support on adolescent false self behavior. *Child Development*, *67*(2), 360–374.

Hesapçıoğlu, S. T., Tural, M. K., & Kandil, S. (2014). Quality of life and self-esteem in children with chronic tic disorder. *Turkish Archives of Pediatrics*, *49*(4), 323–332. <https://doi.org/10.5152/tpa.2014.1947>.

Jacobson, N. S., Dobson, K. S., Truax, P. A., Addis, M. E., Koerner, K., Gollan, J. K., ... Prince, S. E. (1996). A component analysis of cognitive–behavioral treatment for depression. *Journal of Consulting and Clinical Psychology*, *64*(2), 295–304. Available from http://www.ncbi.nlm.nih.gov/pubmed/8871414.

Kovacs, M. (2011). *Children's depression inventory (CDI2): Technical manual*. North Tonawanda, NY: Multi-Health Systems Inc.

Linville, P., & Higgins, T. (1985). Self-complexity and affective extremity: Don't put all of your eggs in one cognitive basket. *Social Cognition*, *3*(1), 94–120.

Living with Tourette syndrome. (n.d.). Available from https://www.tourette.org/about-tourette/overview/living-tourette-syndrome/.

Mangini, S. J. (1986). *Secrets of self-esteem with a 30-day program for self esteem development*. Canoga Park, CA: N.O.V.A Corp.

McGuire, J. F., Arnold, E., Park, J. M., Nadeau, J. M., Lewin, A. B., Murphy, T. K., & Storch, E. (2015). Living with tics: Reduced impairment and improved quality of life for youth with chronic tic disorders. *Psychiatry Research*, *225*(3), 571–579. <https://doi.org/10.1016/j.psychres.2014.11.045>.

McKay, M., Wood, J. C., & Brantley, J. (2007). *The dialectical behavior therapy skills workbook*. Oakland, CA: New Harbinger Publications, Inc.

Miller, W. R., & Rollnick, S. (2002). *Motivational interviewing: Preparing people for change*. New York: Guilford Press.

Mueller, C., & Dweck, C. (1998). Praise for intelligence can undermine children's motivation and performance. *Journal of Personality and Social Psychology*, *75*(1), 33–52.

Murphy, T. K., Lewin, A. B., Storch, E. A., & Stock, S. (2013). Practice parameter for the assessment and treatment of children and adolescents with tic disorders. *Journal of the American Academy of Child & Adolescent Psychiatry*, *52*(12), 1341–1359. Available from https://doi.org/10.1016/j.jaac.2013.09.015.

Piacentini, J., Woods, D. W., Scahill, L., Wilhelm, S., Peterson, A. L., Chang, S., ... Walkup, J. T. (2010). Behavior therapy for children with Tourette disorder: A randomized controlled trial. *Journal of the American Medical Association*, *303*(19), 1929–1937. <https://doi.org/10.1001/jama.2010.607>.

Prochaska, J. O., DiClemente, C. C., & Norcross, J. C. (1992). In search of how people change. Applications to addictive behaviors. *The American Psychologist*, *47*(9), 1102–1114. Available from http://www.ncbi.nlm.nih.gov/pubmed/1329589.

Shirk, S., Burwell, R., & Harter, S. (2003). Strategies to modify low self-esteem in adolescents. In M. R. Reinecke, F. M. Dattilio, & A. Freeman (Eds.), *Cognitive therapy with children and adolescents: A casebook for clinical practice* (2nd ed., pp. 189–213). New York: Guilford Press.

Stark, K., Hargrave, J., Hersh, B., Greenberg, M., Herren, J., & Fisher, M. (2008). Treatment of childhood depression: The ACTION treatment program. In J. R. Z. Abela, & B. L. Hankin (Eds.), *Handbook of depression in children and adolescents* (pp. 224–249). New York: Guilford Press.

Storch, E. A., Morgan, J. E., Caporino, N. E., Brauer, L., Lewin, A. B., Piacentini, J., ... Murphy, T. K. (2012). Psychosocial treatment to improve resilience and reduce impairment in youth with tics: An intervention case series of eight youth. *Journal of Cognitive Psychotherapy*, *26*(1), 57–71.

Woods, D., Piacentini, J., & Walkup, J. (Eds.), (2007). Treating Tourette syndrome and tic disorders: A practitioner's guide. New York: Guilford Press.

Woods, D. W., Piacentini, J. C., Scahill, L., Alan, L., Wilhelm, S., Chang, S., ... Walkup, J. T. (2011). Behavior therapy for tics in children: Acute and long-term effects on psychiatric and psychosocial functioning. *Journal of Child Neurology*, *26*(7), 858–865. <https://doi.org/10.1177/0883073810397046>.

Zinner, S. H., Conelea, C. A., Glew, G. M., Woods, D. W., & Budman, C. L. (2012). Peer victimization in youth with Tourette syndrome and other chronic tic disorders. *Child Psychiatry and Human Development*, *43*(1), 124–136. <https://doi.org/10.1007/s10578-011-0249-y>.

Chapter 7

Talking About Tics With Peers and Coping in Social Interactions

Jack Dempsey[1], Ashlie V. Llorens[2], Rachel Fein[1] and Allison G. Dempsey[3]
[1]*Department of Pediatrics, Psychology Service, Baylor College of Medicine, Texas Children's Hospital, Houston, TX, United States,* [2]*Department of Crisis Intervention, Houston Independent School District, Houston, TX, United States,* [3]*Department of Pediatrics, University of Texas Health Science Center, Houston, TX, United States*

Brian was a 7-year-old male in second grade. In first grade, he had struggled with reading in the classroom and was diagnosed with attention-deficit/ hyperactivity disorder (ADHD), as well as anxiety by his pediatrician. His parents decided to address his symptoms with environmental accommodations rather than medication and worked with the school to create a 504 plan. Midway through his first grade year, Brian began displaying vocal tics, involving making a high pitched squeaking noise with his throat. The tic was predominantly present at school and increased in frequency and intensity when he was about to speak. Over the course of several months, the tic worsened and Brian began displaying a simple motor tic in the form of rapid eye blinking. His teacher at first interpreted the tics as defiance rather than involuntary, making statements such as "Brian, please stop making that noise and get back to your work." His peers also began making statements, asking him "why do you always make that noise?" and "what's wrong with your eyes." He began displaying withdrawal from some activities and resistance to attending school, and so his parents brought him to a psychologist.

Tourette syndrome and related tic disorders (collectively referred to as TDs) by nature position children to have noticeably different behaviors than their peers and can cause significant social stress to the children. The developmental course of tics follows the pattern of the importance of social/peer relationships, as both increase throughout the elementary and middle school years. However, the courses may diverge during adolescence. Whereas the frequency and severity of tics peak in early adolescence (Bloch & Leckman,

The Clinician's Guide to Treatment and Management of Youth with Tourette Syndrome and Tic Disorders.
DOI: https://doi.org/10.1016/B978-0-12-811980-8.00007-8

2009) and then slowly decline in later adolescence in many cases, the influence of peers continues to increase over the high school years. Thus working with a child to respond to peer inquiries and responses to tic behaviors is an important element of treatment, particularly in the elementary and middle school years (Smith, Fox, & Trayner, 2015).

PEER INTERACTIONS AMONG CHILDREN WITH TICS

Beyond the unpredictable nature of the tics themselves, peer reactions to tics represent another area over which children with TDs may feel helpless. Empowering children to not only manage tic behaviors, but also prepare to respond to peer comments and questions is an important element of treatment. Although the majority of children with TDs have close friendships, they comment on problems in their interactions with their broader peer groups (Wadman, Tischler, & Jackson, 2013) and report being treated differently by peers due to their tics (Conelea et al., 2011). Furthermore children with TDs express that tics frequently interfere with their social lives and ability to develop relationships (for a review, see Houghton, Alexander, & Woods, 2016). Specifically, youth with TDs report significantly higher rates of peer victimization than healthy youth, and youth with a chronic medical illness (Storch et al., 2007). Consistent with the perceptions of the youth with tics, classmates generally rate children with TDs as being more withdrawn and less popular than their other classmates (Stokes, Bawden, Camfield, Backman, & Dooley, 1991). Additionally, children with chronic TDs tend to report slightly below average levels of self-concept (Hanks, Mcguire, Lewin, Storch, & Murphy, 2015), and are more likely to experience social deficits than their peers without tics (Lange & Oliver, 1998). Hanks and colleagues (2015) noted that these social difficulties are further exacerbated by comorbidities. Indeed, these social deficits are most common in children with comorbid symptoms, such as inattention and hyperactivity, and can increase the risk of social functioning problems among children with TDs (McGuire, Hanks, Lewin, Storch, & Murphy, 2013).

In a qualitative study (Lee, Mu, Wang, & Wang, 2016) of adolescents with Tourette Syndrome from China, one adolescent described his/her perceptions of peer reactions to tic behaviors by stating, "My classmates look at me in a strange way, and they even impose discrimination on me... I feel that I am not a part of the peer group, and I suffer from discrimination" (p. 467). Recognizing the role that social interactions play is important, not just to understand the social development of a child with TDs, but also because the stress from the negative interactions may directly manifest in an exacerbation of tics (Lin et al., 2007). Reducing tic behaviors and simultaneously identifying ways to engage with peers, particularly in conversations related to tic behaviors, are important therapeutic techniques to interrupt this negative feedback cycle.

Teasing/Bullying

In addition to stressful interactions related to tic behaviors and perceptions of social neglect, children with TDs are more likely to report being teased or bullied than children without tics (Storch et al., 2007; Zinner, Conelea, Glew, Woods, & Budman, 2012). In fact, children with TDs are more likely to experience loneliness and more severe tics when they experience victimization from their peers. Unfortunately, early adolescence is also the time in development when the frequency of peer teasing and bullying is most prevalent (Nansel et al., 2001). Social dominance theory posits that in early adolescence, peers are most likely to victimize someone who seems different or lesser on the social hierarchy so that the perpetrator can demonstrate social dominance (Pellegrini & Long, 2002). Children with chronic conditions that have noticeable aberrant appearances or behaviors are more likely to be victimized by their peers (for a review, see Dempsey & Storch, 2010). Unfortunately, negative peer status and interactions can be stable over time (Coie, Dodge, & Kupersmidt, 1990) and must be managed proactively.

Protective Quality of Friendships

While many children with TDs are at risk for negative peer interactions, friendships can provide a protective barrier that mitigates the negative effects of these adverse peer-experiences. Not only do close friendships provide a buffer against negative experiences, but they are more important for promoting a positive quality of life than being accepted by the peer group as a whole (Goldbaum, Craig, Pepler, & Connolly, 2003; Waldrip, Malcolm, & Jensen-Campbell, 2008). In qualitative accounts of living with TDs, youth often identify that peer acceptance and having friends improves the overall quality of life (Lee et al., 2016). When a child with TDs does not have these friendships, teasing and negative comments from peers can be more destructive to the social world and self-esteem of the child. The accounts of these children who reported being isolated or teased had a despairing/hopeless quality of simply waiting for their tics to inevitably embarrass them when at school (Lee et al., 2016): "I don't want to make odd movements or sounds. My discomfort becomes a joke in my class and my classmates tease me about it. I sure feel sad and humiliated" (p. 468). In contrast, when children with TDs report having friends, their statements suggest improved coping and quality of life: "Being liked and accepted by my classmates makes me feel very happy, which also makes me like myself more. Because I have these close friends, it proves that, although I have TS, I can still be treated like a normal person and as a good friend" (p. 467). Thus an important aspect of treatment for children with TDs is promoting formation and maintenance of quality friendships.

ADDRESSING PEER INTERACTIONS IN THERAPY

When working with children with TDs to promote positive peer interactions, it will be important to create and rehearse scripts for various peer groups and social situations that they are likely to encounter. The way that the children talk with their peer group with whom they have regular contact at school or recurring social activities (i.e., "recurring peers") will be different than how they interact with other children in occasional or new social situations, such as same-aged children that the child may encounter in public but will likely not see again (novel peers). For the recurring peer group the focus will be on helping peers understand tics, creating scripts, and role-playing how to have conversations about tics, and coping with teasing and bullying if it is occurring (McGuire et al., 2015; Storch et al., 2012).

Talking With Recurring Peers

Inevitable questions come up from peers due to the nature of the tics, particularly in middle childhood and adolescence when youth have less social inhibition. Identifying how to address this curiosity will play an important role in the therapeutic process. The overarching goal of improving peer understanding of tics is to create an attitude of acceptance of the tics in the peer group, which is a critical component in establishing friendships for children with TDs. Such an intervention may also reduce the risk of teasing/bullying behaviors toward the child, as understanding the tic behaviors may position the child as an unacceptable target for victimization in the general peer group, and promote the likelihood that the peer group will stick up for the child should bullying occur.

Helping a child with TD move toward this goal will be a fluid process that requires consideration of multiple variables. Examples include the child's willingness to engage with peers on the topic of his/her tics, the developmental level of the child and peer group, the level of support provided by teachers and family, and the social history the individual has with his/her classmates (e.g., bullying). Ultimately, this strategy must be acceptable to the child and cannot be developed without his/her participation in the process. Whether providing information at the classroom level or in informal conversations with peers, it is important to prepare the child to provide a brief explanation of the condition, not just the diagnostic label (i.e., "I have Tourette syndrome"), as psychoeducation of a condition is a critical component to create positive perceptions and knowledge (Nussey, Pistrang, & Murphy, 2014). An important finding to emerge from the limited research conducted on talking to peers about tics is that self-disclosure of the TD is generally well-accepted by others and has been shown to lead to more positive views of the individual with TD (Marcks, Berlin, Woods, & Davies, 2007; Nussey et al., 2014). The following is a sample dialogue of how a clinician may broach the subject of educating the child's peers about his/her condition:

Clinician:	*"When your friends and teammates make comments or ask you questions about your tics, how do you typically respond?"*
Child:	*"I don't really know what to do. It makes me feel uncomfortable, so I usually change the subject."*
Clinician:	*"I can see how you might feel caught off guard, and changing the subject is one option that may make you feel more at ease. Perhaps your friends and teammates make comments or ask questions because they are trying to get a better understanding of what you're going through. I wonder if you would be interested in talking with them outside of school or practice and sharing some information with them about tics. What do you think about that?"*
Child:	*"I could try it, but I wouldn't know what to say to them."*
Clinician:	*"If you're open to it, I'm happy to spend the remainder of our session developing some different talking points with you."*
Child:	*"Sounds like a plan."*

Therapeutic Activity

For younger children, particularly those in elementary school, a classroom presentation on the condition may be appropriate (Nussey et al., 2014). The child and family may wish to work with the school to present a brief presentation to the classroom in which information about TDs is provided and discussed. This can be delivered by the teacher or other school personnel, and the child can select the degree to which he/she wishes to be involved in the presentation and discussion. Several resources are available for this form of education, including books for young children (Krueger, 2002), the Tourette Association of America's Youth Ambassador Program (for adolescents), and educational videos published by the Tourette's Syndrome of America on YouTube, such as "I Have Tourette's but Tourette Doesn't Have Me" (Tourette Association of America, 2015). Educational videos provide information about tics and promotes more positive attitudes and intentions toward children with TDs (Woods, 2002; Woods, Koch, & Miltenberger, 2003; Woods & Marcks, 2005) although these changes are relatively small (Houghton et al., 2016). During this presentation, general information about TDs should be provided, including a brief explanation that tics are part of a medical condition, which is partially inherited (like eye and hair color), but is not contagious. For younger children, it may also be important to help them understand that TDs are not life-threatening conditions. When describing the nature of tics the use of developmentally appropriate comparisons may be helpful to promote understanding. For example, many children (and adults) can relate to having the hiccups and not being able to stop them voluntarily. They can also relate to the frustration (and likely annoyance) when friends, family, and/or others remark on the hiccups, and offer (unsuccessful) solutions to make the hiccups go away. After cultivating this analogy or another similar one (e.g., trying to "hold in a sneeze" or "stop coughing when you have an itchy throat"), unaffected peers can then be coached that the best way to help the child with TDs is to ignore the tics and treat the child as they do the rest of their classmates. When providing this psychoeducation to children, it is essential to allow time for children to ask questions to address any misconceptions that they may have about TDs (see Chapter 2: Psychoeducation About Tic Disorders and Treatment, for information on common misconceptions). However, if the child presents as resistant to the idea of a classroom-based psychoeducation intervention, then it will be important to respect the wishes of the child so as not to increase distress related to peer interactions. In such cases, a greater priority will be placed on preparing the child for informal conversations with peers that promote an understanding of tics.

Additionally, it will also be important for the child to develop language for describing the condition in individual, informal conversations. Scripted responses to common peer questions can be developed and rehearsed in session. Parents and children should be encouraged to continue to practice the conversations outside of sessions, as well. Here are some examples of commonly asked questions:

Q: "Why do you do that?" or "Why do you make that noise?"
A: *"I have a condition called Tourette Syndrome and sometimes I make sounds or movements called tics. It's not contagious and you can't catch it from someone who has it. No one knows the direct cause of Tourette Syndrome."*
Q: "What's it like to have Tourette Syndrome?"
A: *"You can think of tics in the same way that you think of hiccups. You don't know what they are going to show up, and you can't force them to go away. They can be annoying and even uncomfortable at times, but they're not dangerous."*
Q: "How do we respond to you when you do that or make that noise?"
A: *"The best thing that you can do is to just ignore my tics. So this means that when you see one of my tics in action, try not to talk to me about it or look at me while it's happening."*

Promoting Friendships

Previous findings indicate that children with TDs are disproportionately likely to be socially marginalized, meaning that they have fewer friends, and/or viewed as less accepted than other children in the classroom. Thus proceeding with the assumption that the child with TD has little social capital, it is important to differentially target certain peers for friendship overtures. That is, while classroom bullies and/or highly popular children may be the child with TDs initial targets due to their social salience, initial attempts to shift these individuals' attitudes toward tics may yield few results. Instead, more progress will likely be made by targeting children identified as "nice" and/or "accepting" by informants. With regard to the latter, obtaining information on characteristics of individual children in the classroom from multiple informants, such as patient, teacher, siblings, and parents, will greatly aid in identifying appropriate peers for discussion about tics.

Therapeutic Activity

Often, children who are teased/bullied or socially marginalized may have a difficult time identifying peers for potential friendships. In these cases a helpful therapeutic exercise is to ask the child to think of his/her class (or if the child is in middle or high school, to select one of their classes). Then, ask them the following questions:

1. Who are the two or three most popular students in the class?
2. Who are the one or two students who are the meanest?
3. Who are the three or four students you have never seen being mean to someone else?
4. Who are the one or two students you have seen stick up for someone else when they were being picked on?
5. Which student said something neutral or positive to you in the last week (i.e., who did not say something mean to you)?

After the clinician has a rough social map of the child's classroom, the child can easily identify a few students who are potential targets for friendship overtures. Work with the child to identify a list of topics they can talk about with the peer to have a positive interaction. They should explicitly think of the interests (e.g., favorite television shows, sports teams, or video games) of the specific peer. The clinician may need to ask probing questions to elicit this information. If the child still continues to struggle, making a homework assignment to investigate this is appropriate. Once the target peers and their interests are identified the child and clinician will need to explicitly identify questions or comments that allow for to-and-fro social exchange, rather than simply asking a question or making a comment that elicits a yes/no/thank you response. These should be role-played and rehearsed in the session. This should be supplemented by identifying ways to engage with the peers outside of the school setting.

At this point the child's parent will need to be involved in the session to suggest such extracurricular opportunities and agree to support them, such as taking the children to the movies or mini golf. The parent should also be coached to work with the child at home to facilitate regular role-play practice, and encourage implementation of these social strategies on a daily basis. Parents will also need to discuss the assigned interactions and the peer responses, and engage in problem solving with the child on a nightly basis. In cases when the peer group remains unresponsive, or even responds negatively, parents may need to pursue recreational and leisure activities within the community instead to promote positive social activities. Here the child's reputation will not be such an impediment to establishing positive relationships. Examples of community activities include:

- boy or girl scouts,
- sports teams,

- religious groups (choir, youth groups), and
- classes: martial arts, fencing, art, stop-action film, DJ'ing.

In elementary school and early middle school, parents can support their child's attempts to develop friendships, by networking with other parents and establishing opportunities for the children to get together outside of school. More than simply ensuring that another child comes to play, the parent of a child with TD can improve the odds of a successful social interaction by providing exciting activities, items, and food. Parents can also role play/coach their child on how to perform during the scheduled interaction, and allow opportunities for prosocial behaviors. The following is an example of a clinician teaching a parent to lead a role play with the child:

Clinician: *"Let's think about how to provide some opportunities for your child to share and compromise with his friend."*

Parent: *"May be he can let his friend pick what we eat for lunch."*

Clinician: *"That sounds like a great opportunity! You could work with him to identify two specific meals to offer—something that most kids would like, such as pizza or fast food. The two of you could also create a signal you use to remind him to make the offer to his friend."*

Parent: *"Okay, I can call his friend's parents and ask if he likes pizza. If he does, my child and I can work out a pre-arranged signal like a timer going off that would remind him to ask his friend if he wanted to order pizza for lunch and what he wants on it."*

Clinician: *"What if your child thinks his friend's choice of toppings is gross? Think about how you can work with him ahead of time to compromise if needed."*

Parent: *"I will practice with him ahead of time that if his friend wants something on top that he thinks is gross to just say, 'OK, why don't we get half the pizza with that [topping] and half with pepperonis.'"*

For younger children this may involve ensuring that the child has extras of several desirable toys that they could share/give to the friend during play time. Examples of fun/exciting activities to have for a scheduled peer interaction could include:

- opportunities for informal sports at home: basketball hoop (even one to be hung from a door in the house), badminton net or other yard games, foosball/pool/ping-pong table, darts, skateboards;
- opportunities for interactive games and activities at home: crafts, playing cards or board games, two-player video games;
- going to fun stores or shops (comic book or gaming store, mall);
- ordering a pizza or decorating cookies;
- going to community activities: bowling, laser tag, paintball, haunted houses (at Halloween time), batting cages, mini golf, renaissance fairs, water parks.

Novel Peer Contacts

When encountering novel peers the focus of interactions related to tic behaviors is going to be more reactive. Therefore the focus should be on preparing the child to respond to questions and comments from peers. In these cases the responses will be geared toward deflection of attention from the tics rather than promoting acceptance over time.

Therapeutic Activity

In-session activities and homework assignments for addressing interactions with novel peers should include the following:

1. The clinician and the child will work together to list the tics that he/she displays that others may question or comment on and identify specific casual explanations about why the behavior is present in the moment. Identify simple and developmentally appropriate explanations that will be easy for the child to remember. A list of possible explanations for common tics is listed in Table 7.1.

TABLE 7.1 Sample Explanations for Common Tics

Tic Behavior	Excuse
Eye blinking	I have something in my eye.
Nose twitching	My nose is itching.
Shoulder shrugging	I got a chill.
Head Jerking	I thought I felt a bug land on my head.
Humming	I have a song stuck in my head.
Facial grimacing	I was thinking of what my mom made for dinner last night.
Throat clearing	I have a frog in my throat.
Coughing	My throat tickles. OR I might be getting a cold.
Sniffing	I might be getting a cold. OR I have allergies.
Grunting	I just hit my shin/stubbed my toe/got a papercut.
Squatting	My legs are getting tired. OR I am looking for something I dropped.
Back arching	My back is a little stiff.
Leg kicking	I have a cramp in my leg.
Coprolalia	I just realized I forgot something.

2. Rehearse this in session. Encourage the child to simulate the tic in session. The clinician can pretend to be a peer and make comments that the child reports are frequently made to him/her. If willing the child may also have chances to practice with others in the clinician's office.
3. The clinician and child will create a list of the tics and explanations for the child to take home and review and practice. The child and parent should plan outings where the child simulates his/her tic and practices using the explanations in brief, controlled situations (e.g., waiting in line at the movies, coffee shop, or grocery store). This will be critical as the child will need these memorized so they are easily accessible in the moment when comments about the tic behaviors are made.
4. The clinician may also recommend that the parent and child rehearse these responses before entering situations in which novel peers are likely to be present, such as birthday parties and other peer gatherings, family trips, concerts, and community events.

How to Deal With Teasing or Bullying?

If the child is experiencing peer teasing and/or bullying, it will be important to spend some time in session identifying coping strategies and developing techniques for responding. When children are teased it is critical to establish a positive peer group for the child if he/she does not already have a friendship network. As described previously friends provide a protective buffer for children with tics are particularly important if that child is being teased or bullied.

Therapeutic Activity

By first engaging in the activities described earlier to promote peer acceptance and form friendships, the clinician will be engaging in important activities to protect the child from ongoing negative peer interactions, as perpetrators are more likely to target children who do not have friends. However, additional therapeutic activities may be needed to assist the child in developing appropriate responses and coping techniques for teasing.

One well-verified manner of doing this is a technique called tease-the-tease, which is appropriate for verbal teasing from peers (not physical bullying). This technique is more fully described in *The PEERS Treatment Manual* (Laugeson & Frankel, 2011). Briefly the tease-the-tease technique works by countering the attention-seeking function of teasing. That is, in teasing situations, the perpetrator is assumed to provide a teasing statement to elicit a strong reaction from the child with TD. Obtaining this reaction both indicates a form of control for the bully (i.e., I act-you react) and attracts the attention of peer bystanders to the interaction due to the emotional valence. Examples of sought after reactions may include crying, attempting a retort, running to tell an authority figure, or a resumption of tic activity. Teasing in this way also establishes a social norm in the classroom that the child's tics are NOT accepted. Therefore the child can counter this by providing only a very small reaction that clearly establishes the concept that he/she does not care about the teasing and a brief statement that subtly conveys the impression that the bystanders do not care either. Such a response creates an aversive consequence for the teasing. The clinician should work with the child to identify and rehearse an appropriate response in the session. Examples may include teaching the child to respond with a flat facial expression and small shrug of the shoulders or an eye roll. The child could also practice saying "who cares?" Below is an example of a therapeutic interaction incorporating these techniques:

Clinician: *"Has anyone ever teased or bullied you for having tics?"*
Child: *"Most of the kids at school are pretty cool. But there's this one kid who is constantly talking smack to me and basically anyone that is different."*
Clinician: *"What does he say or do?"*
Child: *"He usually laughs at me or calls me names like 'loser' or 'freak' whenever he sees my tics. Sometimes he mocks me by pretending like he has tics. He's really annoying."*
Clinician: *"That sounds pretty annoying. How do you typically respond?"*
Child: *"Well, I used to tell the teacher, but then he started making fun of me for doing that. So, I usually walk away. But then he follows me and won't stop until I get on the bus. Nothing seems to work."*
Clinician: *"I applaud you for staying calm and keeping your cool. It can be really frustrating when you've tried some different strategies to change your situation, but they don't seem to be working. This kid seems like he wants a reaction from you. I wonder if we could give him a reaction, but not the kind he's expecting."*
Child: *"What do you mean?"*
Clinician: *"Telling the teacher and simply walking away from him doesn't seem to work. What do you think about saying something to him that makes it clear that your tics don't bother you so why should they bother him or anyone else?"*
Child: *"Like what?"*
Clinician: *"What do you think you could say to communicate your point?"*
Child: *"I guess I could say 'So what?' or 'May be I am, but who cares?' or 'Nobody cares.'"*
Clinician: *"I think those are fantastic examples. I would even take it up a notch and say one of those statements while shrugging your shoulders or rolling your eyes. Let's practice."*

Quick Reference Clinician Guide: Step-by-Step Guide

1. Ask questions about the social experiences of the child and parent.
   a. What questions do peers ask about tics? What comments do they make?
   b. Who are the child's friends?
   c. Do classmates ever say mean things (tease you) about the tics?

   d. If so, how do you typically respond?
   e. What has worked? What has not worked?
2. Identify and rehearse strategies for deflecting negative peer attention in the moment.
3. Identify and rehearse responses to comments and questions from recurring peers that include psychoeducation about the TD.
4. Encourage the child to advocate for himself/herself by informing his/her teachers or other school staff about the TD. Work with the child, family, and school to determine the appropriateness of a classroom-based psychoeducation session. For older adolescents this may involve directly rehearsing conversations the adolescent may have with teachers and other school personnel about the nature of the disorder and what the teacher can do to help.
5. Identify strategies for forming and maintaining friendships. Involve parents in this activity, as they can support the child by providing opportunities for scheduled peer interactions outside of school.
6. For older adolescents it may be helpful to talk about how tics may interfere with dating and to develop specific strategies for managing tics around peers in dating situations. Specific role-playing sessions for disclosing and responding to peers for whom there is a romantic interest may be particularly helpful.
7. For children with ongoing adverse peer-experiences and bullying, explicitly teach and rehearse responses for teasing. Work with parents to encourage outside of school activities in which opportunities for positive interactions with peers exist.

Problem-Solving Challenging/Complex Issues

Often, social difficulties may be the factor that triggered the family to seek therapeutic intervention for the child. In these cases the negative peer responses and social marginalization may have been going on for quite a while, possibly even years. In such scenarios, intervention targeted at the peer group, particularly in early adolescence will be more challenging and psychoeducation and scripted/rehearsed responses from the child may not be sufficient to alter the pattern of negative peer reactions (Putallaz & Gottman, 1981). The clinician may need to work with the child and family to explore ways for establishing a newer, more positive peer group. This may involve joining new activities outside of the school setting. If teasing or bullying is a problem for the child the clinician and family may need to work with the school to create a safety plan for the child and ensure that school policies related to handling bullying situations are being appropriately enforced.

Furthermore in situations in which the child is displaying significant social deficits that are comorbid with the presence of a TD, intervention to directly target that deficit will likely be necessary. Most likely, children with social deficits will require explicit social skills training in individual or group settings that allow sufficient opportunities for skill implementation. Although beyond the scope of this chapter, Spence (2003) provides an overview of social skills training interventions that may be helpful for these youth.

CONCLUSION

For children with TD the developmental trajectories of peer and social influences coincide with the increase in frequency and severity of tic behaviors. Specifically, addressing peer interactions for youth with TDs is an important component of treatment that has empirical support for reducing impairment, improving quality of life, and high family treatment satisfaction. Peer interactions are often affected by the overt nature of vocal and/or motor tics, and the presence of tics can increase the risk of a child being targeted for teasing and bullying, especially when psychiatric comorbidities are present. These negative peer interactions and social deficits may also affect a child's self-concept. Effective treatment components for addressing peer interactions for children with TDs include providing psychoeducation about the importance of the protective factor of friendships and targeted skills for actively discussing tics with various peer groups. Furthermore children with TDs also benefit from participating in scripted role-play activities to develop active coping strategies for responding to teasing and bullying. Targeting these specific skill sets empowers children with TDs to respond to comments and questions about their tic behaviors in a manner that may reduce perceived stress related to negative feedback from peers, which can indirectly result in reduction in tic severity.

REFERENCES

Bloch, M. H., & Leckman, J. F. (2009). Clinical course of Tourette syndrome. *Journal of Psychosomatic Research, 67*(6), 497–501.

Coie, J. D., Dodge, K. A., & Kupersmidt, J. B. (1990). Peer group behavior and social status. In S. A. Asher, & J. D. Coie (Eds.), *Peer rejection in childhood* (pp. 17–59). New York: Cambridge University Press.

Conelea, C. A., Woods, D. W., Zinner, S. H., Budman, C., Murphy, T., Scahill, L. D., et al. (2011). Exploring the impact of chronic tic disorders on youth: Results from the Tourette Syndrome Impact Survey. *Child Psychiatry and Human Development, 42*(2), 219–242. Available from https://doi.org/10.1007/s10578-010-0211-4.

Dempsey, A. G., & Storch, E. A. (2010). Psychopathology and health problems affecting involvement in bullying. In E. M. Vernberg, & B. K. Biggs (Eds.), *Preventing and treating bullying and victimization* (pp. 107–131). New York: Oxford University Press.

Goldbaum, S., Craig, W. M., Pepler, D., & Connolly, J. (2003). Developmental trajectories of victimization: Identifying risk and protective factors. *Journal of Applied School Psychology, 19*(2), 139–156.

Hanks, C. E., Mcguire, J. F., Lewin, A. B., Storch, E. A., & Murphy, T. K. (2015). Clinical correlates and mediators of self-concept in youth with chronic tic disorders. *Child Psychiatry & Human Development*, *47*(1), 64–74. Available from https://doi.org/10.1007/s10578-015-0544-0.

Houghton, D. C., Alexander, J. R., & Woods, D. W. (2016). The psychosocial impact of tic disorders: Nature and intervention. *Journal of Developmental and Physical Disabilities*, *28*(2), 347–365.

Krueger, T. (2002). *Taking Tourette's syndrome to school*. Plainview, NY: JayJo Books.

Lange, N. D., & Oliver, M. A. (1998). The self-concept of the adolescent suffering from Tourette's syndrome. *Southern African Journal of Child and Adolescent Mental Health*, *10* (2), 126–132. Available from https://doi.org/10.1080/16826108.1998.9632356.

Laugeson, E. A., & Frankel, F. (2011). *Social skills for teenagers with developmental and autism spectrum disorders: The PEERS treatment manual*. New York: Routledge.

Lee, M. Y., Mu, P. F., Wang, W. S., & Wang, H. S. (2016). 'Living with tics': Self-experience of adolescents with Tourette syndrome during peer interaction. *Journal of Clinical Nursing*, *25*(3–4), 463–471.

Lin, H., Katsovich, L., Ghebremichael, M., Findley, D. B., Grantz, H., Lombroso, P. J., … Leckman, J. F. (2007). Psychosocial stress predicts future symptom severities in children and adolescents with Tourette syndrome and/or obsessive-compulsive disorder. *Journal of Child Psychology and Psychiatry*, *48*(2), 157–166.

Marcks, B. A., Berlin, K. S., Woods, D. W., & Davies, W. H. (2007). Impact of Tourette Syndrome: A preliminary investigation of the effects of disclosure on peer perceptions and social functioning. *Psychiatry*, *70*(1), 59–67. Available from https://doi.org/10.1521/psyc.2007.70.1.59.

McGuire, J. F., Arnold, E., Park, J. M., Nadeau, J. M., Lewin, A. B., Murphy, T. K., & Storch, E. A. (2015). Living with tics: Reduced impairment and improved quality of life for youth with chronic tic disorders. *Psychiatry Research*, *225*(3), 571–579. Available from https://doi.org/10.1016/j.psychres.2014.11.045.

McGuire, J. F., Hanks, C., Lewin, A. B., Storch, E. A., & Murphy, T. K. (2013). Social deficits in children with chronic tic disorders: Phenomenology, clinical correlates and quality of life. *Comprehensive Psychiatry*, *54*, 1023–1031.

Nansel, T. R., Overpeck, M., Pilla, R. S., Ruan, W. J., Simons-Morton, B., & Scheidt, P. (2001). Bullying behaviors among US youth: Prevalence and association with psychosocial adjustment. *Journal of the American Medical Association*, *285*(16), 2094–2100.

Nussey, C., Pistrang, N., & Murphy, T. (2014). Does it help to talk about tics? An evaluation of a classroom presentation about Tourette syndrome. *Child and Adolescent Mental Health*, *19* (1), 31–38.

Pellegrini, A. D., & Long, J. D. (2002). A longitudinal study of bullying, dominance, and victimization during the transition from primary school through secondary school. *British Journal of Developmental Psychology*, *20*(2), 259–280.

Putallaz, M., & Gottman, J. M. (1981). An interactional model of children's entry into peer groups. *Child Development*, *52*(3), 986–994.

Smith, H., Fox, J. R., & Trayner, P. (2015). The lived experiences of individuals with Tourette syndrome or tic disorders: A meta-synthesis of qualitative studies. *British Journal of Psychology*, *106*(4), 609–634.

Spence, S. H. (2003). Social skills training with children and young people: Theory, evidence and practice. *Child and Adolescent Mental Health*, *8*(2), 84–96.

Stokes, A., Bawden, H. N., Camfield, P. R., Backman, J. E., & Dooley, J. M. (1991). Peer problems in Tourette's disorder. *Pediatrics*, *87*(6), 936–942.

Storch, E. A., Morgan, J. E., Caporino, N. E., Brauer, L., Lewin, A. B., Piacentini, J., & Murphy, T. K. (2012). Psychosocial treatment to improve resilience and reduce impairment in youth with tics: An intervention case series of eight youth. *Journal of Cognitive Psychotherapy*, *26*(1), 57–70.

Storch, E. A., Murphy, T. K., Chase, R. M., Keeley, M., Goodman, W. K., Murray, M., & Geffken, G. R. (2007). Peer victimization in youth with Tourette's syndrome and chronic tic disorder: Relations with tic severity and internalizing symptoms. *Journal of Psychopathology and Behavioral Assessment*, *29*(4), 211–219.

Tourette Association of America (2015, April 24). HBO "I have Tourettes but Tourette doesn't have me" trailer [Video File]. Retrieved from https://www.youtube.com/watch?v=7_dBRDvkbTU.

Wadman, R., Tischler, V., & Jackson, G. M. (2013). 'Everybody just thinks I'm weird': A qualitative exploration of the psychosocial experiences of adolescents with Tourette syndrome. *Child: Care, Health and Development*, *39*(6), 880–886.

Waldrip, A. M., Malcolm, K. T., & Jensen-Campbell, L. A. (2008). With a little help from your friends: The importance of high-quality friendships on early adolescent adjustment. *Social Development*, *17*(4), 832–852.

Woods, D. W. (2002). The effect of video-based peer education on the social acceptability of adults with Tourette's syndrome. *Journal of Developmental and Physical Disabilities*, *14*(1), 51–62.

Woods, D. W., Koch, M., & Miltenberger, R. G. (2003). The impact of tic severity on the effects of peer education about Tourette's syndrome. *Journal of Developmental and Physical Disabilities*, *15*(1), 67–78.

Woods, D. W., & Marcks, B. A. (2005). Controlled evaluation of an educational intervention used to modify peer attitudes and behavior toward persons with Tourette's syndrome. *Behavior Modification*, *29*(6), 900–912.

Zinner, S. H., Conelea, C. A., Glew, G. M., Woods, D. W., & Budman, C. L. (2012). Peer victimization in youth with Tourette syndrome and other chronic tic disorders. *Child Psychiatry & Human Development*, *43*(1), 124–136.

FURTHER READING

Nussey, C., Pistrang, N., & Murphy, T. (2013). How does psychoeducation help? A review of the effects of providing information about Tourette syndrome and attention-deficit/hyperactivity disorder. *Child: Care, Health and Development*, *39*(5), 617–627.

Chapter 8

Tourette's in the Classroom: Support and Guidance on Education Issues for Clinicians

Kathy Giordano
Tourette Association of America, New York, NY, United States

INTRODUCTION

Children with Tourette disorder or persistent tic disorders (collectively referred to as TD) and their parents face many challenges, one of which includes navigating the education system. Historically, schools rely on consequence-based strategies for motivating and disciplining a student. However, these approaches can increase stress, exacerbate tic symptoms, and contribute to behavioral issues. As school personnel and educators often lack the necessary knowledge to appropriately support a student with TD and its common related challenges, students may be punished for symptoms and do not receive the necessary supports to be successful academically and socially. This chapter discusses the various ways clinicians can assist children with TD and their parents in developing an appropriate educational setting in which the child is able to succeed and achieve his/her true potential.

Identifying Academic Impairment in Youth With TD

Children with TD may experience several educational barriers, some of which parents and clinicians can help address. In order to identify and overcome these barriers, clinicians must first understand how tics and related symptoms impact the patient's educational performance. Indeed, tic symptoms can cause many subtle (and not so subtle) problems in academic performance. For example, children with TD often have eye or head tics. While parents and/or teachers may believe these symptoms to be relatively minor in comparison to other tics, these tics can significantly impact a student's ability to remain focused during reading activities. Thus, a student may postpone his/her reading homework due to tic symptoms, and/or avoid reading

The Clinician's Guide to Treatment and Management of Youth with Tourette Syndrome and Tic Disorders.
DOI: https://doi.org/10.1016/B978-0-12-811980-8.00008-X

activities altogether due to frustration from multiple unsuccessful attempts. Similarly, youth with TD may also have impairments in executive functioning due to TD and/or related conditions (e.g., learning disabilities, attention deficit hyperactivity disorder (ADHD)). As such, these students may struggle with organization, attending to tasks, and writing assignments. These impairments may hinder the child from demonstrating his/her true abilities, and lead to a declining academic performance, increased anxiety and frustration, decreased self-worth, and eventual refusal to engage in homework and/or school-related tasks. Moreover, as some parents and teachers may struggle to fully recognize how TD negatively impacts academic functioning, they may inaccurately perceive the student to be "unmotivated" and just not wanting to "do the work."

Given the academic impairment TD and common co-morbid conditions may cause, it is important that clinicians inquire about the academic performance of youth with TD, and assess how tics and related conditions may impede this performance (see Chapter 1: Introduction to Treatment and Management of Youth With Tourette Disorders and Tic Disorders, for discussion of assessments). While ratings scales (e.g., Child Tourette Impact Scale-Parent Report, Storch et al., 2007) and questions related to academic performance (e.g., "what are your grades in school?") can be useful to start a conversation about current academic and school problems, these initial queries should be supplemented by a detailed investigation of the emergence of academic struggles and evaluate how tics and/or related conditions may play a role over time. For example, it is not uncommon for a student to obtain honor roll in lower grades due to strong intellectual abilities that compensate for a disability. However, as the student advances into older grades, the demands of academic tasks increase in complexity (e.g., require more organizational skills, better time management, increased note taking, greater writing demand). As a result, a student with an above average IQ and a history of good grades may begin to exhibit a seemingly abrupt decline in academic performance and a dislike for school. While clinicians may initially feel out of place by this focus on academic performance, this information is critical to identify educational difficulties, determine whether a diagnosis should be disclosed to school personnel, and will prove helpful in requesting targeted accommodations from school personnel and guiding school educators how to appropriately support the child with TD.

As the symptoms of TD (and related conditions) typically fluctuate and evolve over time, it may be difficult for parents (and school personnel) to understand which educational interventions (if any) are needed. Accordingly, an important first step is to determine the presence, severity, and duration of education-related impairments. When discussing school performance with the child and parents, common signs that school-based interventions may be needed include: (1) difficulty in going to or staying in school, (2) behavior issues at school or at home (around homework), (3) significant reluctance to complete academic assignments, (4) declining academic performance/grades, (5) increasing symptoms, (6) a depressed mood and/or loss of interest in preferred activities, and (7) difficulties with social communication. When these (or similar challenges) are present, it is important to inquire further about the emergence and course of these difficulties. This information can help clinicians better understand factors that may be influencing the child's performance and inform intervention recommendations.

Initial Steps to Support Parents and Children

Some parents have a sense of relief upon learning their child's diagnosis of TD. However, while clinicians are educated on the topic of TD, parents may incorrectly assume that school educators will also be familiar with TD and will readily know which educational interventions are best for their child. Moreover, there may be some confusion that a diagnosis of TD will immediately lead to educational interventions being put in place. Comparatively, other parents may feel overwhelmed (or even ashamed) about their child's diagnosis, and want to "keep it a secret" from the school system. These parents typically express fears that their child will be stigmatized and labeled "intellectually disabled" or "emotionally disturbed." Accordingly, these parents may be resistant to share information with school personnel.

An important first step for clinicians is to help parents and youth understand exactly how tics and related conditions are impacting youth's educational functioning using the information gained from assessments. As parents and youth gain a better understanding of this impact, clinicians can help parents and youth consider the possible benefits and drawbacks of disclosing diagnoses to a school system. Typically, if a child's symptoms are significant enough to lead the family to pursue an evaluation from a health professional, it is most likely time to inform the school in some capacity. Given that parents may have fears regarding stigmatization, it is important for clinicians to validate parents' concerns and also help them balance the cost/benefit of disclosure versus nondisclosure to the school system. For instance, if a child and parent report no overt academic or social impairment and minimal expression of tics in the classroom, disclosure to the school system may not be necessary at the present time. Alternatively, it may be helpful to alert the school professionals about the diagnosis in general terms and provide them with appropriate educational resources to prevent misperceptions, avoid inappropriate teacher reactions (e.g., punishment for an eye rolling tic), and plan ahead for the child's possible academic needs. Many of these educational resources are freely available on the Tourette Association of America (TAA) website. Meanwhile, if the child is struggling academically (e.g., excessive time spent on school activities, declining academic performance), exhibits many tics in the classroom, and/or other related symptoms (e.g., learning disorders, ADHD, sensory integration issues), it is likely beneficial to inform the school system of the child's diagnoses to instill appropriate educational supports.

When parents are prepared to contact the schools, it is important to consider that educators may question the validity of a TD diagnosis as youth often attempt to suppress and disguise their tics at school. Similarly, school personnel may also be perplexed by the diagnosis of common co-morbid conditions as the child may not appear to exhibit overt symptoms in the classroom (e.g., ADHD, obsessive compulsive behaviors, sensory integration, processing delays, and dysgraphia). As a result, educators may initially misperceive parents to be creating "excuses" for the child's "behaviors." Therefore, clinicians may consider providing school personnel (with parental authorization) a brief letter stating the child's relevant diagnoses contributing to educational challenges. As school personnel typically do not have extensive mental health training, clinicians should provide basic information about TD (and other relevant conditions) and describe how these symptoms may be contributing to the child's educational challenges. The clinician letter and its key components are discussed in further detail later in this chapter. This letter will help educators understand that youth's symptoms may vary over time, and may be expressed differently across different settings due to different internal and external factors. Additionally, the TAA offers toolkits for clinicians, parents, and educators that include accurate information regarding TD and related challenges to supplement this letter. This information is helpful to transition school personnel's possible perception that youth's behaviors are "bad" or "purposeful" toward understanding that the child is suffering from a challenging condition that requires individualized educational support. Indeed, a clinician letter can play a pivotal role in discontinuing an ineffective punishment cycle, which can lead students to become frustrated, angry, avoidant of school and/or the entire education process.

Initial Steps to Support Educators/School Personnel

After learning about TD and related conditions from the clinician's letter and related resources from TAA, school personnel are often interested to learn how they can help the child when in a school setting. While teachers are rarely involved in providing habit reversal training (HRT) or the comprehensive behavioral intervention for tics (CBIT), school personnel can be coached to assist the youth in several other ways. First and foremost, teachers (and related school personnel) should be instructed to ignore the child's tics in the classroom unless the tics are very disruptive. While teachers may want to help the child control the tics and encourage them to "stop ticcing," this can set up a challenging situation. For instance, a child might be successful at momentarily stopping his/her tics using behavioral strategies (e.g., HRT, CBIT) or tic suppression strategies. However, this sets the unspoken expectation that the child can "stop ticcing" if enough effort is applied.

Additionally, as concentration is often required to suppress tics, the child may experience diminished attention capacity to direct toward academic activities (Conelea & Woods, 2008). The child may be focused on stopping his/her tics, but now struggles to pay attention to the classroom academic activity. Thus, when possible, the preferred educational practice is to ignore tics.

However, not all tics can be ignored in an educational setting, and as such require some thoughtful planning and accommodation. Consider the case of a child with TD who has a loud disruptive screeching vocal tic, or a compulsive tic that involves inappropriate touching of other students (e.g., poking, prodding). These tics can present a challenge in common school situations such as taking a test or changing classrooms between classes, respectively. In the case of a loud disruptive vocal tic, it can be helpful to allow the student to take tests/quizzes in a separate location. This accommodation would allow the child with TD to express his/her tic as needed, without causing disruption to other students. Moreover, by not suppressing tic symptoms (different than using behavioral strategies covered in Chapter 3: Habit Reversal Training for Tics), the child's energy and attention is focused on the academic task at hand. Similarly, for typical classroom learning, accommodations might include electronic access (e.g., webcam) to the class when tics are extreme. This way, the student can mute/un-mute the electronic connection as needed when the vocal tic is expressed. For the case of touching other students inappropriately during passing period, an accommodation may be allowing the student to change classes when fewer students are in the halls, or by carrying items that require the use of both arms/hands. The intent of accommodations is not to be a "permanent fix." Rather, accommodations are meant to provide the child with support in the school system, as they are learning to manage their tics using behavioral strategies. As children with TD are often aware of tic triggers, it can be helpful to include them (as developmentally appropriate) in identifying potentially useful accommodations based on specific disruptive tic symptoms. Notably, children with TD may initially perceive educational accommodations as punitive, a "punishment," or even a "failure to control my tics." Therefore, when presenting accommodations to children with TD, it is important to present them in a positive manner (instead of a punitive manner). For example, the accommodations can be framed as positive support to help the child manage his/her tics, while he/she is learning behavioral strategies to better manage challenging symptoms.

When considering accommodations and other targeted recommendations for educators and school personnel, it is important to consider scaffolding the proposed interventions. For example, children and parents may initially be reluctant for the child to go to school when tics are bad, or may request that clinicians write a school note so that the child can leave the classroom as needed to release tics. While acceptable as a "quick fix" in the short term, the long-term implications send a message to the child that tics are something to be "ashamed of" and that missing class due to tics is acceptable. Instead, clinicians should discuss scaffolding accommodations and intervention with the child, parent, and (eventually) school personnel. Stated differently, as a child progresses in treatment and develops the skills to manage tics and tic-related impairment, certain accommodations can be withdrawn to empower the youth to practice these skills in school settings.

Whether tics are disruptive or not, it is important to convey early on to school personnel that tic expression should not be punished. That being stated, the school environment is where children learn strategies for being successful adults. This involves academics, but also includes social interactions that prepare them for the "real world." As such, there may be adverse social consequences for tic expression in school settings. For example, sexual or racial phrases in the wrong social group at school could lead to physical fights with other students and/or social isolation from peers. Thus, the clinician has the important role of both coaching school personnel how to respond and/or accommodate the child's tic symptoms and collaboratively developing plans with families to help children have a successful school experience.

RECOMMENDATIONS AND STRATEGIES FOR EDUCATIONAL INTERVENTIONS

The following section presents guidance for clinicians working with children and families who require educational interventions. The section offers recommendations based on expertise, and helps orient clinicians (who in turn would inform patients/families) about key aspects for educational interventions.

Building a Collaborative Relationship Between Parents, Teachers, and Schools

One of the most important components in a child's educational experience is a collaborative relationship between parents, teachers, and support personnel. A collaborative relationship between these three groups is beneficial for several reasons. First, it fosters a safe and supportive environment. While it is not unusual for children to have anxiety related to school attendance and academic performance, children with TD have the added stress of being "different" and struggling with often misunderstood symptoms. Therefore, it is paramount that the child perceives his/her parents, teachers, and school personnel as working together for his/her benefit. If the child perceives an adversarial relationship between these parties (which sometimes happens), it is only natural that the child's anxiety may be increased at school and result in greater impairment. Along these same lines, it is helpful to encourage parents to take an assertive tone (rather than an aggressive tone) toward educational advocacy. While the internet (e.g., social media, web pages, blogs) often encourages parents to "be aggressive" and to "fight for their child's education," this aggressive tone is typically not well received and may cause a contentious relationship. Advocacy works best when school professionals view parents as a resource for information and a partner in the process of educating the child.

Finally, a collaborative relationship reduces misperception and promotes communication. A common misperception by parents and educators (and even some clinicians) is that if an educator has previous experience working with a student with TD, then the educator will already be aware of how to best work with the current student with TD. While there are some common themes across students with TD, the heterogeneity of TD symptoms complicates broad generalizations across all youth with TD. Thus, when a child with TD begins to struggle in school, parents may blame teachers and schools for not appropriately educating their child. Conversely, teachers may attribute a student's disruptive behaviors to "poor parenting," instead of understanding their common occurrence in TD phenomenology (see Chapter 11: Brief Transdiagnostic Parent Training: A Strengths-Based, Parent-Centered Treatment for Youth With Tourette Syndrome and Chapter 12: Assessing and Treating Emotion Dysregulation and Anger Management). Therefore, it can be helpful to remind parents that teaching children with TD can be challenging and that teachers (or other school personnel) will not have all the answers/all the time. This early recognition can help foster direct and nonjudgmental line of communication between parents, teachers, and school professionals.

Effectively Communicating With School Personnel

As noted earlier, parents may assume that teachers have learned effective approaches for educating a child with TD and common related disorders. Unfortunately, this is typically not the case. When discussing the child's educational needs, clinicians may consider reminding parents that TD has historically been seen as a rare disorder. Accordingly, educators normally do not receive even basic information about it during training. Indeed, parents anecdotally report that they must provide information to teachers about TD on a near annual basis, or request that the previous year's teacher briefly speak with the new teacher about their child's specific strengths and challenges.

One way clinicians can help parents effectively communicate with school personnel is to provide them with informational resources from TAA, which parents can in turn provide to teachers and school personnel. The following are resources that have been reported to be the most helpful as an introduction to TD: (1) Educator's Toolkit; (2) "Ten Things Teacher Can Do for Students With TS"; (3) "Red Flags—Identifying Common Education

Difficulties With Tourette"; (4) "Educator's Guide for Developing Plans for Students With Tourette"; and (5) "Tourette is More Than Tics: Understanding Behavioral Challenges and Related Symptoms." This standardized information should eventually be supplemented with information regarding the child's individualized progression and current educational impairment. Together, this information can help educators understand the child's specific needs and reduce the stress (and possible conflict) parents may experience interacting with teachers and school personnel.

Understanding the Child's Educational Team

Multiple individuals are involved in the child's education and mental health care in a school system. While some individuals are easily identified (e.g., teacher, school psychologist), recognizing the different professionals (and their roles) is essential to develop a comprehensive intervention plan, communicate clearly with school personnel, and utilize resources appropriately. Indeed, this understanding helps clinicians provide clear recommendations that can be implemented in an efficient manner. Moreover, clinicians can direct questions to appropriate school personnel based on their expertise, which school staff generally appreciate. However, when this understanding is not present, it can sometimes lead to confusion and frustration for the parents, school personnel, and clinicians. Table 8.1 provides list of common professionals involved in a student's education and mental health care. When parents (or clinicians) are interacting with school professionals during meetings or phone calls, it is often helpful to inquire about the individual's professional role in the school. As noted in Table 8.1, school psychologists and school counselors can serve different functions in the school setting. Thus questions and recommendations directed to a school psychologist would be very different than those questions/recommendations directed toward a school counselor.

Behavioral Differences Between Home and School Settings

When reflecting on the child's behavior, parents and school personnel may have different perspectives. Children with TD are often motivated to suppress tic symptoms at school to minimize negative attention from peers (e.g., teasing, bullying) and pay attention in class to receive positive feedback from teachers. However, when returning home from school, children can sometimes be exhausted from these activities. Moreover, the external reinforcement (e.g., threats of peer teasing for tics, positive praise for attention in class) that helped to suppress tics and promote attention are no longer present. Unsurprisingly, parents often report that children will exhibit an increase in tic frequency and other behavioral issues when returning home from school. Given the child's behavior in the classroom, teachers and

TABLE 8.1 Descriptions of Possible School Professionals on a Child's Educational Team

Teachers are frontline educators with whom parents and children have the greatest amount of interaction. Clinicians (and parents) should consider providing teachers with helpful information regarding TD, without overwhelming them. Striking an appropriate balance between too little and too much education and interaction can be challenging. However, this balance is important as clinicians, parents, and teachers need to work together to develop a positive and respectful relationship and have effective communication.

School psychologists generally provide education evaluations and assessments. These evaluations/assessments are required when characterizing a student's strengths and weakness, which are used in part to determine eligibility for additional academic support. As such, it is imperative that school psychologists have resources regarding the ways in which TD and related disorders impact students' academic abilities. This is essential not only for evaluations/assessments, but also because other school professionals typically turn to school psychologists for information regarding this complex disorder. When evaluations/assessments are involved, parents should ask to meet with the school psychologist prior to IEP or 504 meetings. Clinicians should encourage parents to ask questions as appropriate, especially when education terminologies are unclear.

School counselors typically provide academic guidance (e.g., what classes to take) and supportive therapy to help students with mood (e.g., anxiety, depression) and social issues (e.g., peer conflicts). As such, school counselors are foster a safe and supportive environment for student to discuss personal challenges and academic difficulties. When utilized by students, school counselors can provide insightful information on the student's personal strengths and struggles. However, it is important to note that school counselors generally do not treat clinically significant psychopathology.

School nurses are the "medical specialist" for school settings. School nurses will dispense a child's prescribed medication, but otherwise typically do not have daily interactions with students. However, when interacting with school nurses, providing them with information that depicts TD as a medical condition can be helpful. An example would be the TAA's "Frequently Asked Questions—FAQs."

Behavior specialists are becoming more common in schools. They are professionals who are typically well-versed regarding emotional disabilities and autism spectrum disorder. However, many do not receive any formal education in TD. When involved, it is important that behavior specialists receive information regarding TD and are directed to relevant websites such as Tourette.org and Understood.org websites.

Consultant/resource teachers can provide essential supports for students who have specific learning disabilities such as executive function deficits. These professionals frequently assist students in managing their academic workload by implementing time management strategies and developing life-long organization and study skills.

Aides and paraprofessionals have the most one to one contact with the student. It is important that aids and paraprofessionals have an understanding of the strategies that have worked best for the student, and should know when to allow privacy and when to offer support. The student needs to see this person as a safety net and not as someone whose job it is to keep them in line. Information regarding TD is critical for these important support personnel.

(*Continued*)

TABLE 8.1 (Continued)

Occupational therapists provide essential evaluations regarding sensory integration issues and developing sensory plans that student and school personnel follow. Additionally, occupational therapists provide assistance and technological supports for related challenges. For example, handwriting, organization and reading difficulties may be supported by an occupational therapist.
Speech therapists generally provide support for language and social communication deficits. Speech therapists may also assist with executive function difficulties, understanding and formatting questions, eye contact, language-based challenges, memory, and attention.

school professionals may be skeptical that the child's symptoms are actually interfering with homework activities. Instead, they may attribute the child's difficulties at home to negative environmental factors or "poor parenting." This may lead teachers and school personnel to take parents' requests for accommodations and support less seriously.

When communicating with either parents or school personnel, it can be beneficial to remind either party about the internal and external factors that can influence tic expression. This can help promote an understanding that the child's behavior in one setting may not exactly map onto a different setting. This way, when parents are requesting accommodations for their child (e.g., reduced home, an extra set of books, copies of notes to help studying) or school personnel are raising concerns about a student's behavior in a particular class, they may be more willing and open to hearing these concerns in a nonjudgmental manner.

Punishment Versus Proactive Supports

The root meaning of the word discipline is "to teach." It can be helpful to remind parents (and school personnel) that the goal of disciplinary action should be "instruction and education." In this capacity, positive and proactive approaches are typically more effective in the long term than reactive approaches such as punishment. Although these approaches may take time and additional effort, positive and proactive approaches help the child learn alternative ways of managing challenging situations effectively. For example, a reactive approach for a child with TD who has copropraxia that involves "giving the middle finger" may be detention and/or dismissal from the classroom. In comparison, a positive and proactive approach would involve a few more steps. First, parents (or clinicians at the bequest of parents) might proactively write a letter informing the teacher about the child's symptoms, so that teachers would be aware prior to any incident. This letter might also inform the teacher that the child is learning strategies to control the tic, so that the teacher has some understanding that this behavior would not be a "regular occurrence." Second, children (and parents) would learn behavioral strategies to manage this tic (see Chapter 3: Habit Reversal Training for Tics). For instance, when feeling the urge to do the tic, the student might rub his finger behind his ear that may satisfy the urge and also not offend anyone. Similarly, co-morbid conditions may also cause problems (e.g., "rage attacks," anxiety; see Chapter 11: Brief Transdiagnostic Parent Training: A Strengths-Based, Parent-Centered Treatment for Youth With Tourette Syndrome and Chapter 12: Assessing and Treating Emotion Dysregulation and Anger Management). When acting reactively, school personnel may frequently attempt to calm the child during an episode and/or may even attempt to restrain them. These reactive attempts are typically ineffective, and may even serve to exacerbate the symptoms (i.e., increase rage duration, prolong the anxiety attack). Accordingly, it may be best if parents (and clinicians) are proactive in educating school personnel and developing a plan to effectively help the child. These plans may include steps for the child (and possibly teacher) to deescalate situations, and allow the child to practice skills learned in therapy. Alternatively, it may be identifying a "safe space" for the child to go to when he/she is feeling agitated or anxious, and return when feeling ready. This way, the child can receive positive praise from parents, teachers, and clinicians for using these skills, which promotes learning. While plans should be collaboratively developed and individualized to the child's specific challenges, proactive and positive approaches are strongly recommended instead of reactive punishment.

Supporting a Child's Strengths and Interests

When inquiring about children's academic challenges and related symptoms, it is easy for conversations to only focus on problem behaviors and learning difficulties. However, it is important to identify the child's academic strengths and interests too. Indeed, while many youth may struggle academically, they may also have a substantial interest/talent in specific areas (e.g., music, art, drama, dance, science, sports). This can help parents and school personnel (and clinicians) develop educational interventions that build on a child's interests/strengths, keep a balanced perspective when discussing youth, and help promote children's self-esteem as they are hearing parents and educators praising their strengths and experiencing academic success (see Chapter 6: Improving Self-Esteem for Youth With Tourette Syndrome and Tic Disorders, for further discussion of strategies to build self-esteem).

Consider the anecdotal case of my own child (Matt), who had significant and challenging symptoms as a child. Initially, a few clinicians believed that he would likely require residential placement as an adult due to the severity of his symptoms as a young child. However, our interventions focused Matt's participation in activities that would promote his self-esteem and help him graduate from high school. We cultivated his strong interest (and extraordinary talent!) with percussion instruments. By the age of 8, Matt was accepted as a student by the lead percussionist for the Rochester Philharmonic. We allowed Matt to attend his weekly Saturday lessons (regardless of his practice and/or behaviors that week) because it was important to support his strength/interest. Matt's passion for music led him to establish Drumechoes, Inc. at the age of 21. Drumechoes provides antibullying school assemblies, drum circles, and inspirational presentations. As Matt says at the conclusion of a short documentary (entitled "75 Watts") that was commissioned by the Tourette Syndrome Foundation of Canada, "After I finish drumming, I may still be ticcing, but the drumming really helps me. People look past the Tourette and do not judge me, criticize me, or make fun of me when they see I have an exceptional talent versus a hard struggle and difficult situation." In short, recognizing and cultivating a child's interests and strengths can serve as an important tool to help cope with other academic and social challenges that come along with TD and related conditions.

Consideration of Common Co-morbid Challenges

While tics can be disruptive in an educational setting, children with TD often have several related challenges that may be more disruptive than the tics themselves. Table 8.2 presents a list of common co-morbid challenges and how these challenges may impact a child's learning. When parents (and children) are describing educational difficulties, a careful evaluation of these common co-occurring challenges may reveal other factors beyond tics that are contributing to the impairment of a child's educational performance. These factors should be taken into consideration when supporting parent's request for an education evaluation with a clinician letter (see later in this chapter for further discussion of a clinician letter).

PRAGMATIC STRATEGIES AND CONSIDERATIONS FOR CHILDREN AND FAMILIES

In addition to the general guidance offered earlier, there are several pragmatic strategies and steps that clinicians may consider employing when working with parents and educators. The following strategies are key aspects that have been found to be helpful over the years, but are by no means an exhaustive list.

TABLE 8.2 Common Co-occurring Challenges That Can Impact a Child's Academic Performance

Attention deficit/hyperactivity disorder (ADHD). ADHD is a very common difficulty for students with TD. It often results in problems with concentration, organization, and impulse control.

Executive function deficits. Executive function is the term used to describe the mental processes that assist in learning from past experience and using this knowledge for present action. While there is not a specific "diagnosis" of executive functioning deficits, these challenges are often seen among children with TD.

Areas that might be impacted are planning, organizing, strategizing, paying attention to and recalling details, and time management. For students who are intellectually advanced, executive function deficits can be particularly distressing as these students are unable to produce the quality and quantity of work of which they are capable.

Having clinicians (school personnel) who have familiarity with executive function deficits can help students develop and implement strategies to overcome these deficits (see Chapter 10: ProblemSolving Strategies to Overcome Common Challenges Associated With Tourette Syndrome, for strategies to overcome executive dysfunction challenges).

Learning disabilities. Learning disabilities are characterized by difficulties related to reading, writing, mathematics, and/or processing information that is not related to general intelligence. Many students with TD are impacted by learning disabilities. However, it is not unusual for learning disabilities to remain undetected in lower grades due to the intellectual abilities that initially compensate for these difficulties. However, as intellectual demands increase in higher grades, disabilities become more apparent and academic performance begins to suffer.

Oppositional defiant disorder (ODD). Children with TD may also have ODD and/or exhibit other forms of disruptive behavior (see Chapter 11: Brief Transdiagnostic Parent Training: A Strengths-Based, Parent-Centered Treatment for Youth With Tourette Syndrome and Chapter 12: Assessing and Treating Emotion Dysregulation and Anger, for strategies on managing disruptive behaviors). While some behaviors may be related to aggressive and/or impulsive urges, it is also important to consider that oppositional and defiant behavior may serve as an (intentional or unintentional) attempt to communicate a skill deficit in a specific area or task.

Obsessive compulsive disorder (OCD). OCD is another common co-morbid condition characterized by the presence ofor compulsive repetitive /or compulsive repetitive behaviors. Additionally, many children with TD may describe needing to complete an activity until it feels "just right." Obsessive thoughts can distract students when engaged in classroom learning, and compulsive behaviors such as checking can impede the completion of school assignments. Given that children may become distressed when unable to complete compulsive behaviors (i.e., ability to attain perfection) it is important to consider the context in which disruptive behaviors primarily occur.

Anxiety disorders. Many (if not all) students experience anxiety from academic demands and/or social interactions. Anxiety disorders are among the most common conditions that affect children. Indeed, students who are bullied, embarrassed by teachers, and have tics that are easily noticed may likely experience increased anxiety

(*Continued*)

TABLE 8.2 (Continued)

that could contribute to school avoidance/refusal. Identifying and acknowledging specific individuals and situations that make the child anxious is instrumental for developing proactive and positive intervention plans.
Dysgraphia. It is a common (yet under-recognized) and interfering challenge confronting youth with TD. Dysgraphia is a specific learning disability that affects a child's writing abilities. It can manifest with spelling, poor handwriting, and even trouble transitioning thoughts to paper. As such, students with dysgraphica have difficulty in writing legibly, taking notes, and organizing thoughts onto paper. For those with dysgraphia, many benefit from using a word processor, but this accommodation may not address all symptoms (i.e., putting thoughts onto paper).
Social communication and social functioning deficits. Although traditionally associated with autism spectrum disorders (ASDs), youth with TD may also suffer from social communication and social functioning deficits. These students may experience the following troubles: difficulty using appropriate social skills "in the moment," trouble maintaining social relationships with peers, and/or problems acting in an age-appropriate manner. Children with TD often have some degree of awareness or insight into their deficits, which can be exacerbated by other co-morbid conditions like anxiety. Chapter 7, Talking About Tics With Peers and Coping in Social Interactions, presents strategies to address social difficulties related to tics. When social communication and social functioning deficits include, clinicians should consider whether the diagnostic criteria for Social Communication Disorder or an ASD are met in order to provide appropriate and effective supports.
Sensory processing issues. Sensory processing issues are related to sense of touch, sound, taste, and smells that can affect students with TD. A student struggling with sensory issues may likely be impacted academically (i.e., smells may be distracting in the classroom, specific sounds may seem unbearable). While some students may be hypersensitive to sensory input, others may require more than average sensory input, or even both at different times. When sensory issues are identified, an evaluation by an occupational therapist who has experience with sensory issues can be helpful. The occupational therapist can help characterize the specific nature and extent of the deficit, and develop a sensory program specific to the student. Effective management of sensory issues may positively impact student's attention and/or behavior in the classroom.

A One-Page Introduction Letter From Parents to Teachers

The importance of proactive advocacy cannot be overstated. It helps to frame the student in a positive fashion, provides upfront information to teachers to help educate the student, and introduces the concept of positive/proactive supports for the student early on. One way parents can engage in proactive advocacy is by providing a one-page introduction to teachers at the start of the new academic year (or whenever a new school staff member joins the child's educational team). These letters can provide pertinent information such as the child's strengths, talents, and interests. This is typically followed by a brief list of current symptoms, challenges the student faces, and brief examples of strategies/interventions that have been previously successful. Given the importance of education, the one-page letter concludes with contact information for the parents and links to the TAA website for further education on TD. This letter can help frame the child as a student "with" a problem instead of "being" the problem. Here is a sample one-page letter:

Hello Mr. /Mrs. [Insert Teacher Name]

My son Erik is excited about being in your class this coming year. He excels in math, has an interest in robotics, and hopes to pursue a career as an engineer. While Erik enjoys hands-on learning activities, he sometimes struggles to recognize that other student in a group may not have the same knowledge or abilities. Thus, he (on occasion) may get frustrated during group learning assignments. In these cases, prior teachers have found it helpful to collaboratively discuss with Erik strategies he could use when he begins to feel frustrated (e.g., stepping out to get a drink of water).

As you may know, Erik has Tourette's Disorder. Although his specific tics have changed over time, Erik currently grunts, shakes his head, taps his fingers and sometimes makes rude comments (which may appear to be purposeful, but are not intentional). In the past, we have found that when Erik explains his struggles to control his tics at the start of the school year, there are reduced incidents of bullying and teasing.

In addition to tics, Erik also struggles with attention, has difficulty writing neatly, and also has some sensitivities to certain sounds and noises. While Erik really enjoys learning and going to school, previous teachers have commented that these symptoms can impact Erik's participation in classroom activities.

*I would be happy to meet with you to answer questions regarding Erik's symptoms and discuss strategies and supports to help promote Erik's learning. Additionally, the Tourette Association of American (*www.tourette.org, *or 888-4-touret) has several online educational resources and information about educating children with Tourette Disorders.*

Educational Legal Rights and Considerations

In addition to a one-page introduction letter, it is helpful if parents (and clinicians) are familiar with several pieces of key legislation that pertain to a student's legal rights to an education. This information is essential for parents when preparing to meet with school personnel to discuss educational supports such as accommodations, a "504 Plan," and individualized education program (IEP).

The Individuals with Disabilities Education Act (IDEA). It is a federal special education law that mandates how federally funded public agencies (e.g., public schools) provide special education, early intervention, and related services to youth with disabilities (or suspected disabilities) by way of an IEP. Section 1400(d) of IDEA states:

> *"The main purposes are:...to ensure that all children with disabilities have available to them a free appropriate public education that emphasizes special education and related services designed to meet their unique needs and prepare them for further education, employment and independent living" and "to ensure that the rights of children with disabilities and parents of such children are protected..."*

Section 504 of the Rehabilitation Act of 1973. It ensures that children with disabilities have equal access to an education similar to students who do not have disabilities and prohibits discrimination against those who are enrolled in federally funded programs (Rehabilitation Act of 1973, 1973). This act states that:

> *No otherwise qualified individual with a disability in the United States ... shall solely by reason of her or his disability, be excluded from the participation in, be denied the benefits of, or be subjected to discrimination under any program or activity receiving Federal financial assistance.*

Section 504 of the Act provides the basis for "504 Plans" providing services, accommodations, and modifications allowing students with disabilities to receive equal access to a free and appropriate education from schools that receive federal funding.

Family Educational Rights and Privacy Act (FERPA). It is a federal law that protects the privacy of student education records and applies to all schools that receive public funds (FERPA 20 U.S.C. § 1232g; 34 CFR Part 99). While there are many aspects of this act which parents should familiarize themselves (e.g., rights to student's education records), clinicians should be aware that schools will need parental (or legal guardian) consent to share educational records with the clinician that are protected under IDEA (e.g., educational record), as well as any personal health information (PHI) for which the school might be responsible (e.g., medications the student receives). Without parental consent, schools may only disclose "directory information" about a student (e.g., name, address, telephone number). Therefore, it is essential for clinicians to obtain parental consent to contact the schools when coordinating care.

Understanding the Differences Between a "504 Plan," and an IEP

When navigating the education system, several terminologies may arise such as requests for accommodations, a "504" plan, and an IEP—all of which relate to providing educational supports for the student. While these phrases may seem similar on a surface level for many clinicians (as they are all focused on helping the student perform well in an educational setting), there are subtle (and not so subtle) distinctions.

A "504 plan" refers to accommodations sought under Section 504 of the Rehabilitation Act of 1973 which is a civil rights law. A 504 plan *may* include special education services, but typically these plans provide accommodations and modifications. The term "accommodation" refers to a change in how a student learns the material, whereas the term "modification" refers to a change in what a student is taught and/or expected to learn. For example, an "accommodation" might change where a student sits in a classroom to help him/her learn better, or change the modality of learning from visual (e.g., reading text) to auditory (e.g., listening to an audiotape). In comparison, a "modification" would assign a student shorter and/or easier reading assignments, and not necessarily expect them to achieve the same benchmarks as peers (e.g., doing five math problems instead of the entire worksheet).

In a 504 plan, accommodations and modifications are provided to ensure that the student with a disability has the same access to an education as a student without a disability. For example, if a student's handwriting interferes with a student's ability to take notes, equal access would involve notes being provided to the student to allow them the same access to study materials as a student without disabilities. Common accommodations on a 504 plan include extended time to complete work/tests, access to assistive technology (e.g., computer), separate testing location, preferred classroom seating (i.e., near door, close to board, near teacher), and classroom notes provided. Meanwhile, a common (if not the most common) modification is reduced school work and homework. While these are some examples of common accommodations and modifications, there is no "standard 504 plan" because each plan is individualized to the student to make education accessible.

In comparison, an Individualized Education Program (IEP) falls under IDEA and requires public schools to provide accommodations and special education services to qualified students. While students with TD qualify for these services under the "Other Health Impairment" (OHI) classification, it is important to note that a diagnosis of TD does not automatically make a child eligible for either a 504 plan or IEP. There is a formal process to request a 504 plan and IEP conducted by the school system, and it must be determined that the student's academic, developmental, social/emotional, physical, and/or functional needs are impacted by the identified disability. After starting the process, students will typically undergo an assessment (usually conducted by the schools) in all areas related to the suspected disability (e.g., general intelligence, social/emotional functioning, communication skills, academic performance) in order to determine whether educational performance (not necessarily academic performance) is impacted. As school personnel may not be as familiar with the ways in which TD and its common co-occurring conditions can impact a student's educational performance, a clinician letter can be particularly helpful (see later for further discussion of a clinician letter). An IEP may include access to special education services (e.g., occupational therapy for sensory integration deficits, speech therapy for communication deficits, a classroom aide to help with learning activities, sessions with a school counselor), accommodations (e.g., access to assistive technology like computers, resource room support, extended time for assignments and tests, smaller classroom setting), and modifications (e.g., reduced homework).

While there are similarities between a 504 plan and an IEP in that both come from federal laws and must be adhered to by school personnel, there are at least two noteworthy distinctions. First, accommodations under a 504 plan can be easily modified, augmented, or removed to meet the needs of a student as they change over time. In comparison, the modification of an IEP is a more formal (and sometimes lengthy) process. Second, there may be (and is likely) some federal and/or state funding available to support services provided under an IEP. However, schools must cover all expenses associated with a 504 plan. As such, schools with limited funding may struggle to provide accommodations on a 504 plan, even if they believe them to be beneficial.

Providing Referrals for Additional Educational Support

Navigating the education system can be a challenging process for anyone. Indeed, clinicians are not expected to be an expert in this area, but it does help to be at least knowledgeable of the key items mentioned earlier. As such, it can be helpful if clinicians are aware of additional resources for parents to help navigate them through the processes of seeking education accommodations. For example, local agencies like Parent Training and Information Centers (PTICs) may be a helpful resource. PTICs are funded by the Federal government to provide information regarding special education services and IEPs within a specific state. They are intended to support parents of children with behaviors that interfere with a child's education, irrespective of a specific disability. Further information about PTICs can be found at http://www.parentcenterhub.org/. In addition to PTICs, local chapters of the TAA may be able to provide relevant information to parents based on their knowledge (and experience) with obtaining educational services. In some cases, these organizations may even be able to have an advocate attend the school meetings with parents when 504 Plans and IEPs are discussed. Furthermore, these organizations often have local support groups where parents (and students) can learn from and draw strength from other's experiences navigating the local education system. Beyond attending support groups, parents have also found that reading and hearing about other parents' experiences raising a child with TD to be helpful. Indeed, the book that my son (Matt) and I wrote (*A Family's Question for Rhythm: Living With*

Tourette ADD, OCD and Challenging Behaviors) serves as one such example. Meanwhile for youth, some TAA chapters have a Youth Ambassador Program. TAA Youth Ambassadors have received specialized training on how to engage in self-advocacy and speak with peers about their experiences having TD. Self-advocacy can be important for youth with TD, as it is a skill not only relevant for school, but one that can be used for his/her entire life.

In addition to directing parents to these supports, clinicians may also consider helping parents prepare for educational meetings in some capacity. This may include helping parents consider in what manner symptoms are impacting the child's educational performance, and providing parents with clear information (and handouts) to present to school personnel. These materials can help educators recognize symptoms and related issues, and help parents reflect on specific requests for their meetings. For example, the Educator' provides Guide for Developing Plans as well as Preparing Yourself and Your Child For a 504/IEP Meeting (both found on the TAA website) provides many strategies and may be helpful for parents in preparing for 504 Plan and/or IEP meetings.

A Clinician Letter to the Schools

A clinician letter can be instrumental in helping school personnel understand the child's disability, and provides assistance in youth receiving educational supports (e.g., accommodations, modifications, special education services) in the form of a 504 plan or IEP. While the school system will typically conduct their own assessment to determine whether the student's educational performance is impacted by a purported disability, a clearly written letter can help school personnel understand, appreciate, and integrate how the student's symptoms are impacting their educational performance and interfering with learning processes.

After obtaining the parents'/legal guardians' consent to send this information to the school, the first paragraph should state the child's diagnosis of TD, briefly describe the phenomenology of the condition, and note that these symptoms may cause impairment in academic and social functioning. It can also be helpful to mention that different internal (e.g., stress, anxiety) and external (e.g., classroom, home, sports) factors can influence the expression of tic symptoms. The second paragraph should briefly describe the current tics that the child is experiencing and help school personnel understand how these tics are likely interfering with the child's education. The third paragraph can outline co-morbid conditions that may also be impeding the child's education, if present and necessary. Otherwise, this paragraph can be used to orient the reader to the classification of TD under IDEA as an OHI. Finally, the letter should conclude with some recommendations based on child's current challenges in an educational setting and recommendations for a formal psychological evaluation to be completed by the school. In addition to these recommendations, providing the reader with website link to the TAA for further information and educational resources can be helpful. A sample letter is provided later for a child with TD who has eye movement tics, facial grimaces, sniffing, and throat clearing, but does not experience any co-morbid conditions. It is important to individualized each letter to the child and their current symptom presentation so that educators can understand how best to help the student.

> Dear [**school psychologist and/or school counselor**],
>
> This letter is to document that [**Child's Name**] meets diagnostic criteria for [**Tourette's Disorder**]. This disorder is a long-lasting neurological condition that consists of multiple motor and phonic tics. Tics are rapid, sudden, repetitive, non-rhythmic motor movements or vocalizations. The number, frequency, location and complexity of tics often change during the course of [**Tourette Disorder**]. Tics often wax and wane in presentation and severity, and may be influenced by internal states and external environmental factors. As a result, many children experience impairment in both school and social functioning because of their tics.
>
> [**Child's Name**]'s current tics include, but are not limited to, eye blinking, facial grimaces, sniffing, and throat clearing. These motor tics can cause difficulty with reading, and classroom behavior. For example, [**Child's Name**]'s eye blinking tics can make reading assignments more difficult as children will often have to re-orient themselves after each eye tic. As tics often occur in bouts, this can prove frustrating and time consuming, as well as delay completion of class assignments. Classroom behavior can also be impaired by tics, as unintended facial expressions and sounds like sniffing or throat clearing may disrupt classroom functioning, and draw negative attention from teachers and peers. These are only two examples of tics [**Child's Name**] experiences, which complicate performance in the classroom and on assignments.
>
> Within the reauthorization of Individuals with Disabilities Education Improvement Act (IDEIA, 2004), Tourette syndrome (now called Tourette's Disorder) has been specifically listed as a disability under Other Health Impaired (OHI). From an educator perspective, educational interventions across all tiers are required to manage the symptoms of Tourette's Disorder and secondary problems, including teacher and peer education efforts, direct interventions, and classroom accommodations.
>
> When strategizing classroom accommodations and modifications, it can be beneficial to include the student in developing strategies for managing truly disruptive tics. From a teacher perspective, it is also important to remember that tics wax and wane in intensity and frequency and can change over time, so any identified accommodations and interventions should be flexible. [**Although Child's Name has learned behavioral strategies to suppress/manage some of his/her tics**], it is also important

to note that not all children can suppress tics or suppress them all the time.

Based on [**Child's Name**]'s current tic symptoms, the following strategies and accommodations are recommended:

1. The recommendation for a formal psychological evaluation to assess for the presence of specific learning disability, skills deficits and other difficulties associated with Tourette's Disorder.

[**Insert relevant strategies and recommendations for accommodations based on the child's symptoms and described educational impairment**]

For further information on educational interventions, the Tourette Association of America offers information about educational accommodations that have been useful to youth with Tourette's Disorder.

SUMMARY

While clinicians are not expected (or anticipated) to be experts in the educational system, an appreciation and awareness of the educational system can help children and parents navigate this difficult process. Educational supports for youth with TD can be difficult to ascertain, especially if school personnel have limited experience and/or familiarity with the complexities of TD. However, on a positive note, many of the educational interventions and supports for TD can be provided in the general education setting and require a minimal financial investment by the school. Moreover, the majority of students with TD experience only a mild-to-moderate impact on their educational performance. A "common-sense" approach of ignoring tic symptoms (when possible) and strategies to reduce stress and anxiety may often decrease the level and occurrences of tics in school. However, for students who are more significantly impacted, positive and proactive supports will be essential. Clinicians play a critical role in educating school personnel on the specific challenges of having TD and helping to guide and support parents and children through the process of obtaining needed educational accommodations, modifications, and services.

REFERENCES

Conelea, C. A., & Woods, D. W. (2008). Examining the impact of distraction on tic suppression in children and adolescents with Tourette syndrome. *Behaviour Research and Therapy, 46* (11), 1193–1200.

Family Education Rights: Privacy Act (FERPA) of 1974. (2012) 20 6.S.C. § 34 CFR Part 99.

Individuals with Disabilities Education Improvement Act of 2004.20 U.S.C. § 1400 et seq.

Rehabilitation Act of 1973.Pub. L. 93–112. 26 Sept. 1973. H.R. 8070.

Storch, E. A., Lack, C. W., Simons, L. E., Goodman, W. K., Murphy, T. K., & Geffken, G. R. (2007). A measure of functional impairment in youth with Tourette's syndrome. *Journal of Pediatric Psychology, 32*(8), 950–959.

FURTHER READING

Giordano, K., & Giordano, M. (2013). A Family's Quest for Rhythm: Living with Tourette, ADD, OCD & Challenging Behaviors.

Chapter 9

Managing Avoidance and Accommodation of Tics and Related Behaviors

Joshua M. Nadeau[1,2] and Meme Hieneman[3]

[1]*Department of Pediatrics, University of South Florida, Tampa, FL, United States,* [2]*Rogers Behavioral Health—Tampa Bay, Tampa, FL, United States,* [3]*Positive Behavior Support Applications, Tampa, FL, United States*

INTRODUCTION

Tourette disorder and persistent motor and/or vocal tic disorders (collectively referred to as TD) are neuropsychiatric conditions characterized by repetitive movements and/or sounds that interfere with daily functioning (American Psychiatric Association (APA), 2013). Prevalence estimates for TD range from 3 to 8 per 1000 children, with provisional tic disorders estimated to affect as many as 20% of school-age youth (Scahill, Specht, & Page, 2014). The tics of TD may manifest themselves as "simple" motor or vocal movements (i.e., eye blinking or coughing), or more "complex" behaviors, such as mimicking another person's movements or repeating words and sounds (APA, 2013). While the natural course of TD is well-established, the relationship between tic severity and impairment has been inconsistent. For example, tic severity has at times been associated with academic (Packer, 2005), family (Wilkinson et al., 2001) and social impairment (Storch et al., 2007; Zinner, Conelea, Glew, Woods, & Budman, 2012). However, other studies suggest tic severity and social impairment are either unrelated (Carter et al., 2000), or in some fashion mediated by other variables (McGuire, Hanks, Lewin, Storch, & Murphy, 2013). In addition to—indeed, often as a result of—the tics themselves, youth may develop additional problem behaviors not directly associated with tics (Sukhodolsky et al., 2003; Tabori Kraft et al., 2012). Specifically, reports of social skills deficits (McGuire et al., 2013), psychological and emotional difficulties (Bloch & Leckman, 2009; Kraft et al., 2012), and reduction in quality of life (QOL) (Eddy et al., 2011; Storch et al., 2007) are more commonly reported for this group than for same-age peers without TD.

The Clinician's Guide to Treatment and Management of Youth with Tourette Syndrome and Tic Disorders.
DOI: https://doi.org/10.1016/B978-0-12-811980-8.00009-1

Traditionally, TD has been managed with pharmacological (Murphy et al., 2009) and behavioral interventions (McGuire, Piacentini, et al., 2014), both in which the primary treatment focus is on the reduction of tic frequency and severity. However, such approaches rely upon the assumption that tics are maintained largely by physiological or sensory outcomes. As such, these interventions approaches often neglect indirect functional impairment and QOL concerns. Although it is enticing to focus solely upon reductions in tic severity and assume associated problems are not within a patient's (and/or families') volitional control, evidence suggests that this may not be the case. These assumptions can lead to inappropriate interventions that fail to provide desired and/or durable behavior changes (Ingram, Lewis-Palmer, & Sugai, 2005; Miller & Lee, 2013). For example, an adolescent with TD may be experiencing significant tics in the classroom, which the clinician might assume is causing the adolescent's exclusion from peer social activities and a poor QOL. While a clinician might want to persist with behavior therapy and/or initiate a trial of pharmacotherapy to reduce the adolescent's tic severity, this may (or may not) lead to peer inclusion and a better QOL. In comparison to treatment approaches that entirely focus on tic severity, recent psychosocial interventions have focused on cultivating patient resilience, developing coping skills to minimize tic-related impairment, and improve QOL with early success (McGuire et al., 2015; Storch et al., 2012).

When considering psychosocial interventions to minimize tic-related impairment and improve QOL in patients with TD, it is important to consider that internal and external factors influence the expression of tics and tic-related behaviors. Tics and tic-related behaviors (e.g., inattention, hyperactivity, disruptive behaviors, anxious behaviors, compulsive behaviors) are commonly affected by social contingencies, and may (intentionally or unintentionally) serve the function of escape/avoidance from situations or settings perceived as aversive. In the case of the adolescent with TD mentioned above, it may be that the significant tics expressed in the classroom allowed the adolescent to avoid certain classroom assignments, limited interactions with troublesome peers, and/or provided the adolescent with preferential attention from the teacher or other school support staff. Indeed, tic-related avoidance and accommodation have been directly and indirectly reported in several recent studies (Capriotti et al., 2015; Himle et al., 2014; Storch et al., 2017). In this capacity, avoidance refers to the behavior enabling escape from a situation and/or aversive outcome (e.g., escaping from undesirable academic assignment, escape from peer teasing). Meanwhile, accommodation refers to changes in the environment that the behavior elicits (e.g., receiving attention from a teacher, modification of family routine if tics expressed at home). When examining the relationship between tic severity and accommodation/avoidance, findings also appear to be mixed. One study found greater tic severity was associated with higher levels of child-reported home and public tic-related consequences and accommodations (Capriotti et al., 2015). Meanwhile, another study found that tic severity was not related to accommodation, but instead was predicted by cooccurring anxiety and externalizing behaviors (Storch et al., 2017). In either case, techniques to identify and address avoidance and accommodation of tics and tic-related behaviors can be essential to help patients with TD develop more adaptive behaviors, improve day-to-day functioning, and promote QOL.

This chapter describes a process for identifying tic-related behaviors that commonly serve the function of avoidance and/or accommodation. It describes the design of suitable interventions for these behaviors that promote both positive behavior change and improve QOL. Although the approaches described here are well-established approach for other neurodevelopmental disorders [e.g., autism spectrum disorders (ASD), attention-deficit/hyperactivity disorder (ADHD)], these specific approaches have not been directly evaluated for challenging behaviors associated with TD. Therefore, many of the references are drawn from other sources, making a case that these methods are sensible to address avoidance and accommodation of tics and related behaviors.

AN INTRODUCTION TO POSITIVE BEHAVIOR SUPPORT

For the purposes of this chapter, QOL can be understood as the degree to which an individual is satisfied and fully actualized in terms of the most important aspects of life—health and safety, self-advocacy, social relationship, productive activity, and community participation (Hieneman et al., 2015; Schalock, 2004). As previously noted, TD and related behaviors have the potential to significantly affect (or not affect) any and/or all of these aspects of QOL. For example, the adolescent with TD who is expressing significant tics in the classroom may be allowed to avoid academic assignments and escape peer-teasing. However, by avoiding classroom activities and peer interactions, the adolescent is also missing out on in-class group activities and the opportunity to engage in positive peer interactions—which may lead to friendships and improve the adolescent's QOL.

Applied behavior analysis (ABA) is an evidence-based approach that has been widely used for many neurodevelopmental disorders (Hagopian & Boelter, 2005). Despite its empirical support, some criticisms have been raised with more traditional ABA interventions in regards to treatment effects and QOL. These criticisms include: (1) the perception that many procedurally based behavioral approaches show a lack of concern for the dignity of those displaying problem behaviors; (2) concerns that ABA lacks a mechanism for recognizing the importance of child and family QOL; and (3) beliefs that there is an overall failure to address autonomy and self-determination when designing behavioral interventions (Carr et al., 2002; Horner et al., 1990). Beyond dissatisfaction with narrowly focused applications of ABA, these criticisms illuminate a barrier to intervention in general. Specifically, if interventions are not seen as increasing QOL—whether directly by enhancing participation and success within daily functioning, or indirectly via improving the patient's adaptive behavioral responses within situations that are of the greatest value to the patient and family—the patient (and family) are less likely to implement interventions with fidelity, and the patient will not be motivated to fully engage in the treatment.

The development of positive behavior support (PBS) was due in part to this theoretical deficiency. In PBS, behaviors and impairment are recast as factors that affect QOL (i.e., "*How would life be different if...?*," "*What would you be able to do if...?*"). When problem behaviors are seen as not being goal-oriented (i.e., intentional), youth (and families) are often more motivated to investigate the functional etiology of these behaviors, as well as to work collaboratively on formulating replacement behaviors that are more congruent with patient and family goals. Treatment methods based on this conceptualization involve a three-pronged approach. First, the effectiveness of behavioral intervention rests primarily upon correctly identifying the function of problem behaviors. Therefore, an accurate and reliable method for identifying a behavior's function is a critical first step in PBS. After the function is accurately identified, replacement behaviors can be introduced that serve the same function in a more socially acceptable manner. Second, in order for a behavioral intervention to be effective, the problem behavior must be understood and considered to be relevant in the environment in which a patient exists. For this reason, a second key step is identifying activities and routines that are disrupted by the problem behavior. Third, from a developmental and pragmatic perspective, behavioral interventions must be generalizable to a variety of locations, people, and activities. Therefore, educating the patient and family on strategies to adapt the behavioral intervention to different settings/environments/situations is just a vital as developing the behavioral intervention itself. In order to illustrate and explain the concepts and techniques being introduced here, as well as to better provide guidance on implementing interventions that address avoidant and accommodating behaviors, this chapter makes use of two hypothetical cases: "Joey" and "Stephanie." Joey is a young (elementary school) male student, while Stephanie is an older (high school) female student.

ASSESSING TARGETS FOR INTERVENTION

Prioritization of Problematic Behaviors

Prioritizing problem behaviors is critical to the success of behavioral interventions for at least two reasons. First, it is rare that youth with TD exhibit a single problematic behavior in a single instance. Instead, it is far more common that youth exhibit many tics symptoms and other problematic behaviors across a variety of settings that result in avoidance and/or accommodation (Capriotti et al., 2015; Storch et al., 2017). Second, the perceived level of disruption and interference associated with youth's behaviors may often be quite severe (Barfell et al., 2017; Storch et al., 2007). When taken together, the sheer number of challenging behaviors and the level of interference may often leave some patients and families feeling overwhelmed. Without a systematic approach to prioritizing these challenging behaviors, early intervention efforts may often appear inaccurate, inconsistent, or irrelevant to youth and families.

As a first step, a structured approach is required to list and "rank" disruptive/bothersome tics and associated behaviors. Listing these tics and related behaviors in the context(s) in which they do/do not occur facilitates the process of characterizing baseline impairment and understanding circumstances in which challenging behaviors are present (i.e., shouting tic occurs only at church and just before school, it does not occur during school hours; see Chapter 1: Introduction to Treatment and Management of Youth with Tourette Disorders and Tic Disorders for recommendations on assessments for TD severity and functional impairment). This is critical to later perceptions of "success" (treatment response) by patients and families. Additionally, when making these ratings/ranking, it is also important to inquire about subjective distress and perceived impact on QOL by the patient and family. This can offer insight into the manner and magnitude by which patient's and families' lives are being disrupted by the problem behaviors.

A method commonly used to capture these impressions in behavioral interventions is the subjective units of distress scale (SUDS; see Tanner, 2012 for overview). SUDS ratings are favored in part for their simplicity and ease of implementation across behaviors, patient populations, and intervention settings. Fig. 9.1 provides an example of a SUDS "thermometer," wherein the perceived level of distress is conceptualized as existing upon a scale (typically 0–10 or 0–100) with increasing numbers representing increased distress. When discrepancies exist in reports between patients and families (i.e., parents view a behavior as a problem, but youth do not), it may be helpful to use "difficulty controlling the behavior" or "level of disruption the behavior causes" instead of distress.

Upon introducing the SUDS thermometer (or comparable scale), it is important to familiarize patients (and parents) with its ratings by establishing anchor points. Specifically, youth (and parents) should practice accurately locating the patient's baseline level of distress, and also identify example situations in which the patient would experience minimum and maximum levels of distress. For example, a patient should be able to locate preferred activities (i.e., playing with a favorite toy, watching TV, reading an enjoyable book, drawing or coloring) on the lower end of the SUDS thermometer, as these activities/behaviors would not cause any distress or discomfort.

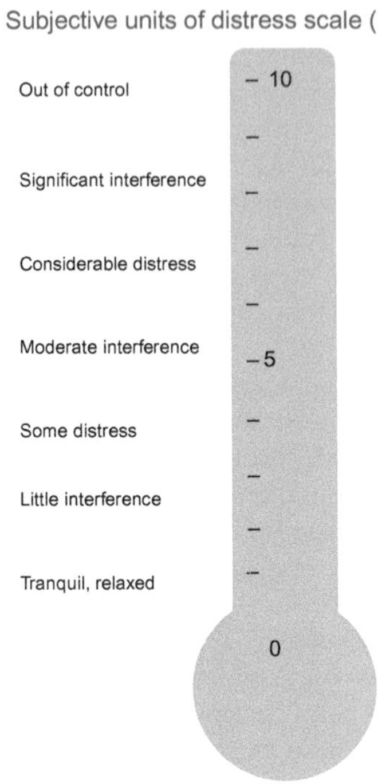

FIGURE 9.1 Feelings thermometer.

However, undesirable activities (i.e., taking a test, being "in trouble" with an adult, being hungry or tired while unable to eat or sleep) should be located on the higher end of the SUDS thermometer. As youth (and parents) show a basic understanding of making accurate SUDS ratings, a behavioral hierarchy can be constructed in preparation for modifying problematic behaviors.

In general, the severity of a problem behavior is considered to be a primary concern when designing behavioral interventions. For example, all other circumstances being equal, self-injurious tics or other related self-injurious behaviors are a more pressing concern than annoying noises or distracting behaviors. Additionally, another important consideration is the family context within which problem behaviors occur. Specifically, an understanding of everyday routines—or activity settings—that occur within the family is critical to designing behavioral interventions that are considered acceptable (and therefore more likely to be effective) to the patient and family (Lucyshyn et al., 2009).

Confirming Functions and Identifying Contexts of Avoidance and Accommodation

Functions of behavior are categorized around four primary patterns (Newcomer & Lewis, 2004): (1) social attention, (2) tangible items, (3) escape/avoidance, and (4) sensory outcomes. Prior to intervening with potentially avoidance or escape maintained behavior, it is essential to confirm the function of the behavior. For example, avoidant behaviors typically occur in certain "demand" circumstances and result in breaks, delays, or complete cessation of activities and/or removal from settings. Meanwhile, problem behaviors may alternatively serve to modify the patient's context and result in accommodation for the patient. In either case, this pattern of delay/cessation/modification needs to be largely consistent in order to conclude that behaviors are maintained by avoidance/accommodation and do not serve another function in that setting.

It is important to note that avoidant behaviors are triggered by particular contexts (Stichter, Hudson, & Sasso, 2005). Specific antecedents (i.e., events immediately preceding the behavior) and setting events (broader or more distal circumstances and conditions) need to be identified to intervene effectively. With regard to avoidant and accommodating behaviors, it is important to determine what specific circumstances patients find unpleasant, difficult, and/or challenging.

Functional Behavioral Assessment

Identifying functions of behavior and the contexts in which these behaviors operate is commonly achieved through a process called functional behavioral assessment (FBA; Hanley, Iwata, & McCord, 2003; O'Neill, Hawken, & Burdock, 2015; Wacker, Berg, Harding, & Cooper-Brown, 2011). FBAs are driven by the following questions (O'Neill et al., 1997):

1. Under what circumstances—immediate antecedents and setting events—are particular behaviors most and least likely to occur (e.g., who, where, when, during which activities)?
2. What consequences does the patient receive (accommodation) or avoid (avoidance) following the behavior that is maintaining the behavior?

Traditionally, the process of conducting a FBA (which answers the above questions) involves three general steps: (1) defining problem behaviors as clearly as possible to ensure that the focus of the FBA is explicit, (2) gathering information through indirect and direct assessment methods, and (3) analyzing and summarizing patterns of behavior to inform intervention (Anderson & Long, 2002; Kern, Hilt, & Gresham, 2004; O'Neill, Albin, Storey, Horner, & Sprague, 2014).

The goal of the FBA process is to confirm avoidance/accommodation functions and identify the immediate antecedents that precipitate the behavior pattern. In addition to these factors, it is also helpful to identify other contributing factors that are referred to as "setting events." Setting events serve to explain variations in behavior under the same immediate circumstances. For example, a patient may predominantly engage in a problematic behavior only when the patient has had a poor night's sleep (i.e., sleep deprivation), or when there has been a disruption in the patient's daily routine (i.e., expecting to go home after school, but finding out they have to run errands with a parent). In this case, sleep quality/sleep deprivation and disruptions in after-school routine would be considered setting events. Returning to the two sample cases of Joey and Stephanie, below are two examples of hypothesis statements illustrating different contexts for avoidance/accommodation behaviors:

- *When Joey is asked to perform lengthy, repetitive tasks such as math problems at school or home, he will fidget and complain. This typically results in his teacher or parent either assisting him or reducing the demands of the assignment.*
- *When Stephanie's friends begin conversing about topics that are unfamiliar to her, she will cough loudly and repeatedly or ask unrelated questions until they shift the conversation. If her friends do not change the subject, she will make an excuse to leave (e.g., needing a drink).*

To test these hypotheses, Joey's parents (under the direction of his clinician) could use simple ratings to record both the difficulty and repetition of tasks, and the intensity of his fidgeting and complaining in the identified circumstances in which the behavior occurs (see later in the chapter for description of ratings). Similarly, Stephanie's clinician (or available confederate) could initiate a conversation focused on unfamiliar topics, while observing and recording the rate of coughing and unrelated questions. Additionally, it can be helpful to obtain Joey's and Stephanie's subjective evaluation of the discomfort/difficulty of the situation using a SUDS rating before, during, and after the task at hand.

The burgeoning hierarchy of problem behaviors can be expanded and refined through a series of questions about triggering stimuli and situations. This encourages hypothesis testing in an imaginal fashion, and thereby limits potential consequences that may occur in actual environmental manipulations. Examples of amplifying question scripts used to build hierarchies are provided below for both sample cases:

JOEY

- *When your teacher gives you a math problem to work on, where are you on this feelings thermometer?*
- *When you have several math problems, does it change where you are (on the SUDS)?*
- *If your teacher or parent is there to help, where are you (on the SUDS)?*
- *Where are you when you do a reading worksheet?*
- *Where would you be if you asked for help?*
- *How hard (on the SUDS) would it be to ask for a break?*

STEPHANIE

- *Let's say your friends are talking about something you've never heard of before; where would you be on the SUDS?*
- *What about when they're discussing things you really don't care much about?*
- *And if the topic is something you all like, or talk about all the time?*
- *Where would you be if you had to ask a question about a topic you don't like (or aren't familiar with)?*

Notably, Joey's and Stephanie's responses to these questions (i.e., higher, lower, or no change) will aid the clinician in designing a more accurate and comprehensive intervention. Specifically, understanding the impact of situational variables facilitates a more gradual, "stepped" approach when helping Joey and Stephanie confront challenging situations that may elicit strong emotional reactions (e.g., anxiety, aggression, frustration) and overcome reliance on problematic avoidant/accommodating behaviors.

It is important to recognize that many behaviors serve more than one function, and that youth may have complex behavior patterns that serve different purposes across different circumstances (Day, Horner, & O'Neill, 1994; Hagopian, Rooker, & DeJoey, 2013). For example, Joey may fidget and complain both when presented with difficult demands and when an enjoyable upcoming event has been delayed—meaning that, under different circumstances, the same behavior serves both avoidance and accommodation functions (i.e., Joey wants the desired event to occur soon). As a result, it is important to define contexts in which functions operate. Specifically, clinicians should identify not only the immediate antecedents and consequences, but also those distal from the immediate circumstance that is affecting behavior.

Indeed, a patient's capabilities, health condition, living circumstances, daily routines or demands, and social relationships can all mediate behavior and motivation. Therefore, avoidance and accommodation functions must be teased out, and some interventions may need to be situation specific.

MODIFYING BEHAVIORS THAT LEAD TO AVOIDANCE AND ACCOMMODATION

After completing the following steps noted above: (1) ensuring the avoidant /accommodation function of problematic behaviors, (2) clearly identifying how these behaviors manifest across settings, and (3) building a comprehensive behavioral hierarchy; designing effective interventions to manage these problematic behaviors is relatively straight-forward using a competing behavior model akin to the one described in Chapter 3, Habit Reversal Training, for tics (O'Neill et al., 1997). In this model, patients are taught

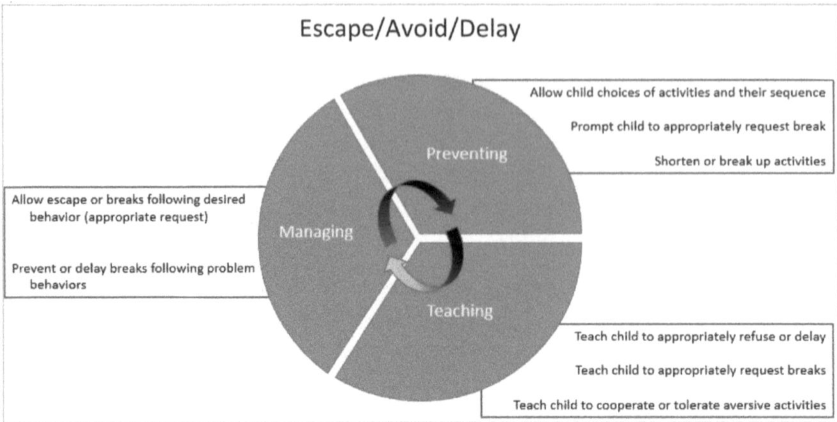

FIGURE 9.2 The escape, avoidance, and delay cycle of tics and problem behaviors.

alternative preferred behaviors to implement instead of the problematic behavior. Reinforcement is provided for the alternative preferred behaviors that "compete" with the reinforcement initially received for the challenging behavior. Concurrently, reinforcement for problematic behaviors is withheld and/or minimized as much as possible (i.e., withhold or minimize avoidance, escape, or accommodation). Importantly, the environment/setting/context in which the challenging behavior occurs is rearranged to support these strategies and facilitate access to reinforcement for the alternative preferred behaviors. This enables the adaptive behaviors to be reinforced to a greater degree than the problematic behaviors. Some potential strategies for avoidant, escape, and/or accommodation behaviors are provided in Fig. 9.2. In each instance, the focus is on reinforcement: (1) reducing or removing reinforcement in response to problem behaviors; (2) establishing or increasing reinforcement in response to more socially acceptable/desirable/preferred competing behaviors; and (3) artificially structuring the immediate environment such that the patients are provided multiple opportunities to display competing preferred behaviors (and thus receive a relatively high rate of reinforcement).

Selecting Replacement Behaviors

When selecting replacement behaviors, it is important to identify replacement behaviors that are acceptable to the patient and appropriate for the settings in which the problematic behaviors occur. Consider the case of a child who makes loud and distracting noises in weekend religious services, which promptly leads to his removal from the service by his parents. An initial preferred replacement behavior for the loud and distracting noises may be to have the child politely ask to excuse himself from the service without making any distracting noise. Alternatively (or at a later point in intervention planning), the child might receive additional reinforcement (i.e., rewards, tokens) for either using therapeutic skills to manage distress in the setting (i.e., relaxation skills) or receive reinforcement for sitting quietly. As the frequency of behaviors is mediated by the quality and schedule of reinforcement maintaining them, adaptive behavior should ideally result in access to reinforcement more quickly and consistently than the problem behavior(s) and also remain salient (Horner & Day, 1991; Reed & Kaplan, 2011). Using the nascent hierarchies developed for the two sample cases, multiple options for replacement behaviors are provided for each case below.

JOEY

- *Ask for explanation*
- *Ask for assistance*
- *Request a 5-minute break*

STEPHANIE

- Ask relevant questions about unfamiliar topics
- Appropriately transition to other conversational topics
- Appropriately excuse self from unfamiliar/uncomfortable conversations

When developing replacement behaviors and considering reinforcement strategies, it is important to note that immediate or complete avoidance (or accommodation) is not always possible or appropriate. For example, a patient who is experiencing significant anxiety/distress about going over to a peer's house for a playdate due to possible questions about her tics, cannot (and should not) avoid all peer social interactions. Therefore, it is essential to teach patients (and parents) skills that help them function within, cope with, and/or anticipate challenging situations. These skills may include coaching in social activities, self-regulation, and/or calming techniques (Carter, Lane, Crnobori, Bruhn, & Oakes, 2011; Gresham, Cook, Crews, & Kern, 2004). While some patients may already know the necessary skills to manage their distress, they may not use them consistently and/or in the right circumstances. In these cases, the previously learned skills would simply be prompted and reinforced in the settings in which challenging behaviors occurs. For instance, a child who is struggling to complete an undesirable activity (e.g., math problems) may be receive reinforcement (i.e., screen time, tokens) for using relaxation strategies when starting to become agitated. Meanwhile, in other cases, a more step-wise and systematic approach may be necessary to teach youth necessary skills. For instance, clinicians may work with a patient (and family) to outline the steps associated with using and implementing these new skills/behaviors and teach them in a more systematic approach via modeling or shaping (i.e., receiving reinforcement for every four math problems that are completed in which desired behavior was observed and problematic behavior was not present).

There are often a variety of skills needed to replace problem behaviors and promote adaptive functioning in a given situation. As such, prioritization and planning to address problematic behaviors is essential. The initial assessment and behavioral hierarchy offers guidance in this area, with skills that allow patients to respond to the most triggering circumstances taking priority. When selecting skills to address problem behaviors, it is important to consider the role of "pivotal skills." These are behaviors that are critical to future social success for three reasons: (1) pivotal skills produce high-rate natural reinforcement; (2) they lead to the development of additional skills; and (3) they generalize easily to other aspects of daily life (Koegel & Frea, 1993). One example of a pivotal skill is teaching a child to ask other people questions about themselves (as opposed to questions about things the child find interesting). Notice that asking people questions about themselves: is almost always naturally reinforced (e.g., people are more likely to engage in longer social interactions when talking about themselves); quickly provides practice for additional higher-level social interaction skills (i.e., showing interest, asking follow-up questions, answering questions about yourself, etc.); and generalizes to almost any social situation (e.g., school, church, stores, parks). Teaching of pivotal skills can thus lead to more rapid behavioral changes, while also positively impacting a youth's QOL. Although pivotal skills may vary from patient to patient, examples of salient pivotal skills are listed for each sample case below, along with a brief description of the sample approaches for teaching each pivotal skill.

JOEY

- Pivotal Skill #1: *Increase ability to remain on-task (boredom tolerance)*
  - Method: *Gradually increase task demands while fading external reinforcement.*
  - Rationale: *Naturally reinforced by decreased teacher prompts and increased behavioral marks; provides scaffolding foundation for higher-level academic and/or study skills; boredom tolerance generalizes to non-academic tasks (waiting in line, completing chores at home, etc.)*
- Pivotal Skill #2: *Increase independent work/study schedule planning*
  - Method: *Introduction of scheduling matrix (planner) and incorporate visual reminder cues.*
  - Rationale: *Naturally reinforced by decreased external prompts, increased productivity, and concretely scheduled "free time"; provides scaffolding foundation for academic and non-academic executive functioning skills, including task analysis/decomposition; independent planning generalizes to school, work, and recreational settings.*

STEPHANIE

- Pivotal Skill #1: *Increase distress tolerance*

- Method: *Using stepped or gradual approach to increasing exposure to undesired or uncomfortable social encounters, while fading reinforcement*
- Rationale: *Naturally reinforced by decreased feelings of anxiety and/or discomfort, and increased opportunities for positive social interactions; provides scaffolding foundation for higher-level social and emotional regulation skills; distress tolerance generalizes across all settings, due to the natural prevalence of anxiogenic situations.*

- Pivotal Skill #2: *Increase fluency with respect to asking relevant questions*
  - Method: *Preparing or planning potential conversational topics; role-playing potential conversations with therapist or peer coach*
  - Rationale: *Naturally reinforced by increased opportunities for social interaction; provides scaffolding foundation for higher-level social interaction skills (showing interest, asking follow-up questions, answering questions about yourself); generalizes to almost any social situation (e.g., school, church, stores, parks).*

Environmental Modifications

In addition to skill- and capacity-building approaches, environment modifications are beneficial (Horner, Vaughn, Day, & Ard, 1996; Kern, Choutka, & Sokol, 2002; Luiselli, 2006). Modifications to the environment may include providing environmental cues to prompt particular skills, or removing/minimizing triggers early on in treatment (if possible). Antecedent-based strategies may include using written or pictorial activity schedules to clarify expectations (Koyama & Wang, 2011; Lequia, Machalicek, & Rispoli, 2012), providing choices between activities (Shogren, Faggella-Luby, Bae, & Wehmeyer, 2004), organizing environments to make expectations more evident (Bullard, 2010), and engaging in behavioral rehearsal prior to particularly challenging circumstances (Donohue & Stowman, 2005). For example, a wallet card could remind patients of steps necessary to exit an uncomfortable situation, or the steps necessary to appropriately start a conversation with a peer.

It is important to clarify that environmental modifications are inherently different than providing accommodation. Accommodation refers to changes in the environment that the problem behavior elicits and are reinforced (i.e., receiving attention from a teacher for tics or disruptive behavior). In comparison, environmental modifications are changes in the environment that promote the use of adaptive, appropriate, and preferred behavior. While some environmental modification may initially involve minimizing (or eliminating) exposure to triggers identified during the assessment, these triggers may be gradually reintegrated into the environment as the patient learns appropriate adaptive skills and behaviors. This affords the patient the opportunity to practice the appropriate skills/behaviors and develop further skill mastery.

JOEY

- *Establish homework area that has all necessary supplies and is free from distractions*
- *Create a work schedule to facilitate task decomposition and goal-setting*
- *Review assignments when preparing schedule to build Joey's understanding of expectations*
- *Arrange to have a peer buddy (at school), sibling, or parent available to help as needed when working*
- *Have timer and task-related resources on hand*
- Create contract to engage in preferred activities once work is completed

STEPHANIE

- *Increase exposure to a broader range of topics through social media—establish topic plan*
- *Increase opportunities to engage in desired topics, and provide context for coping with non-preferred topics*
- *Generate and role-play questioning and redirection techniques to be used in conversations*
- *Set goals for remaining in difficult conversations before exiting*

Managing Access to Reinforcement

As mentioned previously, behavior patterns are maintained by the consequences that follow them. Therefore, if a behavior leads to reinforcement, it will continue—if not, it will diminish. As such, it is critical to manage access to reinforcement following problematic and desired behaviors (Athens & Vollmer, 2010), so that replacement behaviors are acknowledged, respected, and appropriately reinforced—and problematic behaviors do not receive reinforcement. If a youth says "*I need a few minutes to think*" (desirable behavior) instead of storming out and slamming the door (problematic behavior), the youth should be given some space.

However, some desired/preferred behaviors do not offer natural reinforcement (or offer only minimal natural reinforcement). Therefore, it is often necessary to identify other reinforcers that will be effective and compete with the reinforcement the patient receives for the problem behavior. In clinical practice, possible and preferred reinforcers are often selected through sampling procedures (Ruggiero & Acierno, 2005). Reinforcement sampling may be informal (i.e., asking a patient what he or she enjoys) or it may be more systematic. There are a variety of questionnaires and inventories for identifying possible reinforcers that allow respondents (youth or parents) to rate different items, activities, or experiences in terms of preference. Additionally, potential reinforcers may be experimentally presented to youth and effectiveness gauged by the patients' willingness to perform desired activities. As different types and intensities of reinforcers may produce different levels of motivation and response (Beavers, Iwata, & Gregory, 2014), it is often helpful to generate a reinforcement hierarchy where higher quality reinforcers are delivered for more demanding tasks.

In addition to providing reinforcement for replacement and preferred behaviors, it is also necessary to withhold or minimize access to reinforcers following problem behaviors (Janney, Umbreit, Ferro, Liaupsin, & Lane, 2013; Lalli, Casey, Goh, & Merlino, 1994). If the patient's problem behaviors are maintained by avoidance or delay, the patient should be required to remain in the situation until he or she requests termination of the activity appropriately. Similarly, accommodations should be withheld and/or minimized for problematic behaviors. However, when cessation of reinforcement is not possible, the goal should be to minimize reinforcement for problem behaviors, while maximizing reinforcement for positive behaviors. For example, a patient engaging in disruptive behavior might be guided away from onlookers in a public setting to minimize their reactions, while a parent (or clinician) provides differential reinforcement for more adaptive preferred behavior. Examples of reinforcement strategies are provided below for both sample cases.

JOEY

- *When Joey requests assistance (appropriately), teachers should provide assistance without "taking over" for him or lessening the demands*
- *If Joey requests a break after the required work is done, teachers should instruct Joey to set a timer (or otherwise signal his return), then allow him to exit the task.*
- *When Joey is supposed to be engaged in assigned work, teachers (and parents!) should withhold preferred activities (e.g., texting, video games, playing with pets or peers) until his work is completed*
- *If Joey works "extra hard" (e.g., completing more problems than required or working quickly), teachers/parents should reward him by removing one problem from his workload*

STEPHANIE

- *Instruct peers (and other adults!) to respond to appropriate questions and attempts at redirection while continuing to engage Stephanie in conversation*
- *Peers/adults should ignore or redirect coughing or inappropriate questions (e.g., "If you are uncomfortable about what we are discussing, you can...")*
- *Peers/adults should directly (and openly) identify excuses to leave that are not appropriate, while continuing to engage Stephanie socially.*
- *Peers/adults should reward Stephanie for tolerating uncomfortable conversations by providing time to discuss topics (or participate in activities) she enjoys.*

Generalization of Strategies

Generalization and maintenance of behavior change is critical. It is important to identify the situations in which replacement behaviors and therapeutic skills will be needed, as well as the natural cues and contingencies within those situations. For example, a teenager with TD may need to use specific skills (and cues) at school, but different skills (and cues) to manage problematic behaviors at home or in social settings with peers. Notably, each of these situations may require minor adaptations to the settings, contingencies, and behavioral routines (e.g., "taking a break" may be appropriate in some situations, but inappropriate in others). Thus, while helping youth develop appropriate skills and practice implementing adaptive preferred behaviors, clinicians should also help youth (and parents) learn to monitor situational variables and make adaptations as needed.

In treatment, clinicians (and parents or caregivers) may prompt particular behaviors, minimize triggers and arrange circumstances to promote positive behaviors, and use supplemental reinforcers. However over time, it is necessary to transfer control of behavior away from any contrived circumstances and contingencies toward those that are naturally occurring to promote independence and resilience (Harvey, Lewis-Palmer, Horner, & Sugai, 2003; Sprague, 2014). Indeed, the best way to maximize intervention durability and sustainability is through teaching self-regulatory processes (Agran, 2015). This allows youth to monitor their own behavior, implement strategies with minimal guidance and support, and access reinforcers independently.

When designing interventions and planning for generalization and maintenance of behaviors, it is helpful to rely on the most naturalistic and least intrusive procedures. This allow the fading of these procedures much more feasible in real-world settings. A key aspect to utilizing naturalistic and unobtrusive procedures comes an understanding of the patient's regular activities and routines. Through this understanding and appreciation, the clinician can embed strategies within these activities and routines to support positive behavior change.

The Importance of Ecological Interventions

While a clinician's initial tendency might be to focus solely on outcomes specific to the patient and immediate environment, from an ecological perspective, it is important to also consider those endemic to peers, important adults in the patient's life, and the community. The reasoning here—from a behavioral standpoint—is that each ecological "level" represents an independent, yet interconnected, source of potential setting events, triggers, and reinforcement. Accordingly, a failure to account for the involvement of others in the behavioral ecology affects the salience, impact, and durability of the implemented intervention. Additionally, a fundamental aspect of PBS is to focus upon increasing QOL, for the patient as well as the family.

Therefore, in order to design effective and sustainable interventions that improve QOL for the patient and family, interventions should consider the actions of those who interact with the patient on a regular basis and/or meaningful fashion (e.g., parents, teachers, peers, extended family). Indeed, these individuals may be very well positioned to understand circumstances that are contributing to the patient's problematic behaviors, and may also be reacting in a way to the patient's behavior that escalates the problem behavior in an unintentional manner (Patterson & Yoerger, 2002). In addition to intervention at the immediate environmental level, techniques that intervene at higher ecological levels can be categorized as interventions intended to prevent, teach, or manage problem behaviors (see Fig. 9.2). For example, parents may want to adopt particular expectations or routines for their entire family, rather than simply structuring them for identified patient. This way, the same behavioral expectations (and reinforcement) are placed on all family members.

Once the plan is designed, parents and other relevant individuals (e.g., siblings, caregivers) may need training in particular approaches to more effectively support the patient. For example, a clinician might instruct a parent to speak more quietly when making requests to the patient (and other family members), or engage in collaborative problem-solving strategies with the patient instead of criticizing them for perceived mistakes. There are several excellent parenting program such as Parent–Child Interaction Therapy (McNeill & Hembree-Kigin, 2011), Positive Parenting Program (Sanders & Prinz, 2005), and Strengthening Families (Kumpfer, Magalhães, Whiteside, & Xie, 2015) that include specific guidelines for parent interaction with youth to minimize behavioral challenges (see Chapter 11: Brief Trans-Diagnostic Parent Training: A Strengths-Based, Parent-Centered Treatment for Youth With Tourette Syndrome for discussion of parent training). Several example strategies that have been shown to promote positive behavior and strengthen parent–child relationship include: active listening, addressing problems nonconfrontationally, and checking tone and body language. Examples of generalization strategies are provided below for both sample cases.

JOEY

- *If necessary, complete educational assessments to identify strengths and skill gaps to facilitate individualization of task assignments*
- *Increase teacher-parent collaboration to maximize consistency of academic expectations and strategies*
- *Identify future goals (employment and living circumstances) to build motivation*
- *Ask the teacher to provide parents with instruction in how to evaluate the difficulty of academic assignments, organize materials, and provide guidance and respond to questions (while managing frustration) to improve his success with homework*

STEPHANIE

- *Encourage enrollment in clubs/activities that provide interesting social opportunities*
- *Enroll a peer confederate to assist in negotiating the complexities of 'teen girl conversation', while deepening the friendship through mutually reinforcing activities*

Progress Monitoring—Data-Based Decision Making

Effective intervention results in changes in perception, behavior, and/or broader circumstances for patients and families. As such, it is important to monitor these changes to evaluate whether the current intervention is producing the desired change. The term "progress monitoring" generally refers to the patient's progress in responding to an intervention. Stated another way, progress monitoring is an ongoing assessment of whether the problem behavior has changed, and if so, to what extent. The general idea behind progress monitoring is relatively simple: if the current intervention is not changing a problem behavior in a timely fashion and/or improving QOL for the patient and family, then the intervention requires revision.

Progress monitoring is important, as the continuation of an ineffective intervention represents an opportunity cost. Resources and time allocated to an ineffective intervention cannot be regained, and may harm the therapeutic relationship between the patient, family, and clinician. Indeed, youth (and families) do not get a "do-over" for the weeks (or months) that were spent engaged in an intervention that was not effective. However, when using progress monitoring to track and analyze youth's responsiveness to the selected intervention, patients (and families) can have objective markers of the behavioral change and use this information to adapt the intervention accordingly. As clinicians are incorporating patient and family feedback to modify the intervention, this activity has been found to strengthen the therapeutic relationship (especially if the desired behavioral changes are achieved).

The targeted behavior(s) should be tracked throughout the intervention process, such that trends in the behavior (increase or decrease in frequency) can be observed. A reliable and objective way to monitor progress in an individualized manner for youth with TD involves a target problems assessment (McGuire, Sukhodolsky, et al., 2014). In this assessment, the target behavior is described at baseline and the frequency, intensity/duration, and impact are characterized. This behavior is then re-assessed at each visit for frequency, intensity/duration, and impact. This allows the clinician to have an objective assessment of whether the behavior is decreasing (or increasing) from visit to visit, and whether modification to the intervention is warranted. When used in this fashion, a data-driven decision-making model is an effective intervention planning tool, as well as an excellent method for testing the hypotheses gleaned from the FBA.

While measuring changes in targeted behaviors is important, it is also critical to evaluate the extent to which behavioral changes are associated with improvements in functional impairment and QOL. These outcomes can be done informally through self-report of the patient and/or family members, but should also include standardized assessments (see Chapter 1: Introduction to Treatment and Management of Youth With Tourette Disorders and Tic Disorders for recommended assessments for impairment and QOL). Examples of progress monitoring strategies are provided below for both sample cases.

JOEY

- *Percentage of assigned items completed and total time to complete work per day*
- *Engagement ratings for assigned work (e.g., 2 = focused on task, 1 = periods of distraction or repeated fidgeting, 0 = complaining and resisting work)*
- *Grades per reporting periods, as well as standardized test scores*

STEPHANIE

- *Tracking self-rated level of conversational difficulty (SUDS rating) vs. time engaged*
- *Self-monitoring—use of questioning and transition strategies (reliability by therapist and/or confederate peer)*

It should be noted that progress can also be monitored by the patient and family outside of visits with the clinician. Patient and family driven progress monitoring has the potential to increase awareness and adherence to the intervention, provided that it occurs in a non-punitive manner. For example, Joey might maintain an assignment checklist with self-ratings for engagement, and both Joey and his parents might review his grades in the educational portal together on a weekly basis. Similarly, Stephanie may use a daily self-check rating and feedback from friends to monitor her interactions and then debrief with her clinician during psychotherapy sessions.

SUMMARY AND FUTURE DIRECTIONS

This chapter presented an approach for: (1) identifying problematic behaviors that cause avoidance/accommodation, (2) confirming avoidance functions and identifying the context in which these problem behaviors occur, and (3) developing interventions that foster positive behavior changes and lasting improvements in QOL. Although a PBS approach has substantial evidence in the literature among various other neurodevelopmental populations—including youth with ASD, ADHD, and intellectual disabilities—there has been little empirical attention to date on its potential in addressing challenging behaviors that interfere with daily functioning for youth with TD. Given the focus of PBS upon restoring functionality while remediating QOL issues, it is hoped that future research (and practice) among youth with TD will increasingly incorporate treatment methods informed by PBS practices.

REFERENCES

Agran, M. (2015). Strategies for self-management. In F. Brown, J. L. Anderson, & R. L. De Pry (Eds.), *Individual positive behavior supports: A standards-based guide to practices in school and community settings* (pp. 333–346). Baltimore, MD: Paul H. Brookes.

American Psychiatric Association. (2013). *Diagnostic and statistical manual of mental disorders (DSM-5)*. American Psychiatric Publishing.

Anderson, C. M., & Long, E. S. (2002). Use of a structured descriptive assessment methodology to identify variables affecting problem behavior. *Journal of Applied Behavior Analysis, 35* (2), 137–154.

Athens, E. S., & Vollmer, T. R. (2010). An investigation of differential reinforcement of alternative behaviors without extinction. *Journal of Applied Behavior Analysis, 43*, 569–589.

Barfell, K. S. F., Snyder, R. R., Isaacs-Cloes, K. M., Garris, J. F., Roeckner, A. R., Horn, P. S., ... Gilbert, D. L. (2017). Parent and patient perceptions of functional impairment due to tourette syndrome: Development of a shortened version of the child tourette syndrome impairment scale. *Journal of Child Neurology, 32*, 725–730.

Beavers, G. A., Iwata, B. A., & Gregory, M. K. (2014). Parameters of reinforcement and response class hierarchies. *Journal of Applied Behavior Analysis, 47*, 70–82.

Bloch, M. H., & Leckman, J. F. (2009). Clinical course of Tourette syndrome. *Journal of Psychosomatic Research, 67*, 497–501.

Bullard, J. (2010). *Creating Environments for Learning*. Upper Saddle River, NJ: Pearson.

Capriotti, M. R., Piacentini, J. C., Himle, M. B., Ricketts, E. J., Espil, F. M., Lee, H. J., ... Woods, D. W. (2015). Assessing environmental consequences of ticcing in youth with chronic tic disorders: The tic accommodation and reactions scale. *Children's Health Care, 44*(3), 205–220.

Carr, E. G., Dunlap, G., Horner, R. H., Koegel, R. H., Turnbull, A. P., Sailor, W., ... Fox, L. (2002). Positive behavior support: Evolution of an applied science. *Journal of Positive Behavior Interventions, 4*, 4–16.

Carter, A. S., O'Donnell, D. A., Schultz, R. T., Scahill, L., Leckman, J. F., & Pauls, D. L. (2000). Social and emotional adjustment in children affected with Gilles de la Tourette's syndrome: Associations with ADHD and family functioning. *Journal of Child Psychology and Psychiatry, 41*, 215–223.

Carter, E. W., Lane, K. L., Crnobori, M., Bruhn, A. L., & Oakes, W. P. (2011). Self-determination interventions for students with and at risk for emotional and behavioral disorders: Mapping the knowledge base. *Behavioral Disorders, 36*, 100–116.

Day, H. M., Horner, R. H., & O'Neill, R. E. (1994). Multiple functions of problem behaviors: Assessment and intervention. *Journal of Applied Behavior Analysis, 27*, 279–289.

Donohue, B., & Stowman, S. (2005). Behavioral rehearsal. In M. Hersen, J. Rosqvist, A. M. Gross, R. S. Drabman, G. Sugai, & R. Horner (Eds.), Encyclopedia of behavior modification and cognitive behavior therapy. Thousand Oaks, CA: Sage Publications, Inc.

Eddy, C. M., Rizzo, R., Gulisano, M., Agodi, A., Barchitta, M., Calì, P., ... Cavanna, A. E. (2011). Quality of life in young people with Tourette syndrome: A controlled study. *Journal of Neurology, 258*, 291–301.

Gresham, F. M., Cook, C. R., Crews, S. D., & Kern, L. (2004). Social skills training for children and youth with emotional and behavioral disorders: Validity considerations and future directions. *Behavior Disorders, 30*, 32–46.

Hagopian, L. P., & Boelter, E. W. (2005). *Applied behavior analysis and neurodevelopmental disorders: Overview and summary of scientific support*. Baltimore: Kennedy Krieger Institute and Johns Hopkins University School of Medicine.

Hagopian, L. P., Rooker, G. W., & DeJoey, I. G. (2013). Initial functional analysis outcomes and modifications in the pursuit of differentiation: A summary of 176 inpatient cases. *Journal of Applied Behavior Analysis, 46*, 88–100.

Hanley, G. P., Iwata, B. A., & McCord, B. E. (2003). Functional analysis of problem behavior: A review. *Journal of Applied Behavior Analysis, 36*, 147–185.

Harvey, M. T., Lewis-Palmer, T., Horner, R. H., & Sugai, G. (2003). Trans-situational interventions: Generalization of behavior support across school and home environments. *Behavioral Disorders, 28*, 299–312.

Hieneman, M., Yeagley, M., Cessna, T., Smith-Kong, T., Downs, H., Fazzio, D., . . . DeFranco, R. (2015). *Positive behavior support quality of life assessment*. Unpublished tool.

Himle, M. B., Capriotti, M. R., Hayes, L. P., Ramanujam, K., Scahill, L., Sukhodolsky, D. G., . . . Walkup, J. T. (2014). Variables associated with tic exacerbation in children with chronic tic disorders. *Behavior Modification, 38*(2), 163–183.

Horner, R. H., & Day, H. M. (1991). The effects of response efficiency on functionally-equivalent competing behaviors. *Journal of Applied Behavior Analysis, 12*, 719–732.

Horner, R. H., Dunlap, G., Koegel, R. L., Carr, E. G., Sailor, W., Anderson, J., . . . O'Neill, R. E. (1990). Toward a technology of "nonaversive" behavioral support. *Journal of the Association for Persons with Severe Handicaps, 15*, 125–132.

Horner, R. H., Vaughn, B. J., Day, H. M., & Ard, W. R. (1996). The relationship between setting events and problem behavior: Expanding our understanding of behavioral support. In L. K. Koegel, R. L. Koegel, & G. Dunlap (Eds.), *Positive behavioral support: Including people with difficult behavior in the community* (pp. 381–402). Baltimore: Paul H. Brookes.

Ingram, K., Lewis-Palmer, T., & Sugai, G. (2005). Function-based intervention planning: Comparing the effectiveness of FBA function-based and non-function-based intervention plans. *Journal of Positive Behavior Interventions, 7*, 224–236.

Janney, D. M., Umbreit, J., Ferro, J. B., Liaupsin, C. J., & Lane, K. L. (2013). The effect of the extinction procedure in function-based intervention. *Journal of Positive Behavior Interventions, 15*(2), 113–123.

Kern, L., Choutka, C. M., & Sokol, N. G. (2002). Assessment-based antecedent interventions used in natural settings to reduce challenging behavior: A review of the literature. *Education and Treatment of Children, 25*, 113–130.

Kern, L., Hilt, A. M., & Gresham, F. (2004). An evaluation of the functional behavioral assessment process used with students with or at risk for emotional and behavioral disorders. *Education and Treatment of Children, 27*, 440–452.

Koegel, R. L., & Frea, W. D. (1993). Treatment of social behavior in autism through the modification of pivotal social skills. *Journal of Applied Behavior Analysis, 26*, 369–377.

Koyama, T., & Wang, H.-T. (2011). Use of activity schedules to promote independent performance of individuals with autism and other intellectual disabilities: A review. *Research in Developmental Disabilities, 32*, 2235–2242.

Kraft, J. T., Dalsgaard, S., Obel, C., Thomsen, P. H., Henriksen, T. B., & Scahill, L. (2012). Prevalence and clinical correlates of tic disorders in a community sample of school-age children. *European Child and Adolescent Psychiatry, 21*, 5–13.

Kumpfer, K. L., Magalhães, C., Whiteside, H., & Xie, J. (2015). Strengthening families for middle/late childhood. In M. Van Ryzin, K. L. Kumpfer, G. Falco, & M. Greenberg (Eds.), *Family-based prevention programs for children and adolescents: Theory, research, and large-scale dissemination* (pp. 68–86). NY: Psychology Press.

Lalli, J. S., Casey, S., Goh, G., & Merlino, J. (1994). Treatment of escape-maintained aberrant behavior with escape extinction and predictable routines. *Journal of Applied Behavior Analysis, 27*, 705–714.

Lequia, J., Machalicek, W., & Rispoli, M. J. (2012). Effects of activity schedules on challenging behavior exhibited in children with autism spectrum disorders: A systematic review. *Research in Autism Spectrum Disorders, 6*, 480–492.

Lucyshyn, J. M., Binnendyk, L., Fossett, B., Cheremshynski, C., Lohrmann, S., Elkinson, L., & Miller, L. (2009). Toward an ecological unit of analysis in behavioral assessment and intervention with families of children with developmental disabilities. In W. Sailor, G. Dunlap, G. Sugai, & R. Horner (Eds.), *Handbook of positive behavior support* (pp. 73–106). Baltimore: Paul H. Brookes.

Luiselli, J. K. (2006). *Antecedent assessment and intervention: Supporting children and adults with developmental disabilities in community settings*. Baltimore, MD: Paul H. Brookes.

McGuire, J. F., Arnold, E., Park, J. M., Nadeau, J. M., Lewin, A. B., Murphy, T. K., & Storch, E. A. (2015). Living with tics: Reduced impairment and improved quality of life for youth with chronic tic disorders. *Psychiatry Research, 225*(3), 571–579.

McGuire, J. F., Hanks, C., Lewin, A. B., Storch, E. A., & Murphy, T. K. (2013). Social deficits in children with chronic tic disorders: Phenomenology, clinical correlates and quality of life. *Comprehensive psychiatry, 54*(7), 1023–1031.

McGuire, J. F., Piacentini, J., Brennan, E. A., Lewin, A. B., Murphy, T. K., Small, B. J., & Storch, E. A. (2014). A meta-analysis of behavior therapy for Tourette syndrome. *Journal of Psychiatric Research, 50*, 106–112.

McGuire, J. F., Sukhodolsky, D. G., Bearss, K., Grantz, H., Pachler, M., Lombroso, P. J., & Scahill, L. (2014). Individualized assessments in treatment research: An examination of parent-nominated target problems in the treatment of disruptive behaviors in youth with Tourette syndrome. *Child Psychiatry & Human Development, 45*(6), 686–694.

McNeill, C. B., & Hembree-Kigin, T. L. (2011). *Parent–child interaction therapy*. Springer.

Miller, F. G., & Lee, D. L. (2013). Do functional behavioral assessments improve intervention effectiveness for students diagnosed with ADHD? A single-subject meta-analysis. *Journal of Behavioral Education, 22*, 253–282.

Murphy, T. K., Mutch, P. J., Reid, J. M., Edge, P. J., Storch, E. A., Bengtson, M., & Yang, M. (2009). Open label aripiprazole in the treatment of youth with tic disorders. *Journal of Child and Adolescent Psychopharmacology, 19*, 441–447.

Newcomer, L. L., & Lewis, T. J. (2004). Functional behavioral assessment: An investigation of assessment reliability and effectiveness of function-based interventions. *Journal of Emotional and Behavioral Disorders, 12*, 168–181.

O'Neill, R. E., Albin, R. W., Storey, K., Horner, R. H., & Sprague, J. R. (2014). *Functional assessment and program development for problem behavior: A practical handbook* (3rd ed.). Cengage Learning.

O'Neill, R. E., Hawken, L. S., & Burdock, K. (2015). Conducting functional behavioral assessments. In F. Brown, J. L. Anderson, & R. L. De Pry (Eds.), *Individual positive behavior supports: A standards-based guide to practices in school and community settings* (pp. 259–278). Baltimore, MD: Paul H. Brookes.

O'Neill, R. E., Horner, R. H., Albin, R. W., Sprague, J. R., Storey, K., & Newton, J. S. (1997). *Functional assessment and program development for problem behavior: A practical handbook*. Pacific Grove, CA: Brooks/Cole.

Packer, L. E. (2005). Tic-related school problems: Impact on functioning, accommodations, and interventions. *Behavior Modification, 29*, 876–899.

Patterson, G. R., & Yoerger, K. (2002). A developmental model for early- and late-onset antisocial behavior. In J. B. Reid, J. Snyder, & G. R. Patterson (Eds.), *Antisocial behavior in children and adolescents: A developmental analysis and model for intervention* (pp. 147–172). Washington, DC: American Psychological Association.

Reed, D. D., & Kaplan, B. A. (2011). The matching law: A tutorial for practitioners. *Behavior Analysis in Practice, 4*, 15–24.

Ruggiero, K., & Acierno, R. (2005). Reinforcer sampling/assessment. In M. Hersen (Ed.), *Encyclopedia of behavior modification and cognitive behavior therapy: Vol. 2. Child clinical applications* (pp. 981–985). Thousand Oaks, CA: Sage Publications.

Sanders, M. R., & Prinz, R. J. (2005). The Triple P system: A multi-level, evidence-based, population approach to the prevention and treatment of behavioral and emotional problems in children. *The Register Report, 31*, 4245.

Scahill, L., Specht, M., & Page, C. (2014). The prevalence of tic disorders and clinical characteristics in children. *Journal of Obsessive Compulsive and Related Disorders, 3*, 394–400.

Schalock, R. L. (2004). The concept of quality of life: What we know and do not know. *Journal of Intellectual Disability Research, 48*(3), 203–216.

Shogren, K. A., Faggella-Luby, M. N., Bae, S. J., & Wehmeyer, M. L. (2004). The effect of choice-making as an intervention for problem behavior: A meta-analysis. *Journal of Positive Behavior Interventions, 6*, 228–237.

Stichter, J. P., Hudson, S., & Sasso, G. P. (2005). The use of structural analysis to identify setting events in applied settings for students with emotional/behavioral disorders. *Behavioral Disorders, 30*, 403–420.

Storch, E. A., Johnco, C., McGuire, J. F., Wu, M. S., McBride, N. M., Lewin, A. B., & Murphy, T. K. (2017). An initial study of family accommodation in children and adolescents with chronic tic disorders. *European Child & Adolescent Psychiatry, 26*(1), 99–109.

Storch, E. A., Morgan, J. E., Caporino, N. E., Brauer, L., Lewin, A. B., Piacentini, J., & Murphy, T. K. (2012). Psychosocial treatment to improve resilience and reduce impairment in youth with tics: An intervention case series of eight youth. *Journal of Cognitive Psychotherapy, 26*(1), 57–70.

Storch, E. A., Merlo, L. J., Lack, C., Milsom, V. A., Geffken, G. R., Goodman, W. K., & Murphy, T. K. (2007). Quality of life in youth with Tourette's syndrome and chronic tic disorder. *Journal of Clinical Child and Adolescent Psychology, 36*, 217–227.

Sukhodolsky, D. G., Scahill, L., Zhang, H., Peterson, B. S., King, R. A., Lombroso, P. J., ... Leckman, J. F. (2003). Disruptive behavior in children with Tourette's syndrome: Association with ADHD comorbidity, tic severity, and functional impairment. *Journal of the American Academy of Child and Adolescent Psychiatry, 42*, 98–105.

Tabori Kraft, J., Dalsgaard, S., Obel, C., Thomsen, P. H., Henriksen, T. B., & Scahill, L. (2012). Prevalence and clinical correlates of tic disorders in a community sample of school-age children. *European Child and Adolescent Psychiatry, 21*, 5–13.

Tanner, B. A. (2012). Validity of global physical and emotional SUDS. *Applied Psychophysiological Biofeedback, 37*, 31–34.

Wacker, D. P., Berg, W. K., Harding, J. W., & Cooper-Brown, L. J. (2011). Functional and structural approaches to behavioral assessment of problem behavior. In W. W. Fisher, C. C. Piazza, & H. S. Roane (Eds.), *Handbook of applied behavior analysis* (pp. 165–181). New York, NY, USA: Guilford Press.

Wilkinson, B. J., Newman, M. B., Shytle, R. D., Silver, A. A., Sanberg, P. R., & Sheehan, D. (2001). Family impact of Tourette's syndrome. *Journal of Child and Family Studies*, *10*, 477–483.

Zinner, S. H., Conelea, C. A., Glew, G. M., Woods, D. W., & Budman, C. L. (2012). Peer victimization in youth with Tourette syndrome and other chronic tic disorders. *Child Psychiatry and Human Development*, *43*, 124–136.

Chapter 10

Problem-Solving Strategies to Overcome Common Challenges Associated With Tourette Syndrome

Shannon M. Bennett, PhD[1], Renae Beaumont, PhD[1], Corinne Catarozoli, PhD[1] and Alexandra M. Kushman, BA[2]

[1]*Weill Cornell Medicine, NY, United States,* [2]*Tufts University School of Medicine, Boston, MA, United States*

Individuals with Tourette syndrome and chronic tic disorders (collectively referred to as TDs) experience social, academic, and interpersonal problems in day to day life as a result of tics and associated symptoms. Training and practice in evidence-based problem-solving strategies are very useful for many children with tic disorders; particularly, those children who struggle to solve problems independently due to difficulties with emotion and behavior regulation, poor impulse control, and/or deficits in executive functioning skills. Children with TDs have a higher likelihood of impairment in executive functions, in part due to the high comorbidity with attention-deficit/hyperactivity disorder (ADHD) and obsessive–compulsive disorder (OCD). The complex interplay between the symptomatology of these psychiatric disorders and the neuropsychological consequences can be difficult to tease apart, but it is often associated with academic and social difficulties, as well as other emotional and behavioral challenges (McGuire et al., 2015). This chapter provides a detailed description of specific evidence-based approaches to problem solving across child development, and reviews special considerations for working with youth with impairment in executive functioning. Approaches to problem-solving skills from three specific evidence-based treatments [the Unified Protocol for the Treatment of Emotional Disorders in Adolescents, UP-A; Ehrenreich-May et al., 2018; the Secret Agent Society (SAS) social skills program; Beaumont, 2010; and Dialectical Behavior Therapy, DBT; Linehan, 1993a; Miller, Rathus, & Linehan, 2007] will be outlined in detail, including case examples for children and adolescents.

The Clinician's Guide to Treatment and Management of Youth with Tourette Syndrome and Tic Disorders.
DOI: https://doi.org/10.1016/B978-0-12-811980-8.00010-8

EXECUTIVE FUNCTIONING

The skills and aptitudes included under the umbrella of executive functions are those that help human beings to attend, organize, plan, and act in accordance with short- and long-term goals. Executive functions help us to sustain attention, organize activities and behavior, scaffold and plan steps to accomplish a goal, persist with attention and motivation to complete the goal, manipulate information effectively, and manage our thoughts and emotions to appropriately regulate behavior. Dawson and Guare (2010) provide a comprehensive overview of executive functions in children and adolescents. They organize executive skills into those that assist specifically with problem solving, such as planning, organization, time management, working memory, and metacognition. Other executive skills, such as response inhibition, emotion control, attention control, flexibility, and task initiation and persistence, provide the capacity to modulate behavior in response to incoming stimuli and information (Dawson & Guare, 2010). Executive functions follow a developmental trajectory and are shaped and refined over time with biological, genetic, social, and environmental influences. Barkley (1997) proposed a model for the sequential development of executive functions in which several skills begin to emerge and influence development between 5 and 12 months of age, including behavioral inhibition, nonverbal working memory, and self-regulation of affect, motivation, and arousal. The Barkley model further suggests that the internalization of speech and acquisition of language early in development sets the stage for the later development of metacognition, self-monitoring, and problem-solving strategies.

EXECUTIVE FUNCTIONING IN TOURETTE SYNDROME

There is an evidence that some youth with Tourette syndrome may have deficits in domains of executive functioning, such as in the areas of attention, memory, planning, decision making, and perceptual, motor, and visuomotor performance (Brookshire, Butler, Linda Ewing-Cobbs, & Fletcher, 1994; Eddy, Rizzo, & Cavanna, 2009; Channon, Crawford, Vakili, & Robertson, 2003). However, it is difficult to study such impairments in Tourette syndrome due to the high rates of comorbid disorders, including ADHD, OCD, anxiety disorders in childhood, and depressive disorders in later adolescence and adulthood. Thus it is often unclear whether impairments in executive functioning exhibited by youth with Tourette syndrome are due to Tourette syndrome or to a comorbid condition. For instance, the waxing and waning nature of tics, the likelihood that youth may at times actively suppress tics, and the fact that many studies do not control for age, IQ, or medication make it further challenging to discern the clear and specific impact of TDs on executive functions. In fact, one's performance on cognitive tests may change over time depending on the context and severity of the tic symptoms (Eddy et al., 2009).

A variety of neurocognitive and behavioral tasks have been used to evaluate executive functioning in youth with Tourette syndrome. In a study comparing neurocognitive correlates of pediatric OCD (without Tourette syndrome) and those of Tourette syndrome (without OCD), tasks assessing frontal-striatal functions, such as executive, attention/memory, and visuomotor aptitude found that patients with TS showed trends towards impairments in response to inhibition, divided attention, and cognitive flexibility relative to the OCD and healthy controls groups (Chang, McCracken, & Piacentini, 2007). A study using the Purdue Pegboard and Grooved Pegboard tasks demonstrated impaired motor performance in patients with Tourette syndrome (Bohnen, Kuwabara, Constantine, Mathis, & Moore, 2007; Eddy et al., 2009). However, some studies employing a complex figure drawing task found evidence of a fine-motor and visual-motor deficit in youth with TS, while others did not (Eddy et al., 2009; Loring et al., 1990). On attentional tasks, such as the continuous performance test that requires subjects to track targets surrounded by distractors, there is some evidence to suggest patients with Tourette Syndrome show deficits in attention, but it is difficult to draw a strong conclusion due to the high comorbidity with ADHD. Evidence is also mixed for working memory, with TS patients showing only small deficits in verbal working memory on performance in time estimation and digit span tests (Channon, Gunning, Frankl, & Robertson, 2006; Crawford, Channon, & Robertson, 2005).

In everyday practice, clinicians can first use observation and clinical interviewing of youth and parents to assess for the possible presence of executive function difficulties. Obtaining input from teachers and/or other credible reporters of a child's performance, with appropriate consent, is also essential to getting a full picture of a child's behavior in all important domains and environments. Gold standard assessment of executive functions would include a referral for neuropsychological testing, incorporating specific tests targeting executive functions, such as the Delis Kaplan Executive Function System (DKEFS). Meanwhile, the Comprehensive Executive Function Inventory (CEFI; Naglieri & Goldstein, 2004) and Behavior Rating Inventory of Executive Function (BRIEF; Gioia, Isquith, Guy, & Kenworthy, 2000) are rating scales that can be used to measure the broad spectrum of behaviors that represent one's executive functioning, including attention, emotion regulation, flexibility, impulse control, organization, initiation, planning, working memory, and self-monitoring.

Problem-solving strategies are one set of intervention strategies that can address some of the deficits in the executive functions described above (response inhibition, emotion regulation, metacognition, sustained attention, flexibility) with specific skills practice. Below, problem-solving strategies are described from a cognitive behavioral therapy (CBT) framework, with examples from specific evidence-based treatments, including case examples and specific recommendations for working with youth with TDs who have deficits in executive functioning.

PROBLEM-SOLVING STRATEGIES FROM A COGNITIVE BEHAVIORAL FRAMEWORK

The presence of tic symptoms, and comorbid issues with attention, behavior, and/or emotion control, cause impairment in social, academic, and interpersonal functioning (Kofler, Larsen, Sarver, & Tolan, 2015). The goal of problem-solving strategies is to help an individual generate and evaluate possible solutions for managing situations that are emotionally challenging, including situations where they may be worried about or do not like the perceived outcome, or a situation in which they feel stuck. For children with impulse control challenges, there is a particular focus on slowing down behavioral responses long enough to think through the potential consequences of the child's choices (e.g., the Stop and Think Workbook; Kendall, 1992). Children with deficits in executive functioning can benefit from rote practice in brainstorming possible solutions to a real-world problem and then thinking through the potential consequences of each possible solution.

A number of evidence-based interventions include approaches to problem solving. Some target avoidance of solutions due to overwhelming emotion states, such as anxiety or depression, while others may focus more on behavioral impulse control problems where there is little to no thought of potential consequences before enacting a behavioral choice. Cognitive behavioral approaches to problem solving, such as in the Unified Protocol for Emotional Disorders in Children and Adolescents (Ehrenreich-May et al., 2018) emphasize training in identifying and tolerating uncomfortable emotions, while weighing the pros and cons of a variety of possible solutions.

The first step in a cognitive behavioral approach to problem solving is to work with the child to select and define a relevant problem in the child's life (step 1). It is often useful to select situations that are relevant and current for the child's life; however, if the child will not volunteer an example of personal importance, generic examples can also be used for practice, such as:

Possible Situations (Triggers):

Your brother knocks down a tower you spent all morning building with blocks.

A bully picks on you at school for ticcing.

It is raining so your family has to change their plan for the afternoon.

There is a new kid in your class you would like to talk to.

You have a hard homework assignment but you are not sure how to do it.

Once a problem has been selected, start to brainstorm with the child a list of *all* the possible solutions or behaviors the child could use to address this problem (see Table 10.1). During the brainstorming phase (step 2), write down any solution the child comes up with and tell the child there are absolutely no right or wrong answers. You can write down possible solutions

TABLE 10.1 Steps for problem-solving training

1. Define the problem	
2. Brainstorm possible solutions A. B. C. D. E.	3. List possible consequences of each possible solution A. B. C. D. E. What would happen if I chose Solution A? How would I feel? How would the other person feel? What might the other person do in response? Repeat for Solution B, C, D, E
4. Select the best solution based on the possible consequences	5. Try it out and evaluate what happened

regardless of whether the solution is actually something the child would do. Even if a possible solution is not feasible, not appropriate, or not helpful for the defined problem, the goal is to generate many possible solutions, and evaluate them later. For example, punching a bully who is picking on you is a possible solution to stop the bully, so it can be included in the brainstorming phase. The child can evaluate later the potential consequence of the behavior (e.g., hurting someone else and/or getting in trouble for hitting). This step requires the patient to practice cognitive flexibility, sustained attention, metacognition, perspective taking, and task persistence. Encourage the child to come up with at least 3–5 possible solutions, and praise him/her for effort and participation with each solution offered.

Next (step 3), review each possible solution and talk with the child about what would happen if the child actually chose each option. Discuss what the consequences would be for each possible solution. Weigh the pros and cons of the possible positive outcomes of each solution, as well as the potential negative outcomes. It can also be helpful to ask the child to think through how each person involved would feel if a given solution were selected. This step is important to teach perspective taking and for evaluating possible solutions based on the consequences for each person involved in the problem, not just for the child. For example, banning your patient's brother from the playroom after knocking down the block tower is a possible solution, but may not be preferred by the patient's brother or parents if there is limited play space in the patient's home. This step requires practice in theory of mind, organization, working memory, metacognition, planning, flexibility, and perspective taking.

Finally, have the child choose a solution that appears to have the most favorable, and/or least unfavorable, consequences (step 4) for everyone involved. Plan with the child, and the parents if appropriate, the next steps for implementing the selected solution. The implementation plan should be specific, including the when, where, how, and with whom for solving the problem. For example, "*I will go to the store with my parents to purchase a second set of blocks with my allowance on Saturday morning, so my brother and I can each have our own set to play with.*" After the child has chosen a solution and tried it out, talk with the child about the outcome of the solution (step 5). Importantly, praise the child for engaging in the process, even if their chosen solution did not produce their desired response. If a nonfavorable outcome did occur, help the child think through what actions might be better to choose next time.

Here is a brief role play of a clinician introducing the concept of executive functioning difficulties with a patient and his family, and setting up the use of problem-solving strategies to work through family conflict around getting homework done:

Clinician: John, I want to talk today about the difficulty you have had around getting your homework done, and I thought it would be helpful for your parents to join because homework is causing a lot of fighting at home. I am hoping we can all put our heads together to find a way to make homework time go easier for everyone. I have reviewed the report from the neuropsychologist you met with, and one thing she noted in the report is that, although you are very good at arithmetic, doing word problems in math is challenging because it is hard for you to remember and organize the information you have read so that you can answer the question correctly. You have also told me that you hate writing essays for English class because even though you enjoyed the book you read, it is hard for you to plan out how to share your thoughts about it in writing. The problems are not with your aptitude for English or math, but instead with how you approach your work. This is what she called "executive functions" which means things like how you organize, plan, pay attention, remember details, and stick with an assignment until it is done. If these things are tough for you, I wonder if part of the reason you put off starting homework is because these difficulties in figuring out how to approach certain kinds of work makes it that much harder to get started?

John: Well, I do try to put off doing my essays until the last possible moment, but I think that is just because I work better under pressure.

Parents: But John, every time you leave your essay until the last minute, you always complain the next day that you could have gotten a better grade if you had just had a little more time to get it done! That's why we are always on your case about starting it earlier!

John: Dad, it is my homework, so you need to just let me do it my way.

Clinician: The neuropsychologist suggested that strategies like organizing your thoughts in an outline before writing an essay might be very helpful for you, but that will take a little more time than you often leave yourself. So let's brainstorm all the possible solutions that might help you get homework started earlier. There are no wrong answers at this stage. Anyone can share ideas and later we'll think about which ones will work best (see Table 10.2).

TABLE 10.2 Example of using problem-solving steps for solving problem with getting homework started on time

1. Define the Problem: I wait until the last possible moment to start my homework	I fight with my parents about homework and I don't always get the grade I wanted
2. Brainstorm possible solutions	3. List possible consequences of each possible solution
A. Stop doing homework altogether B. Start my homework as soon as I get home C. Make a schedule at the beginning of each week of what I need to get done D. Take a 45 minute break after school and then get started on my homework with short breaks in between subjects E. Make my parents do my homework	A. Cause more fights at home. Get bad grades at school B. I will be too tired and won't do good work C. This will help me stay organized and plan how much time I actually need to set aside each day to get my work done D. Get to have some breaks and still get my work done earlier than I do now E. Never gonna happen.
	What would happen if I chose Solution A? How would I feel? How would the other person feel? What might the other person do in response? Repeat for Solution B, C, D, E
4. Select the best solution based on the possible consequences. C and D	5. Try it out and evaluate what happened Parents rewarded me for sticking to the plan. I felt good about doing better on my work

The type of problems a child will encounter, as well as the sophistication and independence with which they can work through generating, evaluating, selecting, and enacting potential solutions will vary greatly depending on the child's development stage. Below we provide recommendations for tailoring problem-solving strategies to a specific developmental stage (childhood versus adolescence) and provide clinical examples for each.

TEACHING PROBLEM-SOLVING STRATEGIES WITH SCHOOL-AGED CHILDREN

Primary-school-aged children with Tourette syndrome and other tic disorders often present with co-occurring mental health conditions, including ADHD, OCD, and other anxiety-related disorders, which underscore the need for training in problem-solving skills (Lebowitz et al., 2012). Teaching children problem-solving skills at a young age (with parent and school staff support) can help to empower them with the skills and confidence to successfully overcome these challenges, improve their wellbeing, and increase their quality of life. Although the evidence base for teaching problem solving specifically to children with Tourette syndrome and/or other associated disorders is limited, findings from the broader child therapy literature [see Manassis (2012) for further details], together with clinical wisdom, suggest that there are 12 key strategies for effectively teaching problem-solving skills to school-aged children. These steps are not a "recipe" meant to be followed in order, but rather are a collection of recommendations for making problem-solving skills more accessible, desirable, and effective for young children. These 12 strategies are summarized below, followed by a case illustration of how to apply the recommendations when teaching problem-solving skills in individual therapy with a school-aged child.

Twelve Tips for Teaching Problem Solving to School-aged Children

1. Use engaging resources (e.g., books, online clips, apps, video games) to introduce an example problem scenario to a child that is similar to a problem that she/he is facing in a fun, nonthreatening manner.
2. Use the example scenario(s) to encourage the child to discuss the problem that she/he is currently facing. Empathize with the child, and share a personal example of a similar challenge or problem (if possible, appropriate and relevant).
3. Introduce a structured step-by-step problem-solving formula to the child that they can apply to a range of problems (present and future). This formula can help to overcome executive functioning deficits that are common among children with Tourette syndrome and other associated disorders (e.g., ADHD and OCD), such as disorganized thinking, difficulties inhibiting inappropriate responses, challenges generating a range of appropriate solutions to problems and deciding on the optimal solution, particularly in relation to social problems (Channon et al., 2003).
4. Try to use a problem-solving formula that includes visual illustrations of the problem-solving steps for children with reading difficulties and/ or those who learn best from visual information.
5. Include steps that help the child to accurately define the problem and incorporate emotion-regulation strategies as an integral part of the solution. Children with attentional difficulties may fail to notice contextual clues that are important for them to accurately detect, and define problems and those with social anxiety are prone to misinterpreting emotional clues as threatening (Heuer, Lange, Isaac, Rinck, & Becker, 2010).
6. If the child is resistant to learning a problem-solving formula because they associate problem solving with negative life events, initially use the formula to review and celebrate a past situation that he/she successfully coped with. Then, gradually progress to solving a current problem that the child is facing.

7. If the child is likely to only suggest silly and/or unhelpful solutions, explain from the outset that you and the child will take turns proposing solutions to the problem. This ensures that some appropriate solutions will be discussed.
8. For children who are visual learners, consider helping them to draw stick-figure pictures of the possible consequences for each of the solutions that have been suggested. A website or app (e.g., Comics Head, Strip Designer) may also be used to create comic strips to explore the likely outcomes of different solutions, and may increase the child's engagement and motivation.
9. Develop a detailed plan with the child of what they will say and do for their chosen solution.
10. Act out the solution, with you competently demonstrating it in the role of the child first. Then, ask the child to act it out. Help the child to fine-tune and practice the solution multiple times in session and encourage them to continue to practice it at home with parent support before putting it into action in real life. Role play/behavioral rehearsal is a powerful technique to build children's skills and confidence to successfully implement skills and solutions in real life (Sukhodolosky, Golub, Stone, & Orban, 2005). Consider filming the skill demonstrations for later review and evaluation (if possible). The child can review footage of themselves competently demonstrating a target skill multiple times before executing it in real life to further enhance their confidence.
11. Prompt the child to evaluate what you do well and what you could improve on after you demonstrate the solution and to self-evaluate their own performance (both when practicing the solution in session or at home, and when the child puts the solution into action in real life). This self-evaluation process helps to build self-awareness and independent problem-solving skills. Research suggests that children with a range of conditions, including ADHD and Tourette syndrome are less accurate in judging their social competence and in reflecting on the appropriateness of the solutions that they choose for social problems (Channon et al., 2003).
12. Initially engage parents (and where possible, teachers and school support staff) to help the child apply the problem-solving formula to a range of scenarios (to optimize skill generalization), and to offer praise and rewards for their efforts. As the child's problem-solving skills improve, adult support can be gradually phased out.

CASE EXAMPLE

"Nathan" was a 10-year-old boy with Tourette syndrome, ADHD—combined type, and social anxiety disorder who was teased at school for his vocal and motor tics. A group of boys in his class imitated him (eye-rolling, head-turning, and grunting), laughed at him and called him a "weirdo." Nathan tried to stay away from the boys, but when he noticed them imitating him, he would quickly become angry, yelling at them to stop and to leave him alone.

As shown in the therapy session excerpt below, the topic of Nathan's bullying was sensitively broached in therapy by encouraging him to play a computer game activity that illustrated an example of bullying, from the Secret Agent Society social skills program computer game (Beaumont, 2009). The clinician gently asked Nathan for his thoughts about the animated scenario shown, and if he had ever seen or experienced bullying himself. When he described the bullying that he was enduring, she suggested troubleshooting the problem using a step-by-step formula—the D.E.C.O.D.E.R (see Fig. 10.1). Each letter of the word "D.E.C.O.D.E.R" stands for a different problem-solving step.

Except from Therapy Session:

Clinician	Nathan, today we're going to play a computer game to explore different ways of solving social problems. I'd like you to log on to the Secret of the Schoolyard Ghost mission in level 3 of the game.
Nathan	OK, that sounds like fun.

Clinician watches as Nathan logs onto the computer game activity. Nathan reaches the part of the game where his avatar is bullied and he is asked to choose how to cope with the bullying. He chooses 'Tell the bullies to stop calling him names', and watches as the rest of the computer game animation plays out.

Clinician *(At the end of the game activity)*	What do you think of how the bullies reacted to your character in the game when he told them to stop calling him names?
Nathan	That's not what really happens (*looks down*). Bullies don't just stop bullying you when you tell them to stop.
Clinician	Yeah, bullying can be really tough to deal with. You're right - sometimes other kids don't stop bullying you when you tell them to. When have you seen this happen?
Nathan	I've seen lots of kids get bullied at my school.
Clinician	I see... That must be hard to watch. A lot of kids get bullied at one time or another. I know I did when I was at school. I was a slow runner, and the kids used to call me 'turtle'. Have you ever been bullied?
Nathan	Yeah, sometimes. There are a couple of kids in my class who call me names and copy my tics. It makes me so angry and they just won't stop.
Clinician	That sounds really annoying and tough to deal with. I've got something that might help. It's a step-by-step formula called the D.E.C.O.D.E.R which was developed to work through problems like this. Let's go through the steps together and see if we can figure out a game plan to deal with the boys' teasing you at school. As we talk about different solutions, you can tell me what you think will work, and what won't.
Nathan	Ok...

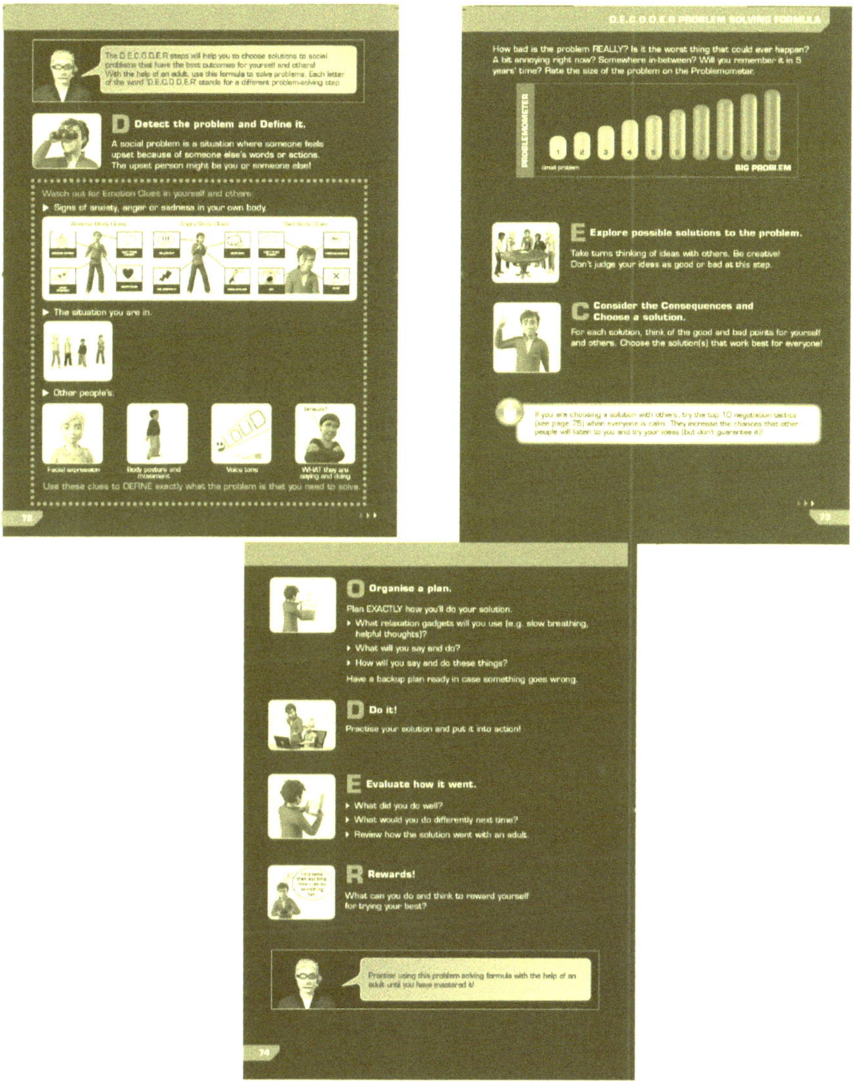

FIGURE 10.1 The D.E.C.O.D.E.R problem-solving formula (excerpt from the Secret Agent Society—Solving the Mystery of Social Encounters Cadet Handbook, Version 2; Beaumont, 2016). Reproduced with author's permission.

The D.E.C.O.D.E.R problem-solving formula emphasizes the importance of children attending to different aspects of a scenario (including their own emotional state, the situation they are in, other people's facial expressions, body postures and movements, voice tones, and what they are saying) to accurately define a problem before attempting to solve it. Each step of the formula is illustrated with visually engaging graphics, and the "problemometer" helps children to put their problem into perspective by thinking about whether it is the worst thing that could ever happen (particularly useful for children with anxiety who tend to catastrophize). As part of the "Organize a Plan" step, children are encouraged to use relaxation strategies or "gadgets" to calmly put their chosen solution into action, and the formula also features an evaluation step to help build children's self-awareness of what they did well and what they could do differently next time.

The clinician helped Nathan to apply each of the D.E.C.O.D.E.R steps to his bullying problem. From the outset, the clinician suggested that Nathan could suggest two solutions and she would suggest two solutions for the "E—Explore possible solutions to the problem" step. Nathan suggested 1) continuing to tell the kids who were teasing him to stop, and 2) trying to stare them down. The clinician suggested that (1) he tell his teacher about the teasing when the other kids were not around and (2) act like he did not really care what they did or said by looking bored, saying "Seriously?" and calmly walking away. The clinician helped Nathan to draw stick-figure pictures with speech and thought bubbles to explore the consequences of each solution for himself and others. Through this process, Nathan discovered that continuing to tell the boys to stop teasing him and staring them down made him more annoyed and seemed to please the boys, because they got a reaction from him. By contrast, acting like he did not care what they said might result in them becoming bored and leaving him alone. Telling the teacher might also lead to the boys being punished for teasing him and therefore being less likely to continue doing it.

The clinician helped Nathan to plan the details of how he would implement his chosen solution (use slow breathing to stay calm, think "they are just doing it to make themselves feel strong," say "seriously" in a bored voice, with a relaxed face and body, calmly walk away, talk to his teacher when others are not around). Then, the clinician acted out the solution steps for Nathan (part of the "Do it" step of the D.E.C.O.D.E.R formula), with her playing the role of Nathan and Nathan playing the role of one of the boys that tease him. The clinician asked Nathan to use her tablet camera to film the demonstration. They then watched the footage and Nathan identified what she did well (looked calm and relaxed) and what she could do differently next time (possibly walk away a little more slowly so that she did not look scared).

Nathan and the clinician then swapped roles, and the clinician filmed Nathan's demonstration of the solution steps. After the demonstration, she prompted him to watch the footage and self-identify two things that he did well (relaxed face and body, walked away slowly), and one thing that he could do differently next time. Nathan struggled to identify anything that he could do differently, so the clinician specifically inquired about the solution step that she believed he needed to improve on (i.e., more clearly communicating to his teacher what the boys were saying to him and when). The clinician praised Nathan for his efforts and encouraged him to repeatedly practice the teacher explanation step of the solution in session to improve on it.

At the end of the session, the clinician invited Nathan's mother to join the session, and Nathan explained the D.E.C.O.D.E.R formula and how it was applied to his bullying problem. Nathan was asked to demonstrate the solution for his mom (Sharon), and she was encouraged to help him to continue practicing the solution at home with her help before putting it into action at school. Sharon was also encouraged to praise and reward her son for his efforts at practicing and attempting the solution (irrespective of the outcome). Nathan requested videogame time as his reward. Nathan and Sharon were warned that Nathan may need to implement the solution multiple times before the boys became bored and stop bullying him.

Sharon was also given a teacher handout of the D.E.C.O.D.E.R formula to share with Nathan's classroom teacher and teacher-aide to try to ensure that everyone was using a consistent approach to help Nathan solve problems. It was explained to Nathan and his mom that the D.E.C.O.D.E.R steps are a review and planning tool that Nathan can initially use with adult support. As Nathan's skill and confidence using the formula improves, adult support can be gradually phased out, and only provided when needed.

At the next week's consultation, the clinician checked in with Nathan to see how the solution worked. Nathan enthusiastically explained that after 3 days, the bullies stopped bothering him and his teacher was very supportive when he spoke to her. She encouraged Nathan to report any bullying incidents to her, and reassured him that there would be consequences if the boys continued teasing him. Nathan was thrilled that he was able to successfully manage the bullying himself, without needing the teacher to intervene. The clinician praised him for his efforts, and suggested that they apply the D.E.C.O.D.E.R formula to another of Nathan's current challenges—his fear of asking the teacher questions in class because of his vocal tics. This helped Nathan to learn how to generalize his newly learned problem-solving skill to a range of life challenges.

USING PROBLEM-SOLVING STRATEGIES WITH ADOLESCENCE

As patients with TDs progress into adolescence, clinician involvement in problem solving ideally shifts to a more consultative role to reflect the increasing independence of this developmental stage. Similarly, while treatment for younger children with TDs includes a great deal of parental participation, the contribution of parents both in session and at home should be modified accordingly with adolescents. The goal at this stage is to foster an increased sense of self-efficacy and autonomy with problem solving and prepare teens as they move through adolescence to eventually transition into young adulthood with confidence in their abilities to manage TD-related challenges alone. Given the numerous challenges that adolescents with TDs face across academic, social, and behavioral domains, and the evidence that suggests children diagnosed with TDs experience worse psychosocial and psychiatric outcomes as older adolescents compared to their nondiagnosed counterparts (Gorman et al., 2010); it is critical to provide these patients with empirically-supported, developmentally appropriate clinical care. Independence in problem solving can be fostered with several empirically-informed techniques, including the implementation of a "consultation to the patient" approach and through the use of behavioral chain analyses and solution analyses. Each of these strategies is discussed in the following paragraphs.

While therapists or parents of younger patients with TDs may engage in direct environmental intervention on behalf of the patient (i.e., speaking with school personnel about academic challenges related to TD, advocating for accommodations, facilitating conflict resolution with peers or siblings), during adolescence direct intervention should be gradually reduced as the youth learns to solve problems on his or her own. This concept, known as "consultation to the patient," is a hallmark approach in DBT, aimed at empowering patients to act autonomously with the support of the clinician, rather than having a clinician act fully on behalf of the patient (Linehan, 1993a; Miller et al., 2007). While directly intervening is appropriate and oftentimes necessary for younger patients, this approach becomes more problematic with teens, as it communicates that they are not sufficiently equipped to cope with everyday challenges. The consultative model sends a message to the teen that they have the capability to manage problems on their own, and that they do not need an intermediary to intervene for them. Rather, problems that arise become opportunities for the adolescent to learn to interact effectively with others, face and overcome obstacles, experience successes, and build mastery (Miller et al., 2007).

Exceptions to this approach may be when the patient's immediate safety is at risk or if the environment is too powerful for a teen to reasonably manage alone (Miller et al., 2007). For example, navigating the Board of Education to obtain a new school placement that is better suited to TD-related academic challenges may continue to require heavy adult involvement. However, as much as possible, providers and parents should be gradually "stepping back" and encouraging patients to initiate the problem-solving process themselves. This approach may be particularly relevant to social challenges, for which it was acceptable for parents to intervene when the patient was younger, but is no longer as appropriate, and patients must thus learn to navigate these difficulties more independently. For example, a clinician of a younger child with TD whose teacher is responding punitively toward tics might reasonably call the patient's teacher to explain his diagnosis and symptom presentation and discuss classroom management strategies. During later adolescence, however, the clinician may instead coach the patient in session on how to speak to his teacher about his condition and advocate for himself. By providing consultation and less direct environmental intervention, clinicians can guide teens with TDs toward autonomy in social problem solving.

An additional problem-solving intervention pertinent to the adolescent stage is the implementation of behavioral chain analyses in session. Behavioral chain analyses (or "chains") are used to break down problematic situations, examine antecedents and consequences of behavioral targets, and offer opportunities to examine behavioral patterns. This strategy, which has roots in behavior therapy and has been adapted and applied within numerous other treatment approaches for adolescents including CBT, applied behavior analysis, and DBT, also allows for a close examination of a real-life scenario, so adolescents learn problem solving in a context relevant to them. This process also elucidates variables that may be cueing or reinforcing problematic behavior, as well as clarifies the function of behavior that hinders effective problem solving. Conducting a chain analysis in session involves eliciting an example of a recent conflict or problematic behavior from the adolescent, and asking him or her to describe this situation in detail, step-by-step, including vulnerability factors, prompting events, and consequences. Each successive step in the given situation serves as a "link" in the chain. The clinician prompts the adolescent to identify thoughts, feelings, and bodily sensations experienced at each step, and may ask questions to clearly define the problem behavior and identify associated emotions. This process is flexible and should be tailored to the individual patient and the TD-related challenge that they identify (see Rizvi & Ritschel, 2014, for example of a chain analysis in DBT).

Particularly for adolescents with executive functioning deficits, drawing out the chain or using a visual handout is a useful tool to concretize the verbal discussion. Drawing arrows on the chain for skill insertion, starring appropriate skill behavior, and underscoring problematic behavior are additional helpful visual cues. Teens with executive functioning deficits may struggle to break down situations in a stepwise manner, and often report that a problematic situation occurred with no trigger. Slowing down the teen's thinking by using the analogy that he or she should describe the situation in tiny pieces, like they are giving actors stage directions, may be helpful in eliciting more detail. Additionally, prompting adolescents for numeric ratings of emotional intensity (i.e., "I was angry at a 7 out of 10") can anchor their descriptions and show how emotions fluctuated throughout the chain. Particularly when working with adolescents who have limited language abilities, clinicians may need to infuse a greater number of prompts to elicit detail. For example, asking, "*What happened next?*" or "*What did you do after that?*"

Following the initial chain analysis, the clinician shifts to the solution analysis, a strategy aimed at identifying the desired outcome of the chain situation and the adaptive or skillful behavior needed to reach this outcome. In essence, this is a discussion of what the adolescent could have done differently and how he or she could respond to a similar challenge more adaptively in the future. Key to the solution analysis is incorporation of both *which* specific skills or alternative behavior should be inserted into the chain, and *where* these should be included. Prompting adolescents to think about how the rest of the chain could have differed, and even drawing a secondary hypothetical chain underneath the original, encourages understanding of the link between behavior and consequences. The solution analysis can further guide treatment in that it highlights what skills to work on for adolescents for whom skills deficits interfere with achieving the desired outcome. For example, a common challenge facing college-bound adolescents with TDs is anxiety about how and when to disclose their diagnosis to the new peers they meet at school. This issue is particularly pertinent to those patients who were diagnosed as young children, when parents were in charge of this disclosure process. A chain might highlight the patient's pattern of avoidance of having a conversation about TD with a peer, and during the solution analysis, the clinician and patient might collaboratively brainstorm alternatives to reduce anxiety and skills to aid the youth in feeling more comfortable with the disclosure.

CASE EXAMPLE

Maria was a 14-year-old female with TD. She had several simple motor tics, such as blinking and a shoulder shrug with a neck tilt, as well as a complex phonic tic of shouting the phrase "Is it really ok" loudly. The volume of her vocal tic caused conflict at home because her younger sister would become easily annoyed, complained that she could not focus on her homework due to the noise, and often yelled at Maria to stop. Maria reported feeling hurt and misunderstood at these comments, as well as frustrated that her sister did not understand that she could not control the tic symptoms. At times, Maria responded to her sister by yelling back or physically pushing or hitting her. In session, Maria reported a recent conflict in which her sister asked Maria to be quiet when Maria ticced while they watched a television show together. Maria explained that this escalated to an argument "out of nowhere" during which she hit her sister and threw her cell phone. Maria's parents punished her by taking away her cell phone for three days, and Maria arrived to session frustrated by the revoked privileges.

The clinician initiated a behavioral chain analysis of this scenario (see Fig. 10.2) by starting with how Maria was feeling leading up to watching television with her sister. How anxious was she beforehand? How frequent and severe were her tics earlier in the day? What kind of day did she have at school? Through this line of questioning, Maria described her vulnerability factors and the antecedents to this situation (i.e., she was already feeling anxious at a 5 out of 10 because she had received a poor grade on a science exam at school; she felt self-conscious because a classmate made a comment

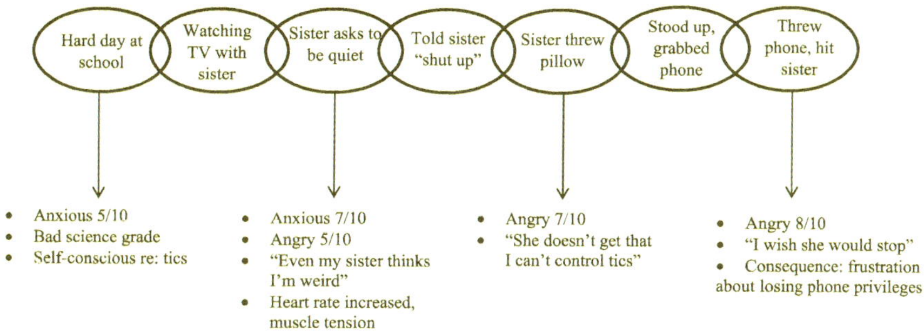

FIGURE 10.2 Chain analysis example.

about her tics that day), and as she shared this information, the clinician drew these as links in the chain. Next, the clinician moved on to the cueing event of Maria's sister's request for her to be quiet, prompting Maria to identify specific thoughts (i.e., "Even my sister thinks I'm weird"), bodily sensations (i.e., increased heart rate, muscle tension), and emotions (i.e., anxiety increased to 7 out of 10). By providing detailed prompts, such as "*How did you get from the couch to the cell phone?*", the clinician highlighted several links in the chain that shed light on the escalation in conflict (i.e., Maria first responded to her sister by telling her to shut up, following which her sister threw a pillow at her, which Maria stood up to dodge, all of which was associated with a further increase in emotion).

During the solution analysis, the clinician assisted Maria in coming up with several potential alternatives to the problem behaviors of hitting and throwing objects, including using skills like deep breathing to manage baseline anxiety, and leaving the room to engage in a distraction activity as she became increasingly emotional. The clinician highlighted how these skills ultimately are in service of Maria's goal of keeping her cell phone, to underscore the connection between her behavior and consequences, and maintain motivation for practicing the skills in real time at home.

Sample Chain Analysis:

Clinician Ok, Maria, let's take a look at this situation more closely.

Maria I don't know what happened, we were just watching TV and I blew up at my sister out of nowhere.

Clinician Hold on, let's rewind. What was going on before the fight with your sister last night? How was your day at school, and how were you feeling in general?

Maria Well, it was a pretty rough day at school. I got a terrible grade on my science test, and during lunch a kid at my table asked why I was moving my neck back and forth. I felt really self-conscious for the rest of the afternoon.

Clinician Wow, what a tough day. Sounds like you were feeling pretty anxious. How would you rate that feeling 1-10?

Maria Probably about a 5 out of 10.

Clinician Ok, so fast forward to the evening, you're already feeling anxious from school, you're sitting watching TV with your sister, and what happens next?

Maria I was ticcing, both doing the neck tic and saying "Is is really ok", and I guess it must have been loud because my sister asked me to be quiet.
Clinician What thought went through your head when she said that?
Maria I thought, oh great, even my own sister thinks I'm a freak.
Clinician Ok, and what happened to your emotions? Did your anxiety level change?
Maria My anxiety got even worse, like a 7 out of 10. I also felt angry because my sister of all people should understand.
Clinician Did you notice any feelings in your body as you felt more anxious and angry?
Maria Yeah, my heart started racing and I felt my muscles get all tight. I think that's why I exploded and hit her.
Clinician Back up a little bit, is that what happened next? She asked you to be quiet and you hit her? Let's think of every little step.
Maria Oh, well first I just said "shut up" and then she threw a pillow at me and I had to duck to get out of that way.
Clinician I see, what was going through your head at that point?
Maria I was thinking that she really doesn't understand that I can't control my tics and it's totally unfair she's telling me to stop.
Clinician Sounds like your anger went up a notch at that point too?
Maria Definitely, I was probably at a 7 out of 10.
Clinician Ok, paint me a picture, what happened after you ducked from the pillow?
Maria Well, I was standing up and I saw my sister's phone sitting on the coffee table, so I picked it up and threw it across the room. She got up to get it and I pushed her out of my way and stormed out of the living room.
Clinician What were you thinking when that happened?
Maria I wished she would stop commenting on my tics and leave me alone. Of course, I'm the one who ended up getting in trouble for breaking her phone.
Clinician Ok, so I think we can both agree that the situation didn't end up how you had hoped it would. At what point in the chain do you think we could do things differently? *(shift to solution analysis).*
Maria I know I shouldn't have hit her.
Clinician True, hitting her ended up getting you in trouble but I can understand that you were really angry and anxious. Is there a place earlier on in the chain where you could have done something differently? How about when you noticed your anxiety rise after she asked you to be quiet? What strategies might have been helpful there?
Maria I could do my deep breathing exercises, or used my helpful thoughts, like "I know my sister doesn't think I'm weird."
Clinician Great ideas. Using strategies to manage your anxiety right after school could also help; I know you typically enjoy listening to music as a distraction. How about towards the end of the chain when you were super angry? How could you react in a way that would be in service of your goal of having your cell phone?
Maria It probably would have been better to leave the room and stop interacting with my sister completely until I cooled off.
Clinician Definitely, that would likely de-escalate everything. Good problem-solving.

EVALUATION, MAINTENANCE, AND RELAPSE PREVENTION

Problem-solving strategies are most often just one intervention approach as part of a larger treatment plan. Evaluation of outcomes specifically in problem solving may not be represented in typical pre/post treatment or symptoms severity measures. Quality of life, social skills, and self-esteem assessment measures may reflect improved capacity for and confidence in problem solving. Newly developed and validated tools for measuring outcomes in problem solving may also be useful (e.g., Caldas, Broaddus, & Winch, 2016). For youth with a variety of situations in need of problem solving help and practice, the clinician may consider creating a "hierarchy" or problem scenarios to address incrementally over the course of treatment. Similar to a standard Fear and Avoidance Hierarchy in CBT, the patient can provide weekly ratings for each item on the hierarchy of how "big" a problem the patient considers the situation to be and/or how strong the emotional reaction is to the situation, tracking changes over time. Repeated practice of problem-solving skills is imperative for the patient to maintain gains over time, particularly in situations evoking strong emotions. Depending on the age and developmental stage of the patient, parents should learn and practice the skills, as well in order to both model effective problem solving in their own lives and to support the child's practice with tough problems during the week or after the therapy has ended. A gradual spacing out of sessions prior to termination (e.g., every other week, every 3 weeks) or a booster session model (scheduling a check-in session every couple of months) may also be useful for maintenance of gains and relapse prevention.

REFERENCES

Barkley, R. A. (1997). *ADHD and the nature of self control*. New York: Guilford Press.

Beaumont, R. (2009). *Secret agent society—solving the mystery of social encounters computer game*. Brisbane, Australia: Social Skills Training Institute.

Beaumont, R. (2010). *Secret agent society—solving the mystery of social encounters – facilitator kit*. Brisbane, Australia: The Social Skills Training Institute.

Beaumont, R. (2016). Secret agent society—solving the mystery of social encounters cadet handbook. *(2nd ed.)*. Brisbane, Australia: Social Skills Training Institute.

Bohnen, N. I., Kuwabara, H., Constantine, G. M., Mathis, C. A., & Moore, R. Y. (2007). Grooved pegboard test as a biomarker of Nigrostriatal denervation in Parkinson's disease. *Neuroscience Letters*, *424*(3), 185–189.

Brookshire, B. L., Butler, I. J., Linda Ewing-Cobbs, L., & Fletcher, J. M. (1994). Neuropsychological characteristics of children with Tourette syndrome: Evidence for a nonverbal learning disability. *Journal of Clinical and Experimental Neuropsychology*, *16*(2), 289–302.

Caldas, S. V., Broaddus, E. T., & Winch, P. J. (2016). Measuring conflict management, emotional self-efficacy, and problem solving confidence in an evaluation of outdoor programs for inner-city youth in Baltimore, Maryland. *Evaluation and Program Planning*, *57*, 64–71.

Chang, S. W., McCracken, J. T., & Piacentini, J. C. (2007). Neurocognitive correlates of child obsessive compulsive disorder and Tourette syndrome. *Journal of Clinical and Experimental Neuropsychology*, *29*(7), 724–733.

Channon, S., Crawford, S., Vakili, K., & Robertson, M. M. (2003). Real-life-type problem solving in Tourette syndrome. *Cognitive and Behavioral Neurology*, *16*(1), 3–15.

Channon, S., Gunning, A., Frankl, J., & Robertson, M. M. (2006). Tourette's syndrome (TS): cognitive performance in adults with uncomplicated TS. *Neuropsychology*, *20*(1), 58–65.

Crawford, S., Channon, S., & Robertson, M. M. (2005). Tourette's syndrome: performance on tests of behavioural inhibition, working memory and gambling. *Journal of Child Psychology and Psychiatry*, *46*, 1327–1336.

Dawson, P., & Guare, R. (2010). *Executive skills in children and adolescents: A practical guide to assessment and intervention*. New York: The Guilford Press.

Eddy, C. M., Rizzo, R., & Cavanna, A. E. (2009). Neuropsychological aspects of Tourette syndrome: A review. *Journal of Psychosomatic Research*, *67*(2009), 503–513.

Ehrenreich-May, J., Kennedy, S.M., Sherman, J.A., Bilek, E.L., Buzzella, B.A., Bennett, S.M., & Barlow, D.H. (2018). Unified Protocols for the Transdiagnostic Treatment of Emotional Disorders in Children and Adolescents: Therapist Guide. New York: Oxford University Press.

Gioia, G. A., Isquith, P. K., Guy, S. C., & Kenworthy, L. (2000). *Behavior rating inventory of executive function*. Odessa, FL: Psychological Assessment Resources, Inc.

Gorman, D. A., Thompson, N., Plessen, K. J., Robertson, M. M., Leckman, J. F., & Peterson, B. S. (2010). Psychosocial outcome and psychiatric comorbidity in older adolescentswith Tourette syndrome: Controlled study. *The British Journal of Psychiatry*, *197*, 36–44.

Heuer, K., Lange, W. G., Isaac, L., Rinck, M., & Becker, E. S. (2010). Morphed emotional faces: Emotion detection and misinterpretation in social anxiety. *Journal of Behavior Therapy and Experimental Psychiatry*, *41*(4), 418–425.

Kendall, P. C. (1992). *Stop and think workbook* (Second Edition). Workbook Publishing.

Kofler, M. J., Larsen, R., Sarver, D. E., & Tolan, P. H. (2015). Developmental trajectories of aggression, prosocial behavior, and social-cognitive problem solving in emerging adolescents with clinical elevated attention deficit/hyperactivity disorder symptoms. *Journal of Abnormal Psychology*, *124*, 1027–1042.

Lebowitz, E. R., Motlagh, M. G., Katsovich, L., King, R. A., Lombroso, P. J., Grantz, H., ... Leckman, J. F. (2012). Tourette syndrome in youth with and without obsessive compulsive disorder and attention deficit hyperactivity disorder. *European Child and Adolescent Psychiatry*, *21*, 451–457.

Linehan, M. M. (1993a). *Cognitive behavioral treatment of borderline personality disorder*. New York, NY: Guilford Press.

Loring, D. W., Martin, R. C., Meador, K. J., & Lee, Gregory P. (1990). Psychometric construction of the Rey-Osterrieth complex figure: Methodological considerations and interrater reliability. *Archives of Clinical Neuropsychology*, *5*(1), 1–14.

Manassis, K. (2012). *Problem solving in child and adolescent psychotherapy: A skills-based collaborative approach*. New York, NY: Guilford Press.

McGuire, J. F., Arnold, E., Park, J. M., Nadeau, J., Lewin, A. B., Murphy, T. K., & Storch, E. A. (2015). Living with tics: Reduced impairment and improved quality of life for youth with chronic tic disorders. *Psychiatry Research*, *225*, 571–579.

Miller, A. L., Rathus, J. H., & Linehan, M. M. (2007). Dialectical behavior therapy with suicidal adolescents. New York: Guilford Press.

Rizvi, S. L., & Ritschel, L. A. (2014). Mastering the art of chain analysis in dialectical behavior therapy. *Cognitive and Behavioral Practice*, *21*, 335–349.

Sukhodolosky, D. G., Golub, A., Stone, E. C., & Orban, L. (2005). Dismantling anger control training for children: A randomized pilot study of social problem-solving versus social skills training components. *Behavior Therapy*, *36*(1), 15–23.

FURTHER READING

APA. (2013). *Diagnostic and statistical manual of mental disorders: DSM – 5*. Washington, DC: American Psychiatric Association.

Arbuthnott, K., & Frank, J. (2000). Executive control in set switching: Residual switch cost and task-set inhibition. *Canadian Journal of Experimental Psychology, 54*(1), 33–41. (Revue canadienne de psychologie experimentale).

Barkley, R. A., Murphy, K. R., & Kwasnik, D. (1996). Motor vehicle driving competencies and risks in teens and young adults with attention deficit hyperactivity disorder. *Pediatrics, 98*(6), 1089–1095.

Barnett, R., Maruff, P., Vance, A., Luk, E. S., Costin, J., Wood, C., & Pantelis, C. (2001). Abnormal executive function in attention deficit hyperactivity disorder: the effect of stimulant medication and age on spatial working memory. *Psychological Medicine, 31*(6), 1107–11015.

Benzina, N., Mallet, L., Burguière, E., et al. (2016). Cognitive dysfunction in obsessive-compulsive disorder. *Current Psychiatry Reports, 18*(2016), 80.

Boot, W. R., Blakely, D. P., & Simons, D. J. (2011). Do action video games improve perception and cognition? *Frontiers in Psychology, 2*, 226.

Bornstein, R. A., & Yang, V. (1991). Neuropsychological performance in medicated and unmedicated patients with Tourette's disorder. *The American Journal of Psychiatry, 148*(4), 468–471.

Boulougouris, V., & Tsaltas, E. (2008). Serotonergic and dopaminergic modulation of attentional processes. In G. Di Giovanni, V. Di Matteo, & E. Esposito (Eds.), *Progress in Brain Research* (Vol. 172, pp. 517–542). Elsevier.

Chan, Raymond C.K., Shum D., Toulopoulou T., Chen, Eric Y.H. Assessment of executive functions: Review of instruments and identification of critical issues. *Archives of Clinical Neuropsychology, 23*(2), 201–216.

Channon, S., Flynn, D., & Robertson, M. M. (1992). Attentional deficits in Gilles de la Tourette's Syndrome. *Neuropsychology, Neuropsychiatry, and Behavioural Neurology, 5*, 170–177.

Clark, C., Prior, M., & Kinsella, G. J. (2000). Do executive function deficits differentiate between adolescents with ADHD and oppositional defiant/conduct disorder? A neuropsychological study using the six elements test and Hayling sentence completion test. *Journal of Abnormal Child Psychology, 28*(5), 403–414.

Colcombe, S., & Kramer, A. F. (2003). Fitness effects on the cognitive function of older adults: a meta-analytic study. *Psychological Science, 14*(2), 125–130.

Doyle, A. E. (2006). Executive functions in attention-deficit/hyperactivity disorder. *Journal of Clinical Psychiatry, 67*(8), 21–26.

Eggenberger, P., Schumacher, V., Angst, M., Theill, N., & de Bruin, E. D. (2015). Does multicomponent physical exercise with simultaneous cognitive training boost cognitive performance in older adults? A 6-month randomized controlled trial with a 1-year follow-up. *Clinical Interventions in Aging, 10*, 1335–1349.

Eisenberg, N., & Morris, A. S. (2002). Children's emotion-related regulation. *Advances in Child Development and Behavior, 30*, 189–229.

Gilbert, S. J., & Burgess, P. W. (2008). Executive function. *Current Biology, 18*, R110–R114.

Goudriaan, A. E., Oosterlaan, J., De Beurs, E., & Van Den Brink, W. (2006). Neurocognitive functions in pathological gambling: a comparison with alcohol dependence, Tourette syndrome and normal controls. *Addiction, 101*, 534–547.

Jeter, C. B., Patel, S. S., Morris, J. S., Chuang, A. Z., Butler, I. J., & Sereno, A. B. (2015). Oculomotor executive function abnormalities with increased tic severity in Tourette syndrome. *Journal of Child Psychology and Psychiatry*, *56*(2), 193–202.

Karatekin, C., & Asarnow, R. F. (1998). Working memory in childhood-onset schizophrenia and attention-deficit/hyperactivity disorder. *Psychiatry Researc.*, *80*(2), 165–176.

Linehan, M. M. (1993b). *Skills training manual for treating borderline personality disorder*. New York, NY: Guilford Press.

Lovden, M., Backman, L., Lindenberger, U., Schaefer, S., & Schmiedek, F. (2010). A theoretical framework for the study of adult cognitive plasticity. *Psychological Bulletin*, *136*, 659–676.

Mannuzza, S., Klein, Rachel G., & Moulton, John L., III (2003). Persistence of Attention-Deficit/Hyperactivity Disorder into adulthood: What have we learned from the prospective follow-up studies?. *Journal of Attention Disorders*, *7*(2), 93–100.

Matthews, M., Nigg, J. T., & Fair, D. A. (2014). Attention Deficit Hyperactivity Disorder. *Current Topics in Behavioral Neurosciences*, *16*, 235–266.

McLean, A., Dowson, J., Toone, B., Young, S., Bazanis, E., Robbins, T. W., & Sahakian, B. J. (2004). Characteristic neurocognitive profile associated with adult attention-deficit/hyperactivity disorder. *Psychological Medicine*, *34*(4), 681–692.

Moreno, S., Bialystok, E., Barac, R., Schellenberg, E. G., Cepeda, N. J., & Chau, T. (2011). Short-Term Music Training Enhances Verbal Intelligence and Executive Function. *Psychological Science*, *22*(11), 1425–1433.

Moreno, S., Marques, C., Santos, A., Santos, M., Castro, S. L., & Besson, M. (2009). Musical training influences linguistic abilities in 8-year-old children: More evidence for brain plasticity. *Cerebral Cortex*, *19*, 712–723.

Muraven, M., & Baumeister, R. F. (2000). Self-regulation and depletion of limited resources: Does self-control resemble a muscle? *Psychological Bulletin*, *126*(2), 247–259.

Nigg, J. T. (1999). The ADHD response-inhibition deficit as measured by the Stop Task: replication with DSM-IV combined type, extension, and qualification. *Journal of Abnormal Child Psychology*, *27*(5), 393–402.

Nigg, J. T. (2001). Is ADHD a disinhibitory disorder? *Psychological Bulletin*, *127*(5), 571–598.

Nigg, J. T., Hinshaw, S. P., Carte, E. T., & Treuting, J. J. (1998). Neuropsychological correlates of childhood attention-deficit/hyperactivity disorder: explainable by comorbid disruptive behavior or reading problems? *Journal of Abnormal Psychology*, *107*(3), 468–480.

Pennington, B. F., & Ozonoff, S. (1996). Executive functions and developmental psychopathology. *Journal of Child Psychology and Psychiatry*, *37*(1), 51–87.

Rathus, J. H., & Miller, A. L. (2015). DBT skills training manual for adolescents. NewYork: The Guilford Press.

Robertson, M. M., Althoff, R. R., Hafez, A., & Pauls, D. L. (2008). Principal components analysis of a large cohort with Tourette syndrome. *The British Journal of Psychiatry*, *193*(1), 31–36.

Schellenberg, E. G. (2004). Music lessons enhance IQ. *Psychological Science*, *15*, 511–514.

Schellenberg, E. G. (2006). Exposure to music: The truth about the consequences. In G. E. McPherson (Ed.), *The child as musician: A handbook of musical development* (pp. 111–134). Oxford, England: Oxford University Press.

Seidman, L. J., Biederman, J., Faraone, S. V., Weber, W., & Ouellette, C. (1997). Toward defining a neuropsychology of attention deficit-hyperactivity disorder: performance of children and adolescents from a large clinically referred sample. *Journal of Consulting and Clinical Psychology*, *65*(1), 150–160.

Smith, P. J., Blumenthal, J. A., Hoffman, B. M., et al. (2010). Aerobic exercise and neurocognitive performance: a meta-analytic review of randomized controlled trials. *Psychosomatic Medicine*, *72*(3), 239–252.

Staiano, A. E., Abraham, A. A., & Calvert, S. L. (2012). Competitive Versus Cooperative Exergame Play for African American Adolescents' Executive Function Skills: Short-Term Effects in a Long-Term Training Intervention. *Developmental Psychology*, *48*(2), 337 -342.

Sukhodolsky, D. G., Landeros-Weisenberger, A., Scahill, L., Leckman, J. F., & Schultz, R. T. (2010). Neuropsychological functioning in children with Tourette syndrome with and without attention-deficit/hyperactivity disorder*Journal of the American Academy of Child and Adolescent Psychiatry*, *49*(11), 1155–1164, e1. Available from doi:10.1016/j.jaac.2010.08.008.

Takeuchi, H., Taki, Y., & Kawashima, R. (2010). Effects of working memory training on cognitive functions and neural systems. *Reviews in the Neurosciences*, *21*, 427–449.

Usami, M. (2016). Functional consequences of attention-deficit hyperactivity disorder on children and their families. *Psychiatry and Clinical Neurosciences*, *70*, 303–317.

Chapter 11

Brief Trans-Diagnostic Parent Training: A Strengths-Based, Parent-Centered Treatment for Youth With Tourette Syndrome

Matthew W. Specht, PhD[1], Kim R. Edwards, PhD[2], Carisa Perry-Parrish, PhD[3] and Kaushalendra Amatya, PhD[3]

[1]Weill Cornell Medical College/NewYork-Presbyterian Hospital-Westchester, White Plains, NY, United States, [2]Department of Psychiatry and Behavioral Neurosciences, McMaster Children's Hospital and McMaster University, Hamilton, ON, Canada, [3]Department of Psychiatry and Behavioral Sciences, Division of Child and Adolescent Psychiatry, The Johns Hopkins Hospital, Baltimore, MD, United States

Tourette syndrome (TS) is a common neurodevelopmental condition affecting approximately 1% of the general population (American Psychiatric Association, 2013; Robertson, 2008; Scahill, Specht, & Page, 2013). As most people with TS experience mild waxing and waning tics that remit or reduce with age, timely, and appropriately titrated intervention for TS is essential (Abi-Jaoude & Gorman, 2012). However, tics rarely occur in isolation. Studies suggest that the majority (i.e., up to 90%) of individuals with TS also meet criteria for comorbid conditions, which commonly include attention-deficit/hyperactivity disorder (ADHD), obsessive-compulsive disorder (OCD), other anxiety disorders (e.g., social anxiety disorder), learning disabilities, and mood disorders (Cavanna & Rickards, 2013; Scahill et al., 2013; Specht et al., 2011). Although there have been variable rates reported for the prevalence of oppositional defiant disorder (ODD) in clinical samples of youth with TS (6%–26%; Bitsko et al., 2014; Specht et al., 2011), outbursts of disruptive/explosive behaviors (commonly termed "rage attacks") occur in higher than average rates (20%–70% of youth with TS; Budman, Rockmore, Stokes, & Sossin, 2003). These comorbid conditions can often cause more distress and impairment than the tics themselves, and should be considered important targets when treating patients with TS (Bernard et al., 2009).

The Clinician's Guide to Treatment and Management of Youth with Tourette Syndrome and Tic Disorders.
DOI: https://doi.org/10.1016/B978-0-12-811980-8.00011-X

The clinical complexity of youth with TS can make tic management, daily functioning, and overall quality of life challenging for patients and parents alike. For example, disruptive and noncompliant behaviors can negatively impact school attendance, homework completion, peer interactions, and parent–child relationships. Moreover, these behaviors can present a considerable challenge to the management of tics using evidence-based treatments (e.g., noncompliance with behavioral and/or pharmacological interventions).

While many interventions focus directly on treating tics (Woods et al. 2008) and/or cultivating skills to managing tic-related problems (McGuire et al., 2015), training and educating parents offers a unique avenue through which to help youth especially children and adolescents who appear disinterested or disengaged in treatment. Parents play an essential role in children's physical, mental, emotional, and spiritual development. While parenting a child without mental illness can be challenging for many, parenting a child with multiple cooccurring psychiatric conditions can seem (at times) near impossible. As parents typically respond reactively (instead of proactively) to children's behavior, a reciprocal and transactional relationship can form between parenting behavior and disruptive psychopathology in youth (Barkley, 2013). For example, a child with TS, ADHD, OCD, and "rage attacks" might begin to elicit a more negative, controlling, and reactive parenting style in his/her caregivers over time. More specifically, parents may gravitate toward more restrictive and repetitive commands and/or corporal punishment in response to outbursts that continue to occur; still other parents may give up, walk away, or even do the chore/task for their child.

Current best practices indicate the importance of involving parents in their children's mental health care (Chovil, 2009). Targeted programs have been developed for parents of youth with ADHD, ODD, and/or conduct disorder (CD). These treatments have considerable empirical support for reducing disruptive behaviors, and have shown promise for improving consistent and nonviolent parenting, enhancing parent–child interactions, and reducing child psychiatric symptoms (e.g., Barkley, 2013; Kazdin, 2005; Webster-Stratton & Reid, 2017). Parent management training has been shown to be a safe, effective short-term treatment for disruptive behaviors is TS-affected youth (Scahill et al, 2006). However, the emphasis of these prior treatment protocols has been on reducing disruptive behaviors and not on increasing parental capacity to identify and appropriately respond to a youth's "in-the-moment" prosocial behaviors. While reducing disruptive behaviors is important, youth with TS often display many problematic behaviors (e.g., tics, inattention, hyperactivity, impulsivity, disruptive behaviors, "rage attacks," compulsive behaviors) and are more susceptible to receiving negative feedback from caregivers, teachers, and/or peers (e.g., Kumar, Trescher, & Byler, 2016; Mautone, Lefler, & Power, 2011). Accordingly, this chapter presents a brief trans-diagnostic parent training (BTPT) program that is designed as a strengths-based parent-centered intervention for parents of youth with TS.

Our clinical experience suggests that this approach is well received by parents and youth alike, and results in positive outcomes.

This chapter provides an overview of BTPT. First, the importance of completing a comprehensive assessment is broadly discussed. Subsequently, the typical "reactive" approach to parenting is juxtaposed with the proactive approach. A case is made for why proactive parenting is considerably more effective and important for youth than reactive caregiving. The remainder of the chapter outlines the six-session BTPT protocol and its overarching aim to increase the child's adaptive and prosocial behavioral repertoire and secondarily, to extinguish maladaptive and noncompliant behaviors. Throughout, a case is made for why BTPT can be useful for any youth with TS who is exhibiting and/or experiencing problematic behaviors. A forthcoming BTPT manual, currently in development, will offer additional guidance for clinicians.

"SETTING THE STAGE" FOR TREATMENT

As described in Chapter 1, Introduction to Treatment and Management of Youth With Tourette Disorders and Tic Disorders, a comprehensive multimodal (e.g., clinical interviews, observations, questionnaires) and multiinformant (e.g., parents, teachers, youth) diagnostic assessment is a critical first step in delineating treatment targets (e.g., Cohen, Leckman, & Bloch, 2014). Assessments provide an opportunity for clinicians to nonjudgmentally assess parenting styles and any factors that might make the implementation of BTPT more challenging (e.g., psychiatric illness, marital discord). It is often useful for clinicians to "set the stage" for a collaborative and comprehensive assessment by informing parents about what is involved (e.g., format, time commitment) and the rationale for participation.

For example, clinicians may wish to use language (drawn from dialectical behavior therapy; Rathus & Miller, 2014) with parents such as:

> *"Although you are here to discuss your child's tics, I have found that it is helpful to tell families upfront that tics rarely occur in isolation. Many children with tics also experience other challenges, such as anxiety and/or impulsivity, which might be causing more problems for them than the tics themselves. Therefore, before we discuss treatment options, I recommend that you and your child participate in a comprehensive assessment. The purpose of this assessment is not to elicit blame or shame regarding your parenting style or to label your child as 'bad or lazy.' Instead, I operate from the perspective that you and your child are currently doing the best you can in very challenging circumstances, because if you knew of better approaches, you would be doing them. I also believe that your child wants to improve and that all parents and youth could benefit from learning strategies to help them do better. It is my hope that through this assessment we can develop a plan for improving your child's functioning."*

It is important to fully evaluate and appreciate parent characteristics as moderators to treatment outcome as these characteristics can lead to suboptimal patient outcomes or may serve to worsen the long-term prognosis by creating treatment resistance and further destabilization of the family. Therefore, it is advisable that clinicians complete a thorough and detailed family history and when appropriate make recommendations for individual therapy, medications, and/or marital therapy before beginning BTPT. Once the assessment is complete, clinicians should offer a comprehensive conceptualization of treatment targets that have led to patient/family problems while also highlighting the strengths of the child and family. The related discussion should be solution-focused and aimed at capitalizing on patient/family strengths.

TYPICAL "REACTIVE" PARENTING

Many parents rely on their own prior learning experiences with their family of origin, their personality, and/or school bus stop conversations to inform their parenting approach. At some time or another, all parents operate from the reactive (i.e., after-the-fact) end of the parenting spectrum. This may take the form of parents yelling at their child when the child has broken a household rule, or parents threatening their child by stating, "*If you don't do your homework, you won't be able to watch television for a week*." This approach can be effective when children are generally compliant, but many caregivers run the risk of unintentionally falling into a reactive, rigid, and inconsistent parenting pattern.

One operant conditioning principle that typifies reactive parenting is *negative reinforcement*. This occurs when an aversive stimulus (e.g., parent nagging) is removed after a particular behavior is exhibited (e.g., child completes his homework) and increases the likelihood of the behavior subsequently. Frequent parent prompts without follow-through can increase ignoring on the part of a child. For instance, if a child ignores his parent and is still allowed to play video games without completing his homework, the child maybe more likely to ignore the parent subsequently. Frustrated parents may become more persistent and repetitive in their prompts as their child's resistance increases. Hence, a cycle of conflict, reactivity, and hostility between the parent and child can emerge over time. This has been termed the *parent child coercive cycle*, which can lead to worsening behavior in youth, reduced effectiveness of parents, and damaged parent−child relationships (Lunkenheimer, Lichtwarck-Aschoff, Hollenstein, Kemp, & Granic, 2016; Patterson, 1982).

Positive punishment also dominates reactive parenting. This involves parents applying aversive stimuli (e.g., parents yelling, scolding, spanking) following a display of problematic behavior (e.g., a child hitting her sibling) with the hope of decreasing future episodes of the behavior. This approach, when used by parents sparingly can admittedly be very effective and may be appropriate in some circumstances. However, frequent utilization can quickly render the approach ineffective and may also contribute to the *parent child coercive cycle*. Moreover, these behaviors model verbal and physical aggression and erode parental authority.

Practice Guidelines

Clinicians often wonder how to talk with parents about the pitfalls of reactively parenting youth. It is important to approach parents in a nonjudgmental and directive manner. This approach is essential as parents often feel as though they are "bad parents" due to their current circumstances, and have children who are "bad or unmotivated." Providing validation and education to parents in a supportive manner are essential during these initially conversations, especially considering the stigma of mental illness and the sense of isolation many parents feel as a result.

Clinicians may wish to remind caregivers:

> *"Parenting is a daunting task, even in the best of circumstances. You are in an unusually demanding situation, raising a child with mental health conditions. As we talk about parenting, I want to emphasize that the all parents have a tendency to engage in reactive or after-the-fact parenting. That's because we are all 'hard-wired' to preferentially respond quickly and decisively to perceived threats in our environment, for example loud noises. Children with psychiatric illnesses tend to more frequently engage in problematic behaviors, which in turn draw more frequent parent attention and prompt more frequent responses like yelling 'Quiet!' The truth is that despite my expertise, I would probably be prone to adopt the same reactive approach to parenting if I was in your current situation. Yet the reactive style of parenting that most parents instinctively use quickly becomes ineffective in the exact circumstances in which you find yourself. My goal is to work together with you to develop a disciplined approach to parenting that all parents could benefit from, but is particularly important in the very challenging circumstance you find yourself in."*

PROACTIVE PARENTING

In contrast to reactive parenting, a better approach for youth with TS is proactive parenting. This approach involves parent anticipation of circumstances in which the child might find him/herself in, and provides the child with concrete guidance for appropriate behavior. Proactive parenting provides predictability, consistency, and warmth, which are at the core of secure parent–child relationships.

As with reactive parenting, operant conditioning principles can be used to describe the essential features of proactive parenting. The principles of *positive reinforcement* and *negative punishment* underlie proactive parenting and are used to supplant reliance on negative reinforcement and positive punishment, which characterize reactive parenting. Positive reinforcement is any favorable consequence to a behavior that increases the likelihood that the behavior will occur again in the future (Powell, Honey, & Symbaluk, 2017). For example, positive reinforcement includes rewarding a child with a treat after he/she takes out the garbage. Negative punishment involves removing access to reinforcing objects or activities following an undesirable behavior in an attempt to reduce the undesirable behavior in the future. For example, a child is sent to time-out on a chair or stair after fighting with his/her sibling. The consistent and contingent use of these two principles can quickly increase adaptive prosocial behaviors, decrease those that are more maladaptive, and are critical to adopting a proactive, strengths-based approach to parenting.

COMMON PITFALLS AND POTENTIAL SOLUTIONS

Most parents have heard of positive reinforcement and time-out. They often report that they have previously used these strategies, "*but they don't work.*" For parents who have "used" these strategies unsuccessfully, it is helpful to review common pitfalls that can minimize and/or negate the effectiveness of these approaches. These pitfalls include: (1) setting the criterion for reinforcement too high, (2) implementing ineffective reinforcement plans, (3) applying reinforcement inconsistently, (4) incorrect implementation of the time-out procedure, and (5) ineffectively managing extinction bursts.

Setting the Criterion Reinforcement Too High

Parents, teachers and even clinicians tend to operationalize an age-appropriate behavioral goal (e.g., a 10-year-old child remaining in his seat during dinner) and develop a behavioral plan with this goal in mind. Unfortunately for a 10-year-old with ADHD, the probability of the child meeting this expectation is low. Setting the criterion for behavior at or above the ceiling of a patient's current range of behaviors drastically limits the probability that the child and target behavior will receive reinforcement. This is often true even if the potential reinforcers are large, appealing, and enticing (e.g., getting a puppy). Reinforcers that are not experienced by the child will have little effect in shaping behavior. Therefore, prior to developing a behavioral plan, it is extremely important that clinicians help parents to first identify and systematically gather data on the patient's current displays of adaptive, prosocial, and functional behaviors (i.e., age-appropriate behaviors). In this way, children can be rewarded for successive approximations to the desired behaviors.

Ineffective Reinforcement Plans

A second pitfall involves the use of ineffective reinforcement plans, which include the use of prize bins, rewarding outcomes (vs effort), and incorrect use of time-out procedures. A "prize bin" is a container housing a number of different rewards that the child can earn contingent upon displaying desirable behaviors. While in theory a prize bin can be useful, children typically choose the most reinforcing objects first. Therefore, as parent expectations increase, the reinforcement generally decreases. Another ineffective plan involves basing the level of reinforcement upon the outcome versus the effort applied toward achieving that outcome. For example, in the case of a child with TS who is practicing competing response exercises (as part of behavioral treatment for tics), the criterion should be the attempt (or effort) to use the competing response to block the tic, instead of the absence of a tic.

Inconsistent Reinforcement

Optimal reinforcement occurs immediately following the target behavior, every time the target behavior occurs. When parents use inconsistent, delayed, and unpredictable reinforcement (i.e., the child is unsure which behavior is desired by the parent or what behavior is being reinforced), a youth's perception of predictability is devalued and children may become less responsive to the behavioral intervention.

Incorrect Use of Time-Out Procedures

Many parents report that they have used time-out as a punishment procedure with varying degrees of success. It is important to ask questions about the way in which time-out is applied. Common mistakes when applying time-out include: (1) providing many warnings to the child prior to the use of time-out, (2) failing to follow through with time-outs, (3) allowing the time-outs to occur in a location where the child has access to reinforcers (e.g., in a bedroom with toys), and (4) giving the child attention during time-out.

Inability to Tolerate Extinction Bursts

In the broadest sense, one of the biggest challenges to effectively implementing positive parenting strategies (e.g., positive reinforcement) is successfully coping with extinction bursts. Extinction bursts refer to the expected and temporary escalations in the frequency, duration, and/or intensity of the maladaptive "target" behavior (i.e., tantrums). Extinction bursts typically occur whenever parents change the contingency of reinforcement (e.g., withhold screen-time until the child has completed his/her homework). As a result, there is often an escalation in the child's more coercive behaviors (e.g., start screaming when the desired item is not achieved). Parents tend to find these escalations aversive, which in turn elicits reactive parenting tendencies and unintentionally reinforces the child's maladaptive behavior. It is important to remind parents that extinction bursts are expected and counter-intuitively serve as a sign that the intervention is working. However, parents will need help and support to "stay-the-course," tolerate the "burst" without reinforcing the child's undesirable behavior, and collaboratively develop a crisis plan with the clinician for responding to urgent/emergent behaviors that may occur in the context of an extinction burst.

PARENT MANAGEMENT TRAINING

BTPT for youth with TS can be characterized as an intervention within the broad domain of parent management training (PMT) approaches (Barkley, 1997; Kazdin, 2005), similar to other interventions including Parent–Child Interaction Therapy (Cooley, Veldorale-Griffin, Petren, & Mullis, 2014), the Incredible Years Parent Training (Menting, Orobio de Castro, & Matthys, 2013), Positive Parenting Program (de Graaf, Speetjens, Smit, de Wolff, & Tavecchio, 2008) and Parent Management Training—Oregon Model (Forgatch, Bullock, & Patterson, 2004). At its core, PMT focuses on helping parents deliver concise, calm, and specific instructions, provide positive reinforcement, improve children's compliance with parent commands, increase the ability of parents to set limits, and reduce family conflict. Indeed, PMT has been shown to be effective in reducing disruptive behaviors in youth with TS, ADHD, and ODD (Kazdin, 2005; Scahill et al., 2006).

BRIEF TRANS-DIAGNOSTIC PARENT TRAINING

BTPT is a strengths-based and parent-centered treatment designed for broad trans-diagnostic application in outpatient mental health settings. The central goals of BTPT are to equip parents with an optimal approach to parenting through (1) identifying current adaptive prosocial behaviors, (2) consistently redistributing parental attention and reinforcement toward adaptive behaviors, and (3) improving parental consistency with time-out and contingency plans. BTPT differs from other PMT approaches in that BTPT adopts a novel instructional method aimed at quickly teaching core operant conditioning principles and their application to parents in a directive and systematic manner. Relative to other forms of parent training, the primary treatment components of BTPT are not implemented sequentially. Instead, BTPT involves four planning sessions with parents before all treatment components are rolled out together.

It is important to keep in mind that BTPT is not intended to directly target a child's tics or specific psychiatric symptoms; however, BTPT may serve to indirectly reduce coercive maladaptive behaviors that are secondary to the emergence of psychopathology and possible family accommodation that may serve to exacerbate tics and/or other psychiatric symptoms. For example, BTPT does not attempt to reduce tics but instead may serve to decrease tic-associated family accommodation (e.g., child being relieved of chores if her tics are exacerbated) by increasing parental attention and reinforcement of adaptive prosocial behaviors (e.g., eating dinner with the family). This may in turn also increase the frequency of more sophisticated functional behaviors (e.g., engaging in conversation), thereby decreasing time spent distracted by irrelevant stimuli (e.g., urges) and associated nonfunctional behaviors (e.g., tics).

BTPT OVERVIEW

The BTPT protocol consists of six 45 minute treatment sessions. Although sessions are typically completed weekly, clinicians are encouraged to be flexible and use clinical judgment when implementing this protocol in practice. For instance, a clinician might consider completing three sessions a week for two weeks to accelerate treatment gains when clinically indicated.

BTPT is a parent-centered treatment. While the child can be in attendance for all six BTPT sessions, it is preferable to conduct sessions without children/adolescents as youth may become overly concerned with hypothetical situations and disrupt the process. Therefore, in most cases, Sessions 1–4 involve parents and Sessions 5 and 6 can involve both parents and their child.

Session 1 involves discussing the treatment rationale, providing instruction on identifying adaptive behaviors and subsequent collection of related baseline data, and emergency planning. *Session 2* involves reviewing collected baseline data, providing parents instruction for developing a behavioral plan, and addressing any barriers to the implementation of the contingency plan discussed in Session 1. *Session 3* involves discussion of a robust reinforcement procedure (i.e., token economy) to be coupled with the behavioral plan discussed in Session 2. *Session 4* involves providing an overview of the time-out procedure and the relation of the time-out procedure to the contingency plan discussed in Session 1. *Session 5* includes presentation of the behavioral plan, token economy, time-out, and contingency plan procedures to the child. Finally, *Session 6* is focused on an implementation review and transition to other symptom-specific, patient-center forms of CBT and related treatment targets (i.e., tics, ADHD, school problems, etc.). Additional follow-up sessions may be required to review the modified procedures and address additional barriers, although generally these goals can be accomplished at the outset of subsequent treatment appointments.

SESSION 1: TREATMENT OVERVIEW, DATA COLLECTION, AND EMERGENCY PLANNING

Goals

The goals of the first session are to establish rapport, offer a treatment rationale, provide parents with instruction on operationalizing and tracking of prosocial behaviors, and teach parents how to identify appropriate responses to urgent/emergent situations.

Treatment Rationale/Overview

Clinicians may wish to present the rationale for treatment by stating the following:

> *"Neuropsychiatric illnesses (e.g., TS) are different than acute medical ailments, such as a stomach virus, in that they are less common, unpredictably wax and wane (i.e., symptoms increase and decrease over time), are chronic, and have no cure. This can be confusing for parents who may respond reactively to neuropsychiatric illnesses in the way they have been socialized to respond to a stomach virus (e.g., let child stay home from school, bring child liquids). Consequently, caregivers are often at a loss regarding how to manage pediatric neuropsychiatric conditions and accompanying, treatment-interfering, disruptive behaviors. Parents may unwittingly fall into the trap of 'over-accommodating' over time (e.g., allowing a child to miss school if he or she has more tics than usual), which unfortunately can serve to further exacerbate symptoms and lead to the child adopting the 'sick role.'*
>
> *It is also important to consider that youth with neuropsychiatric illnesses tend to receive more negative feedback, peer rejection, disciplinary actions, and less praise compared to children without these conditions. This pattern of interacting with the world can impact youth self-esteem and make youth question whether they have any strengths.*
>
> *Therefore, over the course of our sessions together, we are going to discuss a method to shape your child's behavior through a proactive parenting approach, so that over time positive behaviors are rewarded, strengths are identified and acknowledged, and negative behaviors are extinguished.*
>
> *Today, we are going to start to identify all the things that your child is already doing that are adaptive and/or prosocial. Additionally, we are also going to discuss ways to help you to safely 'ride out the storm' when your child displays the most challenging behaviors. More specifically, we will create a protocol for those impromptu 'emergency' situations (e.g., your child threatens to kill himself) so that moving forward you have a consistent plan to follow in the unlikely event that the need arises.*
>
> *It is important to remember that these strategies will not eliminate all your child's negative behaviors or directly target tic symptoms. However, when used*

correctly, this treatment will significantly reduce problematic and disruptive behaviors, minimize treatment interfering behaviors that can impede therapeutic skill acquisition, and likely improve the overall quality of life for your child and family."

Identification and Tracking of Adaptive Prosocial Behaviors

Parents are informed that the first step of BTPT is to identify and monitor prosocial behaviors to promote/reinforce that the child is already engaging in. To elicit these targets, parents should be guided by the clinician in the identification and operationalization of adaptive, prosocial behaviors that the patient displays at an appropriate base rate (i.e., greater than 80% of the time). For illustrating to parents, it is often helpful to focus on the morning routine, as school day mornings are often the most circumscribed and time-delimited. Parents are then asked to choose two or three additional prosocial behaviors that occur during another time frame (e.g., after school routines) and operationally define these behaviors with assistance. Parents are then instructed to operationally define additional adaptive prosocial behaviors that typically occur throughout the afternoon, dinner, and evening routines on their own following the session. Parents should record whether these behaviors occurred, as operationalized, between sessions. Table 11.1 provides an example of the morning routine and the beginning of an afternoon routine.

TABLE 11.1 Operationalizing and Tracking Current Adaptive Behaviors

Time Frame	Behavior	Completed	
		Monday	Tuesday
Morning	Wakes up		
	Eats breakfast		
	Brushes teeth		
	Uses the bathroom		
	Dresses himself		
	Discards paper napkin in the trash		
Afternoon	Eats snack		
	Completes homework		
________	*Additional adaptive behaviors observed*: ________________		

In addition to tracking of the aforementioned behaviors, parents are asked to record any spontaneous positive behaviors that they observe for each subsequent day (e.g., the child helped clean up his toys after school) and note the time frames in which these behaviors occurred (e.g., after school, after dinner). Parents are then provided with some preliminary coaching about how to effectively praise their child for engaging in the adaptive behaviors. Parents are encouraged to consider timing of praise (i.e., immediately following the positive behavior) and to be specific and genuine with verbal praise. For example, "*I really like the way you helped your sister make her breakfast.*"

Development of a Contingency Plan for Emergent/Urgent Behaviors

While a goal of BTPT is to use proactive and planned approaches to behavior modification, there will be times when unsafe, emergent behaviors unpredictably arise. Therefore, following the discussion about identifying, tracking, and labeling prosocial behaviors, the second central component of this session involves helping parents to develop a robust and noncoercive contingency plan/protocol for emergency situations when the child poses risk to self or others (e.g., suicidal ideation, self-harm, physical aggression) or displays sufficiently poor judgment that calls into question their safety. It is important to remind parents that these plans will likely not be needed, but will be developed to proactively ensure the safety of the child and those around him or her.

Most parents are readily able to identify obvious emergencies. While BTPT is not intended to directly address tics, the contingency plan may serve an important function in extinguishing the most severe and harmful tics a child displays. Often the most challenging situation parent's face is when a child displays poor judgment as a result of their condition(s). For example, a mother of a child who displays complex self-injurious tics (e.g., dropping to his knees abruptly whenever he walks on a concrete surface) might be at a loss for how to help her child in this situation. Parents often report that while they have been told that tics are involuntary and to ignore their child's tics if the tics do not cause their child distress, they are nevertheless distressed by watching their child engage in recurrent tics that cause obvious harm (e.g., bruised and bloodied kneecaps) and experience tremendous upset not responding to these behaviors. For youth who have not learned tic management strategies or are unable to appropriately utilize these strategies, parents are encouraged to consider displays of self-injurious tics as an urgent situation, which may require utilization of the emergency procedure. The purpose of the emergency procedure is to assure the child's safety and to concretely demonstrate to the child that these behaviors are unsafe regardless of their cause (i.e., a symptom of TS) and must be responded to appropriately. In this instance, parents would be advised to first encourage the child to move to a soft surface to reduce the potential for harm. However, if the child refuses or is unresponsive to several re-directs, parents would be advised to physically restrain the child and take them to the nearest emergency department (ED). Should they be uncertain about their capacity to safely restrain and/or transport the child to the ED, emergency personnel should be contacted to safely transport the child with parents following behind. When used appropriately and consistently, contingency plans are an important consideration in reducing the potential for subsequent unsafe behavior.

Homework

Session homework includes asking parents to operationally define, surreptitiously record, and verbally praise their child's high-rate adaptive behaviors as well as implement the contingency plan (as needed).

SESSION 2: DEVELOPMENT OF A ROBUST BEHAVIORAL PLAN

Goals

The goals of this session include: (1) review the operational definitions that were arrived at last session and those that were derived by the parents in the interim, (2) review of Session 1 homework (i.e., baseline data collected over the past week) to ensure that the parents appropriately set the criterion for reinforcement and modifying as necessary, (3) provide the rationale and instruction for the development of a daily behavioral routine, and (4) begin discussion of potential challenges foreseen in implementing the behavioral plan.

Homework Review

A review of the homework should elicit successes and challenges that occurred over the previous week, facilitate learning, and encourage parent investment in BTPT (e.g., emphasize that the parent, not clinician, chooses behaviors to track and shape). Clinicians should also review, with parents, the operationally defined prosocial behaviors (from Session 1) and the data collected during the past week.

It is often helpful to provide additional instruction when parents report that the child displayed a prosocial behavior (e.g., "completing all homework") infrequently over the past week. A further discussion might reveal that the child completed *all* his/her homework 50% of the days, but consistently completed all math homework daily. In this situation, parents could be instructed to modify the criterion behavior to "completes math homework" or for younger children and/or those with reduced workloads in the context of an Individualized Education Plan "completes a math problem."

Behavioral Plan Rationale

The first step in helping parents develop a behavioral plan is providing a compelling rationale. Parents may underestimate the importance of structure and routine in a healthy and effective lifestyle. In part, because daily routines can and often do become layered and complex as familiarity with one's environment/roles increases, many adults may not fully appreciate how routine their lives are and how these routines enable them to cope effectively with life demands. In reality most adults have developed modular routines that can and are readily swapped out as needed. For instance, the typical Wednesday evening trip to the gym routine can be easily replaced by the Sunday morning grocery shopping routine to prepare for Thanksgiving.

Most parents benefit from a discussion that highlights how their own routines serve critically important functions and allow them to lead productive and fulfilling lives. Clinicians should appreciate that most parents have not made these links and therefore making the link explicit is an important task. For example, this may include stating:

> *"In addition to knowing what is expected of us, we all benefit from structure and routine. Most successful adults are able to readily impose structure in their lives and often do so by developing behavioral routines, which serve to increase the speed and efficiency with which tasks are completed. The development of structure and routine is especially important for youth with challenging behaviors in part because their behaviors often lead even the most discipline parents to behave reactively and unpredictably. As a result the use of external structures and supports is critically important to increasing predictability for these youth. Moreover, routines structure our activities, facilitate efficiency, and provide a comfort through familiarity. Therefore, today we are going to spend some time discussing your child's daily routine."*

Behavioral Plan Development

After the rationale is discussed, clinicians provide parents with instruction in creating daily routines (e.g., morning, after school, dinner, and bedtime). It is recommended that the discussion begin with the morning routine for illustration. Parents are asked when the child needs to be awake and when the child needs to leave the house for school. The provided times are then used as start-stop times for the morning routine. Behaviors that have been previously operationalized and tracked (e.g., getting dressed) and which correspond to the targeted time frame (e.g., morning routine) are then listed (see Table 11.2), in sequential order.

TABLE 11.2 Behavioral Routine Data Collection

Time Frame	Behavior	Completed	
		Monday	Tuesday
7:00 a.m. to 8:10 a.m.			
Work (required behaviors)	Wakes up with <5 prompts	✓	
	Urinates in the toilet	✓	✓
	Brushes teeth with presented tooth brush with paste applied	✓	✓
	Dresses himself in clothes laid out the night before by parents	✓	✓
	Eats >40% of provided breakfast	✓	✓
	Discards paper napkin in the trash	✓	✓
Play (reward)	Preferred activity (e.g., book, TV)		
8:20 a.m. to 3:20 p.m.	School	–	–
3:20 p.m. to 6:00 p.m.			
Work (required behaviors)	Unpack back pack (trash in garbage)	✓	✓
	Wash hands with soap and water	✓	✓
	Eat snack provided by parents		✓
	Plate in sink/napkin in garbage <3 reminders	✓	✓
	Complete Math homework	✓	✓
Play (reward)	Preferred activity (e.g., book, TV)		
6:00 p.m. to 7:30 p.m.			
Work (required behaviors)	Wash hands with soap and water	✓	
	Set table for dinner	✓	✓
	Clear own dishes	✓	✓
Play (reward)	Preferred activity (e.g., book, TV)		
7:30 p.m. to 9:00 p.m.	Finish remaining homework	✓	✓
Work (required behaviors)	Take shower	✓	✓
	Brush teeth	✓	✓
	Put on pajamas	✓	✓
	Lights out by 8:30 p.m.		
	Additional adaptive behaviors observed:		
	Billy helped his sister make breakfast	✓	
	Billy calmly handled his disappointment when he could not go to the pool		✓

Following implementation (between Session 5 and 6), parents are encouraged to help the child to complete the tasks in sequential order. Only after successful completion of tasks included in each routine, parents should allow their child access to preferred activities (e.g., toys) with the time remaining (such as for 15 minutes between completion of the morning routine and leaving for school). This encourages children to complete the routine more efficiently over time.

Possible Barriers to Implementation

It is recommended that clinicians validate that, in practice, behavior plans can be very challenging to initiate and implement. Consequently, it is important to recognize that many parents will struggle to develop structure and routine in their own lives. Clinicians should carefully consider the degree to which a parent's failure to establish structure and routines is due to their own difficulties versus difficulties that arise from attempting to parent under duress. Parents who have personal histories that suggest they are generally free from impairment typically develop and implement structure with expert consultation easily. Meanwhile, parents with significant personal functional difficulties may require more assistance and/or their own concurrent treatment.

Homework

Similar to homework in Session 1, parents are asked to surreptitiously track, via check marks, the completion of adaptive prosocial behaviors contained within the behavior plan, using a chart akin to Table 11.2. Parents are also encouraged to continue verbally praising their child's displays of adaptive behaviors.

SESSION 3: INTRODUCTION AND DEVELOPMENT OF A TOKEN ECONOMY

Goals

The objectives of this session include: (1) reviewing homework and making changes to operational definitions (as needed), (2) altering the routine and re-sequencing behavior (as needed), (3) providing information regarding operant conditioning principles and their application to shaping children's behaviors, and (4) providing instruction regarding the development and prospective implementation of a token economy.

Homework Review

Homework review is similar to Session 2. Questions regarding the tracking of the operationalized behaviors are addressed. Parents are reinforced for surreptitiously tracking operationalized behaviors, verbally praising the patient, and enacting the contingency plan (as needed).

Rationale for a Token Economy

Prior to introducing the token economy, it can be helpful to teach parents about the concept of positive reinforcement and provide some examples. For example, clinicians may wish to say:

> *"One particularly effective way to motivate and shape behavior is through positive reinforcement. Most parents are aware of this idea although it is often helpful to review exactly what this concept means. Positive reinforcement occurs when someone engages in a behavior (e.g., a car salesperson sells a car) and is then rewarded for that behavior (e.g., commission). When the reward is contingent upon a specific set of behaviors, it consequently reinforces those behaviors, increasing the likelihood that those behaviors will occur in the future."*

Most parents have discretionary funds that are used for entertainment, gifts, etc. To varying degrees, a portion of this spending is directed toward children. However, parents may not fully appreciate the potential of their discretionary spending to shape their child's behavior. While parents may at some level be consciously attempting to reinforce their child's more desirable behaviors, current attempts may fall short due to inadequate implementation of behavioral principles. In fact, when the topic of a token economy arises, parents often report things like "*I've tried that, it doesn't work.*" What most parents do not recognize is that their reward plans were likely insufficient because they were also unknowingly reinforcing a whole host of less desirable behaviors including coercive or maladaptive behaviors. The key issues revolve around inadvertently reinforcing problematic behavior and/or noncontingent reinforcement.

To broach the topic of token economies, it is important to begin by reminding parents that their role as parents and our role as clinicians is centrally to ensure that their child grows up to be a fully functioning, happy, healthy, and productive adult. Most parents are agreeable to this long-term goal. A sample script for introducing the rationale for token economies is:

> *"The job analogy I provided earlier is an example of positive reinforcement in the real world. In our capitalistic society the rules are pretty simple. For the most part, if you do, you get; if you don't do, you don't get. As harsh as it may seem, the real world does not view psychiatric challenges as excuses for inappropriate behavior or reasons why demands should be reduced or diminished.*

While there are exceptions to this rule, such as disability benefits, disability is not a good outcome for your child. Therefore, it is especially important for your child to learn that they can do things despite or in spite of their illnesses. To do this, we like to develop a 'token economy' in which your child will be rewarded via tokens that are 'contingent' on their more desirable behaviors. The tokens will serve as symbolic of the 'currency' by which preferred activities or items are acquired, just like in the real world."

Addressing Common Concerns About Token Economies

Parents often ask, "*Shouldn't children be protected from the harsh realities of the real world?*" The answer is yes, we should protect them, but not in a way that is misleading and ill-prepares them for dealing with the demands of adult life. Noncontingent reinforcement breeds the notion that it does not matter what you do, you will still get the desired outcome. This learning experience can result in ineffective, dissatisfied young adults who persist in the notion that the world should and might change to suit them. Instead, it is suggested that token economies can be used to teach important life lessons, while protecting children from the real world (i.e., if they fail to earn tokens, they will not go hungry).

Parents also raise the notion that token economies are a form of "bribery." Therefore, it is important to remind parents that the goal of the token economy is to create a mechanism to measure progress toward treatment goals and provide reinforcement contingent on that progress. Treatment goals must always be in the best interest of the patient and must never be used to serve the prerogative of another, as then it would constitute bribery. A properly designed token economy serves to reward the patient for meeting an expectation that is ultimately in his/her best interest.

Development of a Token Economy

After providing the rationale and introduction to token economies, the clinician and parents work collaboratively to develop an individualized token economy to parallel the behavioral plan developed between Sessions 2 and 3. It is helpful for parents to determine a metric for reinforcement that will be easy for children to understand. Parents are typically encouraged to use a token economy whereby tokens (e.g., points) are exchanged for *both* an allowance (i.e., money) and screen-time (i.e., television, video games, etc.). For instance, the concept that 1 point is equal to 1 cent *and* 1 minute of screen-time is an easy calculus for most youth. Simple, relatively well-established, behaviors (e.g., brushing teeth) could be associated with fewer points (i.e., 1 point) and more complex behaviors (e.g., making breakfast) should be associated with more points (i.e., 3 or 5 points).

Table 11.3 provides an example for how token economies can be implemented in the context of the previously developed behavioral routine.

TABLE 11.3 Token Economy as Applied to the Behavioral Routine

Time Frame	Behavior	Points	
		(Possible)	(Earned)
			Monday
7:00 a.m. to 8:10 a.m.			
Work (required behaviors)	Wakes up with <5 prompts	(1)	1
	Urinates in the toilet	(1)	1
	Brushes teeth with presented tooth brush with paste applied	(2)	2
	Dresses himself in clothes laid out the night before by parents	(3)	0
	Eats >40% of provided breakfast	(4)	4
	Discards paper napkin in the trash	(5)	5
	Took out the garbage without being asked		20
Sub total		(16)	33
Play (reward)	Preferred activity (e.g., book, legos, or TV for 33 minutes)		
8:20 a.m. to 3:20 p.m.	School	–	–
3:20 p.m. to 6:00. p.m.			
Work (required behaviors)	Unpack back pack (trash in garbage)	(1)	1
	Wash hands with soap and water	(1)	1
	Eat snack provided by parents	(2)	2
	Plate in sink/napkin in garbage <3 reminders	(3)	0
	Complete Math homework	(3)	3
Sub total		(10)	7
Play (reward)	Preferred activity (e.g., book, TV)		
6:00 p.m. to 7:30 p.m.			

(Continued)

TABLE 11.3 (Continued)

Time Frame	Behavior	Points	
		(Possible)	(Earned)
			Monday
Work (required behaviors)	Wash hands with soap and water	(1)	1
	Set table for dinner	(3)	3
	Clear own dishes	(3)	3
Sub total		(7)	7
Play (reward)	Preferred activity (e.g., book, TV)		
7:30 p.m. to 9:00 p.m.	Finish remaining homework	(5)	5
Work (required behaviors)	Take shower	(2)	2
	Brush teeth	(2)	2
	Put on pajamas	(3)	3
	Lights out by 8:30 p.m.	(5)	5
Sub total		(17)	17
	Additional adaptive behaviors observed:		
	Billy dealt with disappointments calmly		15
Grand total		(50)	79

Parents are asked to consider whether the plan appears to be reasonable and their constraints around the use of screen-time (e.g., during certain time frames only). For consistency and predictability for the child, it is also important that parents consider a reliable pay day/time (e.g., Fridays after school) to exchange tokens for money.

Parents are reminded that when they implement the plan (following Session 5), it is vital to provide children with enough reinforcement that the youth "buys-in" to the token economy. In addition to providing points for hygiene and chores listed on the behavior plan, it can be helpful to encourage parents to liberally dispense "bonus points" for identified behaviors which encourages accelerated growth. For instance, a child may receive 15 bonus points for calmly responding to a stressor, which will help the child to understand the relative importance of this behavior compared to others (e.g., 2 points for brushing teeth). Parents are encouraged to write down questions and bring them to future sessions.

Homework

Weekly homework involves modifying the behavioral plan (as needed), determining point values associated with each behavior on the plan, and beginning to surreptitiously track points earned according to the rules of the token economy. Of note, parents do not share the details of these points with their child until the token economy/behavior plan is unveiled to the youth in Session 5.

SESSION 4: DEVELOPMENT OF AN EFFECTIVE AND SUPPORTIVE TIME-OUT PROCEDURE

Goals

The purposes of this session are: (1) to review homework and address any challenges related to the devised token economy and its association with the behavioral plan, (2) to provide instruction on the time-out procedure, and (3) to link the time-out procedure to the contingency plan for urgent/emergent behaviors (discussed in Session 1).

Homework Review

At session outset, the behavioral plan and accompanying token economy are reviewed in detail for content and appropriateness. Consistent with previous sessions, related issues are discussed and parent questions are addressed.

Time-Out Rationale/Overview

Clinicians may wish to introduce the rationale for time-outs by stating

> *"Time-outs can be an effective form of behavior modification when used appropriately, consistently, and in conjunction with the other strategies you are learning in BTPT. Time-outs involve removing all reinforcement for a short period of time because the child is briefly placed in a neutral (i.e., nonreinforcing) environment. Most parents use a child's bedroom for time-out; however, because the child's bedroom often allows the child free access to an array of potential reinforcers (i.e., toys, books, video-games) and escape from the rants of parents, it actually may reinforce and therefore increase the likelihood of the precise behavior it is meant to extinguish.*
>
> *While the spirit of BTPT is to primarily reinforce adaptive prosocial behaviors, there are several categories of intolerable behavior that are unacceptable, regardless of the origin. These include physical and verbal aggression, property destruction, and blatant violation of rules, norms, values, and laws. There is some variability in what is considered unacceptable based on the family environment and culture. Consequently, we will work together to determine*

what constitutes inappropriate behavior for your child, so that your child does not experience perpetual time-outs, which would undermine our efforts.

Overtime, we will be raising expectations for the child's behavior via the behavior plan and token economy. We, likewise, will progressively lower the threshold for time-out. For instance, initially a child may be placed in time-out only when he/she has actually damaged property (e.g., kicked a hole in the wall); however, he/she may eventually receive a similar punishment for slamming a door in anger. In summary, the goal of time-out is to quickly extinguish maladaptive behaviors and provide a space for a child to de-escalate. Time-outs are used in combination with the other BTPT strategies, which attempt to replace maladaptive behaviors with more adaptive, prosocial ones."

Specifications of Time-Out Implementation

Parents are then taught key principles to consider when implementing time-outs to ensure that this popular discipline strategy is not misused. In short, the use of a predetermined time-out chair or stair located where parents can readily observe the child while completing other tasks should be encouraged. It is helpful if parents remember that the time-out location should be devoid of reinforcers and because children often initially escalate when the procedure is enacted, the location should be a safe distance from important and/or fragile objects that could be damaged and/or used to hurt oneself with. With the exception of commands, there are no warnings before the time-out procedure is enacted. It is helpful to recommend that parents adopt a mantra like "*Since you hit your brother, you get a time-out.*" It is important to remind parents that once those words are uttered, a time-out should ensue irrespective of changes in the child's behavior (i.e., he/she stops hitting his/her brother). It is helpful to remind parents that time-outs are most effective if they immediately follow the problematic behavior. Ideally, children will eventually learn to walk themselves to the time-out location; however, in most cases they will initially need to be escorted by parents to the time-out location. Once the child has arrived at the time-out location he/she must not leave until the time-out is complete. After providing the reason, parents should not rationalize with their child or change the plan. Time-outs should be brief. A good rule-of-thumb that considers child development is 1 minute for each year of a child's life (e.g., an 8-year-old receiving an 8 minute time-out). Time-outs should be followed by a return to positive parental attention in the form of "processing out" of time-out, that is, parents inquiring with the child about what he/she did wrong, what he/she might do instead, and formulating/delivering apologies to those affected. It is important for parents to ask the child what he or she did wrong, what he or she should do next time, and for apologies to occur.

Leaving the chair or stair for even a moment should result in the child being escorted to the "back-up room." The back-up room is a predetermined room in the house that has a door and is devoid of potentially reinforcing activities, treasured items (i.e., family heirlooms), objects that could be used to hurt oneself, or that could potentially damage property (i.e., water source). It is important to caution that the back-up room is often used when a child is most upset. Parents may struggle to determine a suitable location. It is important to consider that a child's room can easily become a back-up room if all reinforcers (e.g., toys, video games) are temporarily removed. Back-up rooms are most frequently required when the time-out procedure is initially instituted. With contingent and reliable implementation, children quickly learn to serve their time-out on the chair or stair and the back-up room becomes less relevant. While back-up rooms must have a door, the door should never be locked. Instead, a parent should remain outside the room holding the doorknob if necessary. It is often a good idea to have a chair, water, and reading materials for parents outside of the back-up room.

Hesitation with Time-Out Implementation

Despite three decades of research showing that time-outs can be effective in decreasing aggressive behaviors in youth (see Borduin Quetsch, Wallace, Herschell, & McNeil, 2015 for a review), the use of time-outs remains a controversial strategy. For example, Siegel and Bryson (2014) published a widely distributed article in Time Magazine scorning time-outs by stating that it adversely impacts a child's attachment and neuroplasticity. However, Siegel and Bryson (2014) failed to account for the large volume of scientific research supporting the use of time-outs as a safe and effective method of discipline or acknowledge that time-out procedures have been endorsed by a variety of professional societies including the American Academy of Pediatrics (1998). Time-outs are generally inappropriate for children under three years of age (e.g., Australian Association for Infant Mental Health, 2009) and over the age of 9–12 years. However, developmental age should be considered instead of chronological age (Webster-Stratton, 2017).

Parents often need to be reminded that many of the behaviors that require a time-out happen for a reason, but the reason matters little. Coercive behaviors (physical aggression, verbal aggression, intentional property destruction, and blatant violation of rules, norms, values, and laws) typically serve a function. While often very effective in producing immediate and dramatic change in the environment, they are particularly maladaptive. It is best to assume that initially these behaviors are not calculated, premeditated, or malicious; however, the longer they persist, the more they shape and are shaped by the environment. If left unchecked, these behaviors can become mainstays of a child's behavioral repertoire and are increasingly voluntary responses intended to impact the environment. The goal of the time-out is to quickly extinguish these maladaptive behaviors and to replace them with more adaptive, prosocial behaviors via the behavioral plan and token economies.

It is not uncommon for parents to discount the inappropriateness of even quite egregious behaviors, particularly if they believe it to be related to the child's condition. Too often, the presence of psychiatric conditions pushes against and extends the boundaries of acceptable behavior. The result is that many parents fail to respond appropriately to these behaviors. It is not uncommon to hear "*he does that because he's anxious*" or "*I think it's a tic.*" Confusion on the part of parents leads to a failure to appropriately respond to inappropriate, maladaptive, and even dangerous behavior, which unintentionally encourages more frequent and extreme behavioral displays. It is important to help parents to appreciate that while the child's condition may be associated with the development of coercive behaviors, failure to respond on those behaviors places the child (and potentially others) at considerable risk. For instance, as a practical matter, it matters very little *why* a person screams "bomb!" in an airport or on an airplane. While a diagnosis of TS may ultimately help to mitigate legal ramifications, it does little to protect the individual and/or public at the moment the behavior occurs. While it is true that we have an obligation to educate the public as to the nature of TS and common cooccurring psychiatric disorders, it is neither beneficial nor reasonable to change the public's expectations for acceptable behavior.

Linking the Time-Out Procedure and Contingency Plan

Parents are cautioned that when they implement the behavioral plan with their child following Session 5, they should be prepared for the possibility of an extinction burst (previously described). During the burst, parents may have a tendency to abandon the plan and inadvertently negatively reinforce their child's maladaptive behaviors (e.g., withdraw expectations or demands until the child has been appeased). Therefore, the use of a contingency plan can be especially important for containing extinction bursts. Furthermore, the plan may be necessary for managing unsafe psychiatric symptoms and coping with unsafe behaviors during a time-out procedure. With regard to the latter situation, sometimes youth with challenging behaviors may feel that a given time-out is not warranted and consequently, may engage in self-harm behaviors while in time-out or following the time-out procedure. In these situations, a contingency plan involving emergency personnel could help to interrupt the cycle of maladaptive/unsafe behaviors.

Homework

Homework involves continuing to track prosocial behaviors within the behavior plan and surreptitiously allotting the associated token economy points. Parents are also asked to consider when and how they would apply the time-out procedure with their child. Of note, the time-out procedure and behavioral plan are implemented following Session 5.

SESSION 5: INTRODUCTION OF PLAN TO CHILD AND WEEK 1 FULL IMPLEMENTATION

Goals

The central goal of this session is for the parents to "unveil" the developed behavior plan, token economy, and time-out procedure to the youth and to address the youth's questions and concerns. A plan for implementation is also discussed.

Introducing the Plan to the Youth

Of note, prior to this session, while the youth may be aware that their parent was participating in BTPT, the child is usually not aware of the specific content of the previous four sessions. The clinician may start the session by asking that child what he/she knows about the BTPT sessions that his/her parents have been attending. The clinician could then state, "*We have been meeting about you and better yet, we have almost exclusively been talking about all the wonderful things that you already do*!" The clinician should encourage parents to share with their child what they have learned in the last four sessions and then help ensure that the family has a clear plan for implementation of the strategies over the week (e.g., how the points will be tracked for prosocial behaviors, when the child can trade in points). Clinicians must ensure that families have realistic expectations for the first week of implementation (i.e., expect some challenges as the child adjusts to this new routine/plan).

Implementation Barriers

Prior to this session, parents may be concerned that their child may not "buy-in" to the behavioral plan, especially if the child is already receiving rewards without any behavioral expectations. While this barrier will be discussed further in a forthcoming BTPT manual, the experience of clinicians using BTPT has demonstrated that this concern is usually unjustified. Instead, youth are often pleasantly surprised to hear that their parents have been recording their positive rather than problem behaviors. Typically, children hop on board with the plan especially when told that if they accept the plan, they will receive rewards based on their behavior that parents have tracked surreptitiously over the preceding week. In reality, one of the most appealing aspects of the behavioral plan for youth is the opportunity to have enhanced and predictable access to reinforcers (e.g., the child knows that every time he/she completes a behavior, he/she can expect a specified amount of allowance and screen-time).

Homework

Homework involves the implementation of the behavioral plan, token economy, time-out procedure, and when necessary, the emergency plan. Parents are encouraged to record any questions, concerns, or challenges that arise over the interim for discussion at the outset of Session 6.

SESSION 6: REVIEW AND ADDRESS BARRIERS

Goals

The purpose of this session is to review implementation of the plan and address any questions, concerns, or challenges that arise over the interim.

Homework Review/Session Content

Clinicians should provide an opportunity for the parents and the child to reflect on how the implementation of the plan went over the past week. Clinicians are encouraged to validate efforts at using new approaches and model appropriate use and delivery of praise. During the homework review, clinicians should be listening for fidelity and adherence to the plan. Although there are times that the child may refuse to comply with the plan, parents should be encouraged not to abandon their efforts thereby reinforcing higher levels of coercive behaviors.

The content covered in this session can occur at each subsequent appointment until the parents and the clinician agree that the parent has the capacity to successfully shape the patient's behaviors. Any additional sessions should involve both the parents and youth. Generally, additional sessions focus on implementation support and the consideration of other adaptive behaviors to shape.

EVALUATING TREATMENT OUTCOMES

The most proximal measure of BTPT success is when the child is earning more points each subsequent week for the successful completion of prosocial behaviors, while time-outs/removal of privileges are reduced substantially. Clinicians could also consider use of the parent-rated Home Situations Questionnaire (Barkley, 1997), Behavior Management Self-Assessment (August, Realmuto, Crosby, & MacDonald, 1995), Disruptive Behavior Rating Scale (Barkley, 1997), and/or the clinician-rated Clinical Global Impression-Severity scale (Guy, 1976) as pre–post outcome measures.

CONCLUSION

In summary, this chapter presented an overview of BTPT, an intervention inspired by the lack of trans-diagnostic treatment options for youth with TS. One goal of BTPT is to help caregivers recognize that typical and reactive approaches to parenting can be ineffective for youth with TS who are exhibiting problematic behavior. Accordingly, BTPT empowers parents to use a more proactive, strengths-based parenting approach and to become experts in shaping youth behaviors toward prosocial responses and away from maladaptive behaviors. The results of this technique include increased capacity of parents to shape their child's complex behavior including psychiatric symptoms.

ACKNOWLEDGMENTS

The authors would like to express their gratitude to Dr. Laura Skriner for her review of an earlier draft of this chapter.

REFERENCES

Abi-Jaoude, E., & Gorman, D. (2012). 5 things to know about Tourette Syndrome. *Canadian Medical Association Journal, 185*(3), 236.

American Academy of Pediatrics: Committee on Psychological Aspects of Child and Family Health. (1998). Guidance for effective discipline. *Pediatrics, 101*(4 Pt 1), 723–728.

American Psychiatric Association. (2013). *Diagnostic and statistical manual of mental disorders: DSM-5*. Washington, DC: American Psychiatric Association.

August, G. J., Realmuto, G. M., Crosby, R. D., & MacDonald, A. W. (1995). Community-based multiple-gate screening for children at risk for conduct disorder. *Journal of Abnormal Child Psychology, 23*, 521–544.

Australian Association for Infant Mental Health. (July 2009). *Position Pager 3: Time Out*. Retrieved from http://www.aaimhi.org/inewsfiles/Position%20Paper%203.pdf.

Barkley, R. A. (1997). *Defiant children: A clinician's manual for assessment and parent training* (2nd ed.). New York: Guilford Press.

Barkley, R. A. (2013). *Taking charge of ADHD: The complete, authoritative guide for parents*. New York: Guilford Press.

Bernard, B., Stebbins, G., Siegel, S., Schultz, T. M., Hays, C., Morrissey, M. J., ... Goetz, C. G. (2009). Determinants of quality of life in children with Gilles de la Tourette syndrome. *Movement Disorders, 24*, 1070–1073.

Bitsko, R. H., Holbrook, J. R., Visser, S. N., Mink, J. W., Zinner, S. H., Ghandour, R. M., & Blumberg, S. J. (2014). A national profile of Tourette Syndrome, 2011–2012. *Journal of Developmental and Behavioral Pediatrics, 35*(5), 317–322.

Borduin Quetsch, L., Wallace, N., Herschell, A., & McNeil, C. (2015). Weighing in on the time-out controversy: An empirical perspective. *The Clinical Psychologist, 68*(2), 4–19.

Budman, C., Rockmore, L., Stokes, J., & Sossin, M. (2003). Clinical phenomenology of episodic rage in children with Tourette Syndrome. *Journal of Psychosomatic Research, 55*, 59–65.

Cavanna, A. E., & Rickards, H. (2013). The psychopathological spectrum of Gilles de la Tourette Syndrome. *Neuroscience & Biobehavioral Reviews, 37*, 1008–1015.

Chovil, N. (2009). *Engaging families in child and youth mental health: A review of best, emerging, and promising practices.* Retrieved from http://heretohelp.bc.ca/sites/default/files/images/FamilyEngagement_LitRev.pdf.

Cohen, S., Leckman, J., & Bloch, M. (2014). Clinical assessment of Tourette syndrome and tic disorders. *Neuroscience Biobehavioral Review, 37*(6), 997–1007.

Cooley, M., Veldorale-Griffin, A., Petren, R., & Mullis, A. (2014). Parent–child interaction therapy: A meta-analysis of child behavior outcomes and parent stress. *Journal of Family Social Work, 17*(3), 191–208.

de Graaf, I., Speetjens, P., Smit, F., de Wolff, M., & Tavecchio, L. (2008). Effectiveness of the triple p positive parenting program on behavioral problems in children: A metaanalysis. *Behavior Modification, 32*(5), 553–566.

Forgatch, M. S., Bullock, B. M., & Patterson, G. R. (2004). From theory to practice: Increasing effective parenting through role-play. The Oregon Model of Parent Management Training (PMTO). In H. Steiner (Ed.), *Handbook of mental health interventions in children and adolescents: An integrated developmental approach* (pp. 782–814). San Francisco: Jossey-Bass.

Guy, W. (1976). *Clinical Global Impression Scales (CGI). ECDEU assessment manual for psychopharmacology (Publication 76-338).* Washington, DC: Department of Health, Education, and Welfare.

Kazdin, A. (2005). *).* Parent management training: Treatment for oppositional, aggressive, and antisocial behavior in children and adolescents. New York: Oxford University Press.

Kumar, A., Trescher, W., & Byler, D. (2016). Tourette syndrome and comorbid neuropsychiatric conditions. *Current Developmental Disorders Reports, 3*(4), 217–221.

Lunkenheimer, E., Lichtwarck-Aschoff, A., Hollenstein, T., Kemp, C., & Granic, I. (2016). Breaking down the coercive cycle: How parent and child risk factors influence real-time variability in parental responses to child misbehavior. *Parenting, Science and Practice, 16*(4), 237–256.

Mautone, J., Lefler, K., & Power, T. (2011). Promoting family and school success for children with ADHD: Strengthening relationships while building skills. *Theory Into Practice, 50*(1), 43–51.

McGuire, J. F., Arnold, E., Park, J. M., Nadeau, J. M., Lewin, A. B., Murphy, T. K., & Storch, E. A. (2015). Living with tics: reduced impairment and improved quality of life for youth with chronic tic disorders. *Psychiatry Research, 225*(3), 571–579.

Menting, A., Orobio de Castro, B., & Matthys, W. (2013). Effectiveness of the incredible years parent training to modify disruptive and prosocial child behavior: A meta-analytic review. *Clinical Psychology Review, 33*(8), 901–913.

Patterson, G. (1982). *Coercive family processes.* Eugene, OR: Castalia.

Powell, R., Honey, P., & Symbaluk, D. (2017). *Introduction to learning and behavior* (5th ed.). Boston, MA: Cengage Learning.

Rathus, J., & Miller, A. (2014). *DBT skills manual for adolescents.* New York: The Guildford Press.

Robertson, M. (2008). The prevalence and epidemiology of Gilles de la Tourette syndrome. Part 1: The epidemiological and prevalence studies. *Journal of Psychosomatic Research, 65*, 461–472.

Scahill, L., Specht, M. W., & Page, C. (2013). The prevalence of tic disorders and clinical characteristics in children. *Journal of Obsessive Compulsive Related Disorders, 3*(4), 394–400.

Scahill, L., Sukhodolsky, D., Bearss, K., Findley, D., Hamrin, V., Carroll, D., & Rains, A. L. (2006). Randomized trial of parent management training in children with tic disorders and disruptive behavior. *Journal of Child Neurology, 21*, 650–656.

Siegel, D.J., & Bryson, T.P. (2014, September 23). *Time-outs' are hurting your child.* Time Magazine. Retrieved from http://time.com/3404701/discipline-time-out-is-not-good/.

Specht, M. W., Woods, D. W., Piacentini, J., Scahill, L., Wilhelm, S., Peterson, A. L., ... Walkup, J. T. (2011). Clinical characteristics of children and adolescents with a primary tic disorder. *Journal of Developmental and Physical Disabilities, 23*, 15–31.

Webster-Stratton, C. (2017). *Incredible years time-out works because of quality time-in.* Retrieved from incredibleyears.com/.../IY-Time-Out-Works-Because-of-Quality-of-Time-In-Web.pdf.

Webster-Stratton, C., & Reid, M. J. (2017). The incredible years parents, teachers and children training series: A multifaceted treatment approach for young children with conduct problems. In J. Weisz, & A. Kazdin (Eds.), *Evidence-based psychotherapies for children and adolescents* (3rd ed., pp. 122–141). New York: Guilford Press.

Woods, D. W., Piacentini, J., Chang, S., Deckersbach, T., Ginsburg, G., Peterson, A., ... Wilhelm, S. (2008). *Managing Tourette syndrome: A behavioral intervention for children and adults therapist guide.* Oxford University Press.

FURTHER READING

Greene, R. (2010). *The explosive child: A new approach for understanding and parenting easily frustrated, chronically inflexible children.* New York: HarperCollins Publishers.

Ladnier, R., & Massanari, A. (2000). Treating ADHD as attachment deficit hyperactivity disorder. In T. Levy (Ed.), *Handbook of attachment interventions* (pp. 27–66). CA, USA: Academic Press.

Miltenberger, R. (2008). *Behavior modification.* Belmont, CA: Wadsworth Publishing.

Patterson, G., & Reid, J. (1970). Reciprocity and coercion: Two facets of social systems. In C. Neuringer, & J. Michael (Eds.), *Behavior modification in clinical psychology* (pp. 133–177). New York, NY: Appleton-Century-Crofts.

Chapter 12

Assessing and Treating Emotion Dysregulation and Anger Management

Justyna Piasecka, MD, Emilie J. Bertschinger, BA, Megan E. Tudor, PhD and Denis G. Sukhodolsky, PhD
Child Study Center, Yale School of Medicine, New Haven, CT, United State

Tourette syndrome and other tic disorders (collectively referred to as TS) are a neuropsychiatric disorder characterized by motor and vocal tics, which first occur in childhood (American Psychiatric Association, 2013). TS is often associated with psychiatric comorbidity, with a lifetime prevalence of any one psychiatric disorder over 85% and over half of the population with two or more disorders. The time of greatest risk of onset for most psychiatric comorbidities is early childhood, between the ages of 4 and 12 years (Hirschtritt et al., 2015). The high rates of comorbidity in TS with obsessive-compulsive disorder (OCD) and attention-deficit hyperactivity disorder (ADHD) are well described. In additional, TS can cooccur with mood disorder, anxiety disorder, autism spectrum disorder (ASD), and impulse-control disorder (Robertson, 2015). Disruptive behavior disorders (DBDs), which include oppositional defiant disorder (ODD) and conduct disorder (CD), also represent a significant portion of the comorbidities associated with TS, affecting approximately 30% of individuals with TS (Hirschtritt et al., 2015). In clinical samples, up to 80% of children and adolescents with TS can meet criteria for cooccurring ADHD, ODD, or CD (Coffey et al., 2000a). In addition, of all comorbidities affecting individuals with TS, ADHD and DBDs have both the youngest age at onset (5 years old) and earliest ages of highest risk (Hirschtritt et al., 2015).

While psychiatric diagnosis of ODD and CD are typically categorized together as DBDs, "disruptive behaviors" can encompass aggression, anger, noncompliance, and span across multiple psychiatric conditions including TS (i.e., a child with TS may exhibit disruptive behaviors but not meet diagnostic criteria for ODD). Disruptive behaviors represent a significant cause of impairment in children and adolescents, and are one of the most common

The Clinician's Guide to Treatment and Management of Youth with Tourette Syndrome and Tic Disorders.
DOI: https://doi.org/10.1016/B978-0-12-811980-8.00012-1

reasons for outpatient mental health referrals (Armbruster, Sukhodolsky, & Michalsen, 2004). Indeed, as many as 80% of clinically referred children with TS exhibit disruptive behaviors (Coffey et al., 2000a). In addition to irritability, anger, argumentativeness, and noncompliance, explosive outbursts of physical and verbal aggression have also been reported among youth with TS, with 35% of clinically referred children having experienced such outbursts (Budman, Bruun, Park, Lesser, & Olson, 2000).

This chapter reviews the literature on the phenomenology, assessment, and treatment of emotion dysregulation, including irritability, anxiety, and mood disorders, as it pertains to TS. The chapter provides practical strategies for behavioral intervention for emotion dysregulation in TS, and concludes with a case illustration of a child with TS and disruptive behavior who was treated with both pharmacologic and behavioral therapies.

PHENOMENOLOGY OF ANGER AND DISRUPTIVE BEHAVIOR IN TOURETTE SYNDROME

Disruptive behavior has long been recognized as a common clinical feature of TS. In fact, several of the original cases described by Gilles de la Tourette in 1885 include phrases that evoke what would later be termed "rage attacks," including one individual with "ferocious fits of rage" and another who was "immediately thrown into a turmoil... by an unpleasant event" (Martino & Leckman, 2013, p. 92). Several types of disruptive behavior are commonly seen in TS: anger, noncompliance, and aggression. These behaviors overlap and can be difficult to disentangle from one another. Moreover, these terms are often used interchangeably in research, contributing to an incomplete understanding of the phenomenology of anger outbursts within TS. Anger is a negative affective state and subjective feeling, which can include experiences of physiological arousal and thoughts about harm or blame (Kassinove & Sukhodolsky, 1995). Comings and Comings (1985, p. 444) commented upon the importance of this basic human emotion in TS, writing, "If there was a single word that best characterized the behavioral problems in TS it would be 'anger.'" Noncompliance and aggression are two common ways in which anger can be inappropriately expressed by children and adolescents. Noncompliant behavior is a refusal to follow instructions or established rules (Mcmahon & Forehand, 2003). Although frequently reported in children in the general population, it is more common in clinic-referred children, especially those with DBDs (Keenan & Wakschlag, 2004). Noncompliance is a central feature of ODD, a pattern of defiant, disobedient, and hostile behavior toward those in authority (American Psychiatric Association, 2013). In comparison to noncompliance, aggression is defined as behavior that results in harm or poses risk of harm to self, others, or property. It is a normal part of development and is commonly seen in very young children in the form of temper tantrums. However, aggressive behaviors recede as children mature and acquire the ability to self-regulate and manage their impulses. Pathological aggression refers to aggression that is no longer within the realm of normal development (Budman, Rosen, & Shad, 2015).

Disruptive behavior, anger, and aggression are characterized in different ways in the literature, including diagnosis with CD/ODD, clinical reports of aggression, and scores on "dimensional measures" of aggression. This had led to some difficulty in disentangling the phenomenology and etiology of anger, aggression, and disruptive behavior within TS. However, many studies have shown higher levels of disruptive behavior in children with tics as compared to children without tics (Gadow, 2002; Scahill, Williams, Schwab-Stone, Applegate, & Leckman, 2006c; Snider et al., 2002).

Of the forms of disruptive behavior seen in TS, both the most dramatic and debilitating are explosive outbursts, also referred to as "rage attacks." These "rage attacks" are unpredictable episodes of intense verbal and/or physical aggression that are out of proportion to the offending situation; in fact, they can appear entirely unprovoked to the bystander (Budman et al., 2000; Chen et al., 2013). Explosive outbursts are often accompanied by a feeling of complete loss of control, as well as autonomic activation including symptoms such as increased heart rate, sweating, shortness of breath, and hot flashes. These outbursts can last from minutes to as long as an hour, and are usually grossly out of character for the child (Budman, Rockmore, Stokes, & Sossin, 2003). A child experiencing an explosive outburst often either threatens or causes actual physical harm to property, others, or even to him/her. Most commonly, these outbursts occur at home and are directed toward a family member. Many individuals have also described phenomena associated with explosive outbursts that are reminiscent of tics themselves. For example, there may be feelings of increasing tension prior to the outburst, followed by relief once the outburst is complete (Budman et al., 2000). Individuals often feel a profound sense of regret or shame afterward, amplified by the perception that these outbursts are out of their control. When present, explosive outbursts are distressing and quite impairing to individuals affected by them, disrupting family relationships and both academic and psychosocial development (Budman et al., 2015). In fact, parents have described explosive outbursts in their children as one of the most impairing symptoms in TS (Dooley, 1999).

Explosive outbursts occur in 23%–40% of clinically referred individuals with TS (Budman et al., 2015). Although past studies have often not differentiated between anger, disruptive behavior, and explosive outbursts, recent research have noted the similarity between intermittent explosive disorder (IED) and explosive outbursts in TS and have used IED criteria in their methodology (Chen et al., 2013). A small exploratory study of 31 adults with TS found that 51.6% of them met criteria for IED (Frank, Piedad, Rickards, & Cavanna, 2011). The etiology of explosive outbursts in TS is poorly understood. However, it is clear that it is complex and likely multifactorial. In a study of 218 children and adolescents with TS that were recruited from the United States and Costa Rica (Chen et al., 2013), researchers found that 20% of participants reported experiencing explosive outbursts, and that explosive outbursts were strongly associated with ADHD. Freeman and colleagues (2000) examined a large, international database of 3500 individuals with TS across 22 countries and found that anger control problems were strongly correlated with comorbidity. In this study, 10% of individuals with TS only had anger control problems, compared to 40% of individuals with TS and at least one comorbid psychiatric condition. These findings suggest a complex interplay between TS, its associated comorbidities including ADHD, and anger and explosive outbursts that should be explored further.

The significant rate of comorbidity between TS and ADHD was well established. It is estimated that between 30% and 50% of individuals with TS in the community also have ADHD, with the rate in clinically referred patients slightly higher at about 60% (Robertson, 2015). Children with TS and cooccurring ADHD are at higher risk of having disruptive behavior problems, relative to children with TS without ADHD. In addition, even in the presence of another comorbid psychiatric condition other than ADHD, disruptive behaviors are far less commonly seen than in TS + ADHD. In a study examining 5080 children and adolescents with TS, CD/ODD was observed at significantly higher rates—around 40%—in children and adolescents with TS and ADHD compared to those without ADHD (Roessner et al., 2007). The authors hypothesized that the combination of TS and ADHD might reduce behavioral inhibition, and thus contribute to the externalizing behaviors seen in these youth. These findings highlight the importance of effectively treating ADHD symptoms in TS.

Diagnoses of ODD and CD are often associated with disruptive behaviors that have been described earlier. In fact, many studies in the literature examining the relationship between TS and disruptive behavior use the diagnostic criteria of ODD and CD to stratify their subjects. The literature suggests that CD and ODD are related to other comorbidities occurring in TS, most notably ADHD, rather than being associated with TS itself. A study by Robertson, Cavanna, and Eapen (2015) examined the prevalence of CD in 578 patients with TS, and found that 14.5% of patients in the sample met criteria for CD. In this study, CD was strongly associated with ADHD in the probands, as well as with a family history of forensic encounters. Similarly, another study of over 1300 individuals with TS found a lifetime prevalence rate of 29.7% for CD/ODD, with the highest rates occurring in individuals with TS + OCD + ADHD, followed by TS + ADHD (Hirschtritt et al., 2015).

It is also important to note the potential role of anxiety and mood disorders in disruptive behavior and emotion dysregulation in TS, both of which are often seen as comorbidities in TS. Hirschtritt and colleagues (2015) have reported the lifetime prevalence in TS of anxiety disorders as 36.1% and that of mood disorders, including both depression and bipolar disorder, as 29.8%, with depression accounting for 26.1%. Elevated levels of anxiety symptoms or cooccurring anxiety disorder are more common in individuals with TS relative to prevalence rates in the general population (Coffey et al., 2000b). If present, anxiety can contribute to subjective distress in the individual and have deleterious effects on quality of life beyond impairments associated with tics (Lewin et al., 2011). In a recent study, anxiety also emerged as a predictor of poorer response to treatment for tics with either behavior therapy or supportive psychotherapy (Sukhodolsky et al., 2017). Specifically, participants with a cooccurring anxiety disorder showed less tic reduction after 10 weeks regardless of treatment with either CBIT or supportive therapy. This is consistent with reports that stress can disrupt tic suppressing efforts (Conelea, Woods, & Brandt, 2011). Therefore, a careful evaluation of anxiety should be part of a comprehensive clinical assessment for individuals with TS.

Depression in children and adolescents differs from depression in adults, where depression is often present with irritability, aggression, or behavior problems (Gurnani, Ivanov, & Newcorn, 2016). The prevalence rates of depression in TS populations was estimated to range between 20% and 30% in clinically referred samples, and 10% and 15% in population samples (Piedad & Cavanna, 2016). Of note, depression in children and adolescents with TS appears to also be correlated with an increased incidence of irritability (Budman et al., 2015). Successful behavioral or pharmacological treatment of depression can improve these symptoms; therefore, as detailed in the next section, careful psychiatric evaluation of disruptive behavior is critical in correctly identifying any comorbidities that can be contributing to disruptive behavior and aggression.

ASSESSMENT OF DISRUPTIVE BEHAVIOR AND AGGRESSION IN TOURETTE SYNDROME

Given the complex nature of TS in youth, a thorough clinical assessment is needed to identify or rule out the presence of other commonly cooccurring disorders (Scahill et al., 2006a). As mentioned earlier, the likelihood of disruptive behavior in this population is high and, notably, the risk for such behavior increases with the number of diagnoses in addition to TS (Freeman et al., 2000). Disruptive behavior in youth takes many forms, ranging from noncompliance (e.g., refusal to clean one's room) to physical aggression (e.g., kicking a parent); variability regarding other components of presentation, such as frequency, duration, and intensity, is to be expected. As such, no single parent or self-report measure is accepted as the "gold standard" for screening or assessment of disruptive behavior in children. Nevertheless, in addition to in-depth diagnostic child and parent interviews, some useful supplemental measures exist that may help a clinician screen for and conceptualize disruptive behavior in youth with TS.

To date, only one measure of disruptive behavior specific to TS exists. The Rage Outburst and Rating Anger Scale (ROARS) was initially developed to specifically assess rage attacks in youth with TS (Budman et al., 2008). The measure is brief, consisting of three items rated on a 4-point Likert scale, with total scores ranging from 0 to 9 (scores equal to or over 7 are considered clinically elevated). The three items assess the frequency, intensity, and duration of outbursts demonstrated by the youth with TS in the past week. The ROARS has demonstrated good psychometric properties in a sample of youth with OCD (Storch et al., 2012) and general clinic sample of youth (Nadeau et al., 2016). While additional study is warranted to identify the uses of this measure in the population of youth with TS, it is likely an ideal "starting point" in assessing disruptive behavior in youth with TS and can be easily added to a standard clinical evaluation.

The child behavior checklist (CBCL; Achenbach & Rescorla, 2001a) is well known as an age- and gender-normed parent-report measure of various childhood behavioral problems. The measure consists of 116 items which are rated on a 0 ("Not True") to 2 ("Very True or Often True") Likert scale. Broadband factors include externalizing problems, though the syndrome subscale of aggressive behavior may provide more specific information about disruptive behavior to the clinician. In addition, the CBCL includes DSM-oriented scales that can be used to predict the likelihood of specific diagnoses, such as ODD. The simultaneous interpretation of all subscales will likely be most useful in clinicians' ongoing assessment (Bellina et al., 2013). Elevated aggressive behavior subscale scores have been demonstrated in youth with TS (Ghanizadeh & Mosallaei, 2009), especially those with cooccurring ADHD (Sukhodolsky et al., 2003). The CBCL is particularly useful to a clinician's toolbox, given that a Teacher Report Form is also available and lends itself to comparison of data across informants.

The Home Situations Questionnaire (HSQ; Barkley, 2013) is a brief parent-report measure wherein parents report on 16 situations that may coincide with disruptive, especially noncompliant, behavior. Parents mark "yes" or "no" to the occurrence of disruptive behavior in these settings and then provide a severity rating (1 = mild to 9 = severe) for endorsed situations. Like the CBCL, the HSQ has extensive evidence of preferred psychometric properties (e.g., Dupaul & Barkley, 1992). While the HSQ has recently become synonymous with the assessment of problem behavior in ASD (Chowdhury et al., 2015), it is still a useful measure across diagnostic categories, including youth with TS. In particular, the HSQ can lend itself to identifying specific antecedents of disruptive behavior that can be targeted in treatment.

Youths' self-report of behavior may also be informative for clinicians. Two unique measures that have been integrated into treatment studies of disruptive behavior are the Children's Inventory of Anger (ChIA; Nelson & Finch, 2000) and the State-Trait Anger Expression Inventory (STAXI; Spielberger, 1988). The ChIA is standardized for ages 6–16 and presents youth with 39 hypothetical situations that may provoke anger. For example, "Somebody says 'I told you so' after something goes wrong." Children are asked to imagine that the situation is actually happening and then rate their anger reactions on a Likert scale with numerical and pictorial scores (cartoon faces depicting different levels of anger). The STAXI is a well-validated measure of anger experience which includes 44 items that have been normed for 12–16 year olds. The STAXI evaluates youths' anger based on their general everyday feelings of anger versus anger that is a reaction to specific circumstances (state). As such, the measure provides information about the control that children report exerting in order to control their anger across on a daily or circumstance-specific basis (e.g., "When angry or furious I tend to harbor grudges that I don't tell anyone about"). One study did not detect significant differences between youth with TS and healthy controls on the STAXI (Cavanna et al., 2015), suggesting that it may not generally be a useful screening measure but, rather, useful for youth with TS that have already been identified as experiencing elevated levels of anger or aggression. Both the ChIA and STAXI may also provide clinicians with a unique perspective that may facilitate discussion about anger experience and, subsequently, treatment planning with youth with TS.

In addition to these questionnaire measures, clinicians may wish to supplement their thorough diagnostic interview with the Overt Aggression Scale (OAS) (Silver & Yudofsky, 1991; Yudofsky, Silver, Jackson, Endicott, & Williams, 1986). The OAS consists of specific aggressive behaviors, including verbal aggression, aggression against objects, self-directed aggression, and aggression toward others. Clinicians rate the frequency and severity of aggressive behaviors based on child and parent report. Each category of aggressive behavior corresponds with a respective weighted score, with physical aggression toward self or others receiving the highest relative scores, ultimately yielding an overall severity score. The OAS has been demonstrated as useful for youth with TS (Steinberg, Shmuel-Baruch, Horesh, & Apter, 2013) sensitive to behavioral changes in children with aggressive behavior posttreatment (Armenteros & Lewis, 2002; Malone, Delaney, Luebbert, Cater, & Campbell, 2000). Clinicians may find the OAS useful in assessing the specific nature of disruptive behavior, especially given that DSM-5 disruptive behavior diagnoses (e.g., ODD) can met by a wide spectrum of behavioral profiles. Using the OAS as a measure of frequency, duration, and intensity of aggressive behavior may be especially meaningful in identifying targets symptoms (Mcguire et al., 2014) and assessing change over the course of treatment.

Ultimately, each evaluation of a child with TS and disruptive behavior will be slightly different, and should be tailored according to the presentation of the child and the clinician's best clinical judgment as to what may be causing or exacerbating the behavior. A thorough psychiatric assessment will provide the foundation of the interview, and can then be complemented by other modalities of assessment when identifying and treating disruptive behavior, including parent-report and self-report measures, as well as supplemental aggression-specific interviewing. In general, the CBCL can be most useful for broadband screening of multiple diagnostic categories. The ROARS, on the other hand, is best for more targeted evaluation and for measuring and monitoring changes in behavior. Before using formal assessment measures, basic open-ended questions can help a clinician get a better sense of what the child and the family are experiencing; e.g., "What do the outbursts look like?" and "When are they most likely to happen?" can help pinpoint the severity, frequency, and triggers of the behaviors.

A careful and thoughtful psychiatric assessment can be critical in identifying the underlying cause for disruptive behavior in TS, and thus selecting the most appropriate treatment. For example, a child with TS and a very "short fuse," whose disruptive behaviors seem rooted in impulsivity and an inability to think before acting may have their behavior improve substantially through identification and treatment of ADHD. If a child with TS has severe social anxiety, he/she might become extremely irritable and lash out mainly in anticipation of situations that puts him/her at risk for perceived judgment or criticism by others, such as schoolwork that requires oral participation. Addressing social anxiety through therapy, rather than disruptive behavior in isolation, might result in better treatment outcomes. Effective psychiatric assessment, through a combination of clinical interview of both parents and child and supplemental questionnaires and measures, can help target behavioral treatment and pharmacotherapy.

There is also a wide range of measures of anxiety and depression that can be used to evaluate these symptoms in individuals with TS. One of the most commonly used measures of anxiety is a Multidimensional Anxiety Scale for Children, which is now in its second edition (MASC-2) (March, 2013; March, Sullivan, Stallings, Conners, & Parker, 1997). The scale consists of 50-items such as "feels tense or uptight" and "gets scared when parents go away" that are rated on a 4-point Likert scale with 0 = never, 1 = rarely, 2 = sometimes, and 3 = often. The parent-rated MASC is highly reliable and provides age- and gender-normed scores for total anxiety as well as for the subtypes of anxiety such as social, separation, and generalized anxiety. Child version of the MASC-2 can be used to obtain child self-report of anxiety. The *Children's Depression Inventory (CDI)* is a 27-item questionnaire of depressive symptoms (Kovacs, 1992, 2011). Similarly to the MASC, the CDI is now in its second edition and both parent and child versions are available. The items are rated on a scale from 0 to 2 and grouped into five major factor areas such as depressed mood and interpersonal problems. The CDI was developed for children by using the Beck Depression Inventory (BDI)

(Beck, Steer, & Brown, 1996), which has been a gold standard for assessing depression in adults. The CDI is widely used assessment of the severity of depressive symptoms in children with well-established reliability and validity. Other common measures of anxiety and depression include the screen for child anxiety related emotional disorders (Birmaher et al., 1999) and mood and feelings questionnaire (Costello & Angold, 1988). Broadband measures of psychopathology such as the CBCL (Achenbach & Rescorla, 2001b) and the Child and Adolescent Symptoms Inventory (CASI) (Gadow & Sprafkin, 2002) also contain reliable and norm-referenced subscales of anxiety and depression.

BEHAVIORAL INTERVENTIONS FOR ANGER AND AGGRESSION IN TOURETTE SYNDROME

Two psychosocial interventions have been shown to be effective in treating disruptive behavior and aggression in children and adolescents with TS: anger control training (ACT) and parent management training (PMT). Both of these interventions have also been studied rigorously across diagnostic categories to treat the symptoms of anger, aggression, and irritability (Sukhodolsky, Smith, Mccauley, Ibrahim, & Piasecka, 2016a). PMT has been used extensively to treat disruptive behavior in children across diagnoses (Michelson, Davenport, Dretzke, Barlow, & Day, 2013). As discussed in Chapter 11, PMT aims to improve parents' understanding of their child's disruptive behavior and noncompliance and to provide strategies for changing behaviors, such as giving positive reinforcement for desired behaviors, setting clear expectations, and the appropriate use of time-outs (Kazdin, 2005). PMT is based on extensive research of parent–child interactions that can inadvertently reinforce child disruptive behavior via the mechanisms of escape and avoidance conditioning (Patterson et al., 1992). Please see Chapter 11: Brief Transdiagnostic Parent Training: A Strengths-Based, Parent-Centered Treatment for Youth With Tourette Syndrome for a more detailed discussion and guidance on PMT (referred to as brief parent training in Chapter 11: Brief Transdiagnostic Parent Training: A Strengths-Based, Parent-Centered Treatment for Youth With Tourette Syndrome).

While parent training focuses on educating parents to manage children's behavior, ACT is a type of cognitive-behavioral therapy (CBT) delivered directly to youth. It targets disruptive behaviors by improving emotion regulation and providing coping skills to better manage anger (Sukhodolsky et al., 2016a). A study on ACT for adolescents with TS and disruptive behavior included 26 participants between the ages of 11 and 16 years who were randomized to either ACT or a treatment-as-usual (TAU) control condition (Sukhodolsky et al., 2009). Participants randomized to ACT were provided 10 one-hour sessions based on a structured manual, with sessions grouped into modules focused on management of emotional arousal, cognitive restructuring, and behavioral practice of assertive behavior. Those in the TAU arm continued to see their previous treating clinicians, but were not provided with any new therapies. At the conclusion of the study, a 52% reduction in disruptive behavior was observed in the ACT group, compared with an 11% reduction in the TAU group.

In conducting trials examining the effects of CBT on anger and aggression in children and adolescents across multiple diagnoses including the study in TS described earlier, Sukhodolsky and Scahill (2012) a manual for clinicians titled "Cognitive-Behavioral Therapy for Anger and Aggression in Children." Application of this treatment in children with TS complicated by anger and disruptive behavior is illustrated in a case illustration below. The CBT approach described in the manual consists of 10 sessions grouped into 3 modules: emotion regulation, problem solving, and social skills. It can be used by clinicians with experience in child behavioral interventions, and allows for enough flexibility to tailor the sessions to more specifically address symptoms that might be unique to a patient with TS. Sessions 1–3 include psychoeducation about anger, including common triggers for outbursts and physiological cues associated with anger, as well as practice of anger-management skills such as deep breathing, positive imagery, and relaxation. Sessions 4–6 involve cognitive restructuring and practicing problem-solving skills, including identifying the consequences of choices taken in common anger-provoking situations and generating alternate solutions based on those consequences. Sessions 7–10 continue practicing the core skills learned through role play of typical situations, including with peers, parents, and teachers. After each session, children are asked to practice the skills they have learned and complete logs describing their experience of successfully managing their anger over the previous week using the skills they have learned. Parents also participate in the treatment, with each session including a parent check-in during which the week is discussed, contents of the session are reviewed, and the clinician troubleshoots any stumbling blocks the family may be encountering. Parenting skills, including identifying observable behaviors and learning about antecedents and consequences that can be used to strengthen appropriate behavior, are also taught to maximize the child's opportunities for success in decreasing the frequency and intensity of their aggression and angry outbursts.

Although there have been no specific treatment studies for anxiety in TS, CBT has demonstrated considerable empirical support for the treatment of anxiety and would likely be helpful for anxiety and emotion dysregulation experienced by individuals with TS. CBT for anxiety has been evaluated in over 40 randomized studies and is considered to be an evidence-based treatment (Seligman & Ollendick, 2011). CBT is usually effective for 50%–60% of participants and shows moderate-to-large effect sizes (Compton et al., 2004). Theoretical underpinnings of CBT assume that pathological anxiety is the result of an interaction between excessive physiological arousal, cognitive distortions, and avoidance behavior. Accordingly, the core components of CBT include teaching emotion regulation skills aimed at the reduction of physiological arousal and maladaptive thinking in conjunction with systematic exposure tasks to feared situations in order to eliminate avoidant behavior. Most CBT programs for childhood anxiety include teaching cognitive emotion regulation skills followed by in vivo exposure (facing feared situations repeatedly while using the emotion regulation skills that have been learned, and remaining in the situations until habituation occurs). After a hierarchy is created in which feared situations are ordered from least to most distressing to confront, children work their way up the hierarchy and are rewarded as they attempt increasingly fearful activities. The parent component of CBT for anxiety focuses on supporting in vivo exposures, using positive reinforcement, and encouraging children's independence in daily routines. Excellent treatment manuals and training programs are available for clinicians (Kendall & Hedtke, 2006; Wood, Piacentini, Southam-Gerow, Chu, & Sigman, 2006).

For a child with TS who experiences any of the aforementioned symptoms of emotion dysregulation (e.g., anger, irritability, aggression, anxiety, disruptive behavior), the individual skills or concepts used in ACT can be helpful in targeting problematic behaviors and improving outcomes, with a full course of ACT recommended. One of the great benefits of all types of CBT is that the skills learned are generalizable, not only within the particular symptom cluster that the CBT is targeting, but also across both diagnostic categories and periods of development. A child who practices and implements deep breathing as a tool to "dial down anger" can use the same skill to decrease his level of anxiety. A 10 year old who learns about the importance of identifying triggers for his/her feelings when he/she always has outbursts around his/her younger sibling taking his/her toys can apply the same concept of identifying triggers as a teenager when experiencing anger every time he/she is asked to do a chore by his/her parents. When faced with a child or adolescent with both disruptive behavior and TS, a clinician familiar with the overall concepts and skills used in CBT can help the child implement strategies that will decrease anger outbursts.

As discussed earlier, many individuals with TS will experience "rage attacks," where anger outbursts feel unprovoked and out of their control. Skills dealing with emotion regulation can be among the most helpful for both children and adolescents. They are simple, concrete, and relatively easy to practice and implement. Deep breathing is a skill that is taught in countless CBT manuals, and is similarly useful in this context. Anger and aggression provoke a "fight or flight" response through the autonomic nervous system, and deep breathing uses physiologic mechanisms to decrease blood pressure and heart rate, and thus cause the individual to feel less angry or aroused. The clinician can introduce deep breathing in several different forms, so that the child can experiment with them and use whichever one works best for him/her. For example, deep breathing can be done in combination with counting backward or with positive imagery. As with all the skills and concepts in CBT, it is important for the child to practice daily and when feeling calm and relaxed, so that the skills feel natural and can be more readily applied during stress-provoking situations.

Recognizing physiological cues for anger is another emotion regulation skill, which is especially helpful in children with TS and disruptive behavior and is discussed further in the case illustration later on in this chapter. Similarly to deep breathing, recognition of physiological cues is a concept that can be useful not only in anger, but also across a range of emotions including anxiety and irritability. While feelings like anger or rage can feel to a child or adolescent as if they "come out of nowhere," there are often subtle (or not-so-subtle) cues that can warn an individual that an anger outburst is imminent. Children might initially deny that any warning signs are present; a discussion of changes that commonly occur in people experiencing anger (increased heart rate, flushing or feeling hot, clenched fists, furrowed brows, etc.) can facilitate identification of relevant physiological and physical cues. Once the child has identified one or two cues that let him/her know that he/she is becoming angry or irritated, he/she can then apply other CBT skills, such as deep breathing or distraction techniques, to stop or at least limit the angry outburst.

Parental involvement is an important part of behavioral therapy, but can be titrated according to factors which may include availability, the child's buy in to treatment, and the relationship between parent and adolescent. One of the most crucial ideas that the clinician should relay to the parent at the beginning of ACT or related treatments is that of "catching the child being good." Often the tendency of the parent is to take note of and draw attention to negative behaviors, which can in turn reinforce these behaviors. By noticing a child's attempts at practicing CBT skills and changing his/her behavior, even when these attempts are unsuccessful, the parent provides positive reinforcement to the child. This can be done through methods both subtle, such as singling out and praising a child for walking away from an argument, or more overt, such as a rewards chart or behavioral contract (see Chapter 11: Brief Transdiagnostic Parent Training: A Strengths-Based, Parent-Centered Treatment for Youth With Tourette Syndrome for further discussion of reinforcing prosocial behaviors).

PHARMACOTHERAPY FOR AGGRESSION AND DISRUPTIVE BEHAVIOR IN TOURETTE SYNDROME

While pharmacotherapy for TS is well covered in Chapter 4, Pharmacological Management of Tic Disorders in Youth, this section briefly covers pharmacotherapy for aggressive and disruptive behaviors. Despite the prevalence of anger, aggression, and disruptive behavior in TS, few studies have examined the pharmacologic treatment of these symptoms within this population. The studies that do exist are mainly open-label or retrospective studies, with small sample sizes, and thus offer limited guidance on treatment. In addition, the studies use different criteria for defining aggressive symptoms and/or explosive outbursts (Martino & Leckman, 2013).

Two studies have assessed the efficacy of olanzapine on tics and aggressive behaviors in TS. The first study enrolled 10 subjects between the ages of 7 and 13 in a single-blind trial (Stephens, Bassel, & Sandor, 2004). Olanzapine was titrated biweekly, as tolerated. All of the subjects completed the trial, and at the end of 8 weeks, there was both a clinically and statistically significant reduction in tics and aggressive behaviors. Even with a relatively short-treatment duration, weight gain was a significant adverse effect in the group. A second study examining olanzapine was an open-label trial conducted in 2008 (Mccracken, Suddath, Chang, Thakur, & Piacentini, 2008). Twelve patients with TS, nine of whom also met criteria for ADHD, ODD, and/or CD, and were between the ages of 7 and 14 years, were enrolled in the 6-week study. A significant reduction in measures of disruptive behaviors such as hyperactivity and aggression was observed, in addition to a reduction in tic severity. Weight gain was noted as a side effect in this study as well.

In addition to the earlier studies on atypical antipsychotics, there has been one study which assessed the effectiveness of paroxetine, an SSRI, on the episodic rages associated with TS (Bruun & Budman, 1998). The open-label study included both children and adults, with the 45 participants' ages ranging from 6 to 55 years, and paroxetine was intended solely to address episodic rages. Seventy-six percent of the patients who completed the 8-week study reported either rages that were significantly decreased or completely absent at the end of treatment.

Alpha-adrenergic agonists, such as clonidine and guanfacine, are used to treat tics in TS; they are often considered first-line treatment due to their more favorable side-effect profiles as compared to the atypical antipsychotics (Murphy, Lewin, Storch, & Stock, 2013). These medications can also be used in the treatment of ADHD, often comorbid with TS, and are thought to be useful in specifically addressing impulsivity and hyperactivity (Pliszka & Issues, 2007). Although no studies have examined the effects of alpha-2 agonists on aggression in TS, there is evidence that these medications may improve disruptive and aggressive behaviors (Gurnani et al., 2016). A meta-analysis of stimulants, alpha-2 agonists, and atomoxetine for oppositional behavior, conduct problems, and aggression in children with ADHD, ODD, and CD found evidence of some effect of guanfacine on problematic behaviors (Pringsheim, Hirsch, Gardner, & Gorman, 2015). However, the meta-analysis noted that there are a limited number of studies of alpha-agonists for the treatment of oppositional behavior, conduct problems, and aggression. Despite the lack of trials specific to aggression in TS, it is reasonable to hypothesize that treatment of tics or comorbid ADHD with an alpha-agonist might have the additional benefit of improving symptoms related to anger and aggression. If future studies of antipsychotics and alpha-agonists for management of tics include measures of anger and aggression, they could provide much-needed understanding and knowledge to clinicians. After many years of controversy regarding the use of stimulants in children with tics, studies and meta-analyses have confirmed their safety and efficacy in comorbid ADHD/TS (Bloch, Panza, Landeros-Weisenberger, & Leckman, 2009).

For the clinician considering whether a child with comorbid TS and disruptive behavior might benefit from pharmacological treatment, the relative risks and benefits of medication should be weighed carefully, especially given the limited studies described earlier. The American Academy of Child and Adolescent Psychiatry recommends behavioral therapies as a starting point for anger and rage outbursts in TS, as identifying and addressing triggers for behaviors and implementing anger-management techniques can be helpful for many children and adolescents (Murphy et al., 2013). For individuals who have attempted behavioral therapies and failed, or whose behavior is severe enough that it interferes with their ability to participate in therapy, a medication trial may be indicated. Although no specific guidelines exist for pharmacological treatment of disruptive behavior in youth with TS, it is reasonable to use the same approach one would use for a child with aggression without TS. As Gurnani et al. (2016) have described, treatment "is based on a comprehensive understanding of the nature, severity, and context of the symptoms; a confluence of psychological, behavioral, and cognitive considerations; and the profile of risk and protective factors that characterize the individual patient and family. In addition, the intensity and developmental course of symptoms must be considered, as well as the potential consequences (e.g., harm to self or others) that could arise from the aggressive behaviors and how likely this is to happen" (Gurnani et al., 2016, p. 66). Current guidelines recommend the first step of pharmacological therapy to be treatment of any underlying comorbid disorder which may be causing or exacerbating aggression or disruptive behavior, including ADHD, anxiety/depression, or CD (Gurnani et al., 2016). If the tic disorder is impairing enough to warrant pharmacological treatment, a medication which treats both the comorbidity and tic disorder, such as alpha-agonists for ADHD or risperidone for severe aggression, may be worth trying as first-line to minimize polypharmacy.

CASE ILLUSTRATION

"Will" was an 11-year-old boy who was diagnosed with TS as well as cooccurring ODD and ADHD. He participated in a randomized controlled trial for children with anger and aggression (Sukhodolsky et al., 2016b) in order to address his defiance, anger, and aggressive outbursts, some of which could be characterized as rage attacks. As a participant in the study, he received 12 sessions of CBT with a child psychiatrist (the first author) that followed a manualized approach and included both child and parent sessions (Sukhodolsky & Scahill, 2012).

He lived at home with his mother and father. He had been adopted by his parents in infancy, so any family history of psychiatric illnesses including TS or ADHD was unknown. According to his mother, he had first demonstrated motor tics at around age 5 and vocal tics a year later. Motor tics mainly included shoulder-shrugging, eye-blinking, facial grimaces, and head-tossing, while vocal tics consisted of throat-clearing, squeaking, and sniffing. When he started treatment, he was prescribed an alpha-agonist (guanfacine), as well as a low-dose antipsychotic (aripiprazole).

Will's CBT treatment started in the middle of the summer, and at the time his parents reported that his explosive outbursts most often occurred when he was not allowed to engage in activities that were highly desirable to him, such as having a playdate or sleepover with a friend. The outbursts would consist of screaming, cursing, crying, and often selectively destroying things that were precious to his parents, such as photo albums or paintings on the wall. In fact, his parents had put many of their most cherished items in storage for fear of them being destroyed during an outburst. These extreme episodes occurred one to two times per week and usually lasted for about an hour. He was typically a friendly, sweet, and outgoing boy; so these outbursts were quite dramatic and represented a significant change from his baseline personality. He was very remorseful following his outbursts and was an enthusiastic participant in treatment, as he wanted these episodes to stop but felt that they were out of his control.

Will's first three CBT sessions were structured around emotion regulation and anger management. These sessions began with psychoeducation about the nature of anger and aggression, as well as about TS and the relationship between TS and disruptive behavior. His anger outbursts had escalated over the summer, and at the same time, he and his parents had also noticed an increase in the frequency of his tics. This was distressing to him, as he found some of his tics embarrassing and they had been infrequent prior to the summer. Psychoeducation, which was supplemental to the usual treatment manual, included discussing the relationship of tics to stress, and their tendency to be exacerbated during periods of intense emotion, anxiety, or stress. In addition, he had started swearing over the summer, and his parents were uncertain as to whether this was an involuntary tic or purposeful misbehavior, as he had never exhibited this tendency before. The clinician discussed with them at length the clinical presentation of TS, including its waxing and waning course and the fluctuating nature of the tics themselves. As part of this discussion, the great majority of his swearing was determined to be a voluntary part of his angry outbursts. At the same time, he was also experiencing coprolalia independently of anger outbursts. Sometimes, when coprolalia occurred in the context of an underlying irritable mood, it could be mistaken for an angry outburst. He, his family, and his clinician spent time distinguishing the characteristics of both, so that coprolalia could be seen as a tic and treated as such, while being effectively ignored in the discussion of angry and explosive outbursts. He was also educated about tic-management strategies that can be used to replace an involuntary coprolalia tic such as focusing on slow, rhythmic breathing or taking a "hard swallow."

Sessions 1–3 also involved identification of anger triggers and monitoring the physiological cues of anger, as well as practicing strategies to prevent or reduce angry outbursts, such as verbal reminders, distracting oneself from anger, and deep breathing techniques. Verbal reminders resonated with him because, as an athlete, he was able to identify with the concepts of "self-coaching" and "positive self-talk," especially after a conversation on the difference between good and bad coaching techniques. He also found the discussion on monitoring physiological cues particularly helpful. When having an explosive outburst, he had previously experienced himself as going into "Beast Mode," as he described it, without any warning, lending to his feeling of being completely out of control in these instances. He and his clinician discussed physiological changes that started to occur just before an angry outburst took place, including racing heart, clenched fists, and a reddened, hot face. He began using these cues to alert him to his rising anger and as a signal that he needed to intervene; e.g., by using the verbal reminder he had chosen, "Just walk away..." and distracting himself with an enjoyable activity such as drawing until his anger decreased to a more manageable level.

Will's next three CBT sessions dealt with social problem-solving strategies including problem identification, brainstorming alternate solutions, and recognizing potential consequences for each solution he generated. Many of his outbursts had a similar trigger, which he had identified in an earlier session—i.e., being told "no" by a parent when he asked for a playdate or sleep-over with a friend. During a session covering others' perspectives and hostile attribution bias, he was able to provide alternative reasons that his parents might be saying no rather than, "they just don't care if I have friends or not," such as "they might be tired after being at work all day," or "I have soccer practice in the morning and they want me to get enough sleep." Following a discussion on compromises that took into account both perspectives in an argument, he independently introduced the idea of a rewards system to the clinician and his parents, where he would have one playdate scheduled each week, with the possibility of earning up to two additional playdates based on good behavior (completion of chores, responding to parents in a calm and pleasant tone of voice, etc.). His parents were impressed with his initiative and willingness to compromise (as he was previously requesting playdates nearly daily), and a rewards chart was successfully implemented for the duration of treatment.

The final CBT sessions centered on social skills training for preventing and resolving conflicts with both adults and peers. These sessions consisted of role play and acting out various scenarios for assertive behaviors during anger-provoking episodes. He was given the opportunity to generate and then "test out" different solutions to the problems that he most commonly faced with peers, parents, and teachers. During role play, the clinician would take the part of the offending peers or adults, and he was often pleasantly surprised when an interaction ended in a positive way rather than in the manner that he had anticipated. One particularly useful scenario explored ways to respond to peers who were not aware of his TS and stared at him or made fun of him when he was experiencing tics (see Chapter 7: Talking About Tics With Peers and Coping in Social Interactions). He was an accomplished soccer player on a youth travel team, and most often experienced this with members of opposing teams. In the past, he had reacted by becoming verbally aggressive and confrontational with the peer, or sometimes even targeting him with foul play on the soccer field. During CBT, he practiced addressing such peers in an assertive way, with good eye contact and in a calm voice, and standing up for himself while also treating the other person respectfully. This included using "I" statements to address the peer, such as "I don't like it when you do that," to reduce the confrontational and accusatory nature of his usual reply, "You're a jerk!" he also wrote and rehearsed a short script where he explained to an unknown peer that he has TS like the renowned American soccer goalie Tim Howard, after talking with his clinician about the fact that most of his friends had not known what tics or TS were prior to befriending him. This in turn led to a conversation about how his role model might have dealt with and been able to ignore similar barbs when he was growing up, and how his strengths and abilities might allow him to do the same.

Throughout his treatment, parent sessions played an important role in the success of the therapy. One or both of his parents attended each of his sessions and took part in a check-in at the end of the session. In addition, three parent-only sessions were held during which parenting techniques were discussed and strategies specific to his outbursts were drawn up. During check-ins, his progress over the previous week was discussed, with parents encouraged to provide positive feedback on conflicts that he had either handled well or situations that could have escalated into an outburst that he been able to walk away from. After the third session, his mother had described an angry outburst that occurred after his father had told him that they couldn't go to a diner together that night like he had hoped. He became enraged, swearing, hitting the furniture, and holding up a baby picture of him as if about to rip it up. However, he was able to stop himself from ripping the photograph, and instead threw it in his father's direction before going to his room and slamming the door. Despite the fact that an outburst had occurred with multiple maladaptive behaviors attached to it, during the session his mother was able to comment instead on the fact that he had been able to restrain himself from destroying the photograph, which had never happened before. His pride in response to his mother's compliment was apparent, and there were no further outbursts where he destroyed something precious to his parents throughout the duration of the treatment.

The CBT approach used for addressing his disruptive behavior allows for enough flexibility to make some adaptations to specifically address the role of tics and TS in a child's presentation. As discussed in his case, psychoeducation on TS and its relationship with disruptive behavior is an integral component of behavioral interventions. Both children and parents should be reminded of the clinical course of TS, namely its waxing and waning nature, its likelihood to be at its worst between the ages of 10 and 12, and the manner in which tics can change in type, intensity, and location. As in his case, the waxing and waning course of TS can lead to confusion with disruptive behaviors, as can the appearance of a new, previously unseen tic. Reviewing the differences between tics and disruptive behaviors can be helpful in distinguishing between the two: namely, tics are involuntary, repetitive, and children often try to suppress them, as compared with disruptive behaviors which are often performed in response to antecedents such as parental demands or peer provocations. Children and parents should be educated on the role of stress and emotional arousal in exacerbating tics, and the dual benefit that can be gained from learning and practicing relaxation techniques, i.e., a decrease in both anger and tic frequency and/or intensity.

The monitoring of physiological cues during the early sessions of CBT can be quite helpful when treating a child with TS or tics. As discussed in the section on explosive outbursts and "rage attacks," his description of his angry outbursts is not unique. Many children and adolescents with TS will describe feeling out of control during an episode, as well as heightened physiological arousal, including having an increased heart rate, sweating, and/or feeling hot or red. By monitoring such symptoms and becoming aware of them earlier, children can more effectively interrupt an angry outburst before it escalates to the level of feeling out of the child's control.

In addition, for many children with TS, their explosive outbursts can stem directly from frustration, anger, or anxiety in dealing with their tics. Suppressing tics can be draining and exhausting, leaving a child with little emotional reserve remaining to effectively deal with conflicts or anger-provoking situations. For this reason, it is important that behavioral therapy for anger outburst is provided in context of competent clinical care for TS that may include behavioral interventions for tics such as habit reversal training (see Chapter 3: Habit Reversal Training for Tics) and/or pharmacotherapy (see Chapter 4: Pharmacological Management of Tic Disorders in Youth) for tics and associated disorders such as ADHD, OCD, and anxiety (Murphy et al., 2013).

CONCLUSION

Anger, irritability, and aggression are common forms of emotion dysregulation in children with TS. Careful clinical assessment is needed to characterize the frequency and severity of these disruptive behaviors and their impact on child's functioning. Most research studies show that the risk of disruptive behavior and associated deficits in cognitive control are conferred by the presence of cooccurring ADHD. However, in some children anger outbursts or rage attacks may be associated with tic severity, complex tics, or with other forms of cooccurring disorders such as OCD and anxiety. Behavioral interventions for anger and disruptive behavior in TS have been tested in small randomized trials. These interventions should be conducted in the context of comprehensive treatment of tics and cooccurring psychopathology.

REFERENCES

Achenbach, T. M., & Rescorla, L. (2001a). *ASEBA school-age forms & profiles*. Burlington, VT: Aseba Burlington.

Achenbach, T. M., & Rescorla, L. A. (2001b). *Manual for the ASEBA school-age forms & Profiles*. Burlington, VT: University of Vermont, Research Center for Children, Youth, and Families.

American Psychiatric Association. (2013). *Diagnostic and statistical manual of mental disorders (DSM-5®)*. Washington, DC: American Psychiatric Pub.

Armbruster, P., Sukhodolsky, D., & Michalsen, R. (2004). The impact of managed care on children's outpatient treatment: A comparison study of treatment outcome before and after managed care. *American Journal of Orthopsychiatry*, *74*, 5–13.

Armenteros, J. L., & Lewis, J. E. (2002). Citalopram treatment for impulsive aggression in children and adolescents: An open pilot study. *Journal of the American Academy of Child & Adolescent Psychiatry*, *41*, 522–529.

Barkley, R. A. (2013). *Defiant children: A clinician's manual for assessment and parent training*. New York: Guilford Press.

Beck, A. T., Steer, R. A., & Brown, G. K. (1996). *Beck depression inventory manual*. San Antonio, TX: Psychological Corporation.

Bellina, M., Brambilla, P., Garzitto, M., Negri, G. A., Molteni, M., & Nobile, M. (2013). The ability of CBCL DSM-oriented scales to predict DSM-IV diagnoses in a referred sample of children and adolescents. *European Child & Adolescent Psychiatry*, *22*, 235–246.

Birmaher, B., Brent, D. A., Chiappetta, L., Bridge, J., Monga, S., & Baugher, M. (1999). Psychometric properties of the screen for child anxiety related emotional disorders (SCARED): A replication study. *Journal of the American Academy of Child and Adolescent Psychiatry*, *38*, 1230–1236.

Bloch, M. H., Panza, K. E., Landeros-Weisenberger, A., & Leckman, J. F. (2009). Meta-analysis: Treatment of attention-deficit/hyperactivity disorder in children with comorbid tic disorders. *Journal of the American Academy of Child and Adolescent Psychiatry*, *48*, 884–893.

Bruun, R. D., & Budman, C. L. (1998). Paroxetine treatment of episodic rages associated with Tourette's disorder. *Journal of Clinical Psychiatry*, *59*, 581–584.

Budman, C. L., Bruun, R. D., Park, K. S., Lesser, M., & Olson, M. (2000). Explosive outbursts in children with Tourette's disorder. *Journal of the American Academy of Child and Adolescent Psychiatry*, *39*, 1270–1276.

Budman, C. L., Rockmore, L., Stokes, J., & Sossin, M. (2003). Clinical phenomenology of episodic rage in children with Tourette syndrome. *Journal of Psychosomatic Research, 55*, 59–65.

Budman, C., Coffey, B. J., Shechter, R., Schrock, M., Wieland, N., Spirgel, A., & Simon, E. (2008). Aripiprazole in children and adolescents with Tourette disorder with and without explosive outbursts. *Journal of Child and Adolescent Psychopharmacology, 18*, 509–515.

Budman, C. L., Rosen, M., & Shad, S. (2015). Fits, tantrums, and rages in TS and related disorders. *Current Developmental Disorders Reports, 2*, 273–284.

Cavanna, A. E., Selvini, C., Luoni, C., Eddy, C. M., Ali, F., Blangiardo, R., ... Termine, C. (2015). Measuring anger expression in young patients with Tourette Syndrome. *Children's Health Care, 44*, 264–276.

Chen, K., Budman, C. L., Diego herrera, L., Witkin, J. E., Weiss, N. T., Lowe, T. L., ... Mathews, C. A. (2013). Prevalence and clinical correlates of explosive outbursts in Tourette syndrome. *Psychiatry Research, 205*, 269–275.

Chowdhury, M., Aman, M. G., Lecavalier, L., Smith, T., Johnson, C., Swiezy, N., ... Bearss, K. (2015). Factor structure and psychometric properties of the revised Home Situations Questionnaire for autism spectrum disorder: The Home Situations Questionnaire-Autism Spectrum Disorder. *Autism*, 1362361315593941.

Coffey, B. J., Biederman, J., Geller, D. A., Spencer, T. J., Kim, G. S., Bellordre, C. A., ... Magovcevic, M. (2000a). Distinguishing illness severity from tic severity in children and adolescents with Tourette's disorder. *Journal of the American Academy of Child & Adolescent Psychiatry, 39*, 556–561.

Coffey, B. J., Biederman, J., Smoller, J. W., Geller, D. A., Sarin, P., Schwartz, S., & Kim, G. S. (2000b). Anxiety disorders and tic severity in juveniles with Tourette's disorder. *Journal of the American Academy of Child & Adolescent Psychiatry, 39*, 562–568.

Comings, D. E., & Comings, B. G. (1985). Tourette syndrome: Clinical and psychological aspects of 250 cases. *American Journal of Human Genetics, 37*, 435–450.

Compton, S. N., March, J. S., Brent, D., Albano, A. M. T., Weersing, R., & Curry, J. (2004). Cognitive-behavioral psychotherapy for anxiety and depressive disorders in children and adolescents: An evidence-based medicine review. *Journal of the American Academy of Child & Adolescent Psychiatry, 43*, 930–959.

Conelea, C. A., Woods, D. W., & Brandt, B. C. (2011). The impact of a stress induction task on tic frequencies in youth with Tourette Syndrome. *Behaviour Research and Therapy, 49*, 492–497.

Costello, E. J., & Angold, A. (1988). Scales to assess child and adolescent depression: Checklists, screens, and nets. *Journal of the American Academy of Child and Adolescent Psychiatry, 27*, 726–737.

Dooley, J. M. J. (1999). Parent perceptions of symptom severity in Tourette's syndrome. *Archives of Disease in Childhood, 81*, 440–441.

Dupaul, G. J., & Barkley, R. A. (1992). Situational variability of attention problems: Psychometric properties of the Revised Home and School Situations Questionnaires. *Journal of Clinical Child Psychology, 21*, 178–188.

Frank, M. C., Piedad, J., Rickards, H., & Cavanna, A. E. (2011). The role of impulse control disorders in Tourette syndrome: An exploratory study. *Journal of the Neurological Sciences, 310*, 276–278.

Freeman, R. D., Fast, D. K., Burd, L., Kerbeshian, J., Robertson, M. M., & Sandor, P. (2000). An international perspective on Tourette syndrome: Selected findings from 3,500 individuals in 22 countries. *Developmental Medicine & Child Neurology, 42*, 436–447.

Gadow, K. D. (2002). Tics and psychiatric comorbidity in children and adolescents. *Developmental Medicine and Child Neurology, 44*, 330–338.

Gadow, K. D., & Sprafkin, J. (2002). *Child symptom inventory-4 screening and norms manual.* Stony Brook, NY: Checkmate Plus.

Ghanizadeh, A., & Mosallaei, S. (2009). Psychiatric disorders and behavioral problems in children and adolescents with Tourette syndrome. *Brain and Development, 31*, 15–19.

Gurnani, T., Ivanov, I., & Newcorn, J. H. (2016). Pharmacotherapy of aggression in child and adolescent psychiatric disorders. *Journal of Child and Adolescent Psychopharmacology, 26*, 65–73.

Hirschtritt, M. E., Lee, P. C., Pauls, D. L., Dion, Y., Grados, M. A., Illmann, C., ... Tourette Syndrome Association International Consortium for, G. (2015). Lifetime prevalence, age of risk, and genetic relationships of comorbid psychiatric disorders in Tourette syndrome. *JAMA Psychiatry, 72*, 325–333.

Kassinove, H., & Sukhodolsky, D. G. (1995). Anger disorders: Basic science and practice issues. *Issues in Comprehensive Pediatric Nursing, 18*, 173–205.

Kazdin, A. (2005). *Parent management training: Treatment for oppositional, aggressive, and antisocial behavior in children and adolescents.* New York, NY: Oxford University Press.

Keenan, K., & Wakschlag, L. S. (2004). Are oppositional defiant and conduct disorder symptoms normative behaviors in preschoolers? A comparison of referred and nonreferred children. *American Journal of Psychiatry, 161*, 356–358.

Kendall, P., & Hedtke, K. A. (2006). *Cognitive-behavioral therapy for anxious children: Therapist manual.* Ardmore, PA: Workbook Publishing.

Kovacs, M. (1992). *Children's depression inventory.* North Tonawanda, NY: Multi-Health Systems.

Kovacs, M. (2011). *Children's depression inventory 2nd edition (CDI-2).* Toronto, Canada: Multi-Health Systems.

Lewin, A. B., Storch, E. A., Conelea, C. A., Woods, D. W., Zinner, S. H., Budman, C. L., ... Murphy, T. K. (2011). The roles of anxiety and depression in connecting tic severity and functional impairment. *Journal of Anxiety Disorders, 25*, 164–168.

Malone, R. P., Delaney, M. A., Luebbert, J. F., Cater, J., & Campbell, M. (2000). A double-blind placebo-controlled study of lithium in hospitalized aggressive children and adolescents with conduct disorder. *Archives of General Psychiatry, 57*, 649–654.

March, J. S. (2013). *Multidimensional anxiety scale for children 2nd edition (MASC 2).* Toronto, Canada: Multi-Health Systems.

March, J. S., Sullivan, K., Stallings, P., Conners, C. K., & Parker, J. D. A. (1997). The Multidimensional Anxiety Scale for Children (MASC): Factor structure, reliability, and validity. *Journal of the American Academy of Child and Adolescent Psychiatry, 36*, 554–565.

Martino, D., & Leckman, J. F. (2013). *Tourette syndrome.* Oxford; New York: Oxford University Press.

Mccracken, J. T., Suddath, R., Chang, S., Thakur, S., & Piacentini, J. (2008). Effectiveness and tolerability of open label olanzapine in children and adolescents with Tourette syndrome. *Journal of Child and Adolescent Psychopharmacology, 18*, 501–508.

Mcguire, J. F., Sukhodolsky, D. G., Bearss, K., Grantz, H., Pachler, M., Lombroso, P. J., & Scahill, L. (2014). Individualized assessments in treatment research: An examination of parent-nominated target problems in the treatment of disruptive behaviors in youth with Tourette Syndrome. *Child Psychiatry & Human Development, 45*, 686–694.

Mcmahon, R., & Forehand, R. (2003). *Helping the noncompliant child. New York: Guilford.*

Michelson, D., Davenport, C., Dretzke, J., Barlow, J., & Day, C. (2013). Do evidence-based interventions work when tested in the "real world?" A systematic review and meta-analysis of parent management training for the treatment of child disruptive behavior. *Clinical Child and Family Psychology Review*, *16*, 18–34.

Murphy, T. K., Lewin, A. B., Storch, E. A., & Stock, S. (2013). Practice parameter for the assessment and treatment of children and adolescents with tic disorders. *Journal of the American Academy of Child & Adolescent Psychiatry*, *52*, 1341–1359.

Nadeau, J. M., Mcbride, N. M., Dane, B. F., Collier, A. B., Keene, A. C., Hacker, L. E., ... Storch, E. A. (2016). Psychometric evaluation of the rage outbursts and anger rating scale in an outpatient psychiatric sample. *Journal of Child and Family Studies*, *25*, 1229–1234.

Nelson, W. M., & Finch, A. (2000). *Children's inventory of anger: ChIA manual*. Los Angeles, CA: Western Psychological Services.

Patterson, G. R., Reid, J. B., & Dishion, T. J. (1992). *A social learning approach: IV. Antisocial boys*. Eugene, OR: Castalia.

Piedad, J. C. P., & Cavanna, A. E. (2016). Depression in Tourette syndrome: A controlled and comparison study. *Journal of the Neurological Sciences*, *364*, 128–132.

Pliszka, S., & Issues, A. W. G. O. Q. (2007). Practice parameter for the assessment and treatment of children and adolescents with attention-deficit/hyperactivity disorder. *Journal of the American Academy of Child & Adolescent Psychiatry*, *46*, 894–921.

Pringsheim, T., Hirsch, L., Gardner, D., & Gorman, D. A. (2015). The pharmacological management of oppositional behaviour, conduct problems, and aggression in children and adolescents with attention-deficit hyperactivity disorder, oppositional defiant disorder, and conduct disorder: A systematic review and meta-analysis. Part 1: Psychostimulants, alpha-2 agonists, and atomoxetine. *Canadian Journal of Psychiatry*, *60*, 42–51.

Robertson, M. M. (2015). A personal 35 year perspective on Gilles de la Tourette syndrome: Prevalence, phenomenology, comorbidities, and coexistent psychopathologies. *The Lancet Psychiatry*, *2*, 68–87.

Robertson, M. M., Cavanna, A. E., & Eapen, V. (2015). Gilles de la Tourette syndrome and disruptive behavior disorders: Prevalence, associations, and explanation of the relationships. *Journal of Neuropsychiatry and Clinical Neurosciences*, *27*, 33–41.

Roessner, V., Becker, A., Banaschewski, T., Freeman, R. D., Rothenberger, A., & Tourette Syndrome International database, C. (2007). Developmental psychopathology of children and adolescents with Tourette syndrome—impact of ADHD. *European Child & Adolescent Psychiatry*, *16*(Suppl. 1), 24–35.

Scahill, L., Erenberg, G., Berlin, C. M., Budman, C., Coffey, B. J., Jankovic, J., ... Lang, A. (2006a). Contemporary assessment and pharmacotherapy of Tourette syndrome. *NeuroRx*, *3*, 192–206.

Scahill, L., Williams, S., Schwab-Stone, M., Applegate, J., & Leckman, J. F. (2006c). Disruptive behavior problems in a community sample of children with tic disorders. *Advances in Neurology*, *99*, 184–190.

Seligman, L. D., & Ollendick, T. H. (2011). Cognitive-behavioral therapy for anxiety disorders in youth. *Child Adolesc Psychiatr Clinics of North America*, *20*, 217–238.

Silver, J. M., & Yudofsky, S. C. (1991). The Overt Aggression Scale: Overview and guiding principles. *Journal of Neuropsychiatry and Clinical Neurosciences*, *3*, S22–S29.

Snider, L. A., Seligman, L. D., Ketchen, B. R., Levitt, S. J., Bates, L. R., Garvey, M. A., & Swedo, S. E. (2002). Tics and problem behaviors in schoolchildren: Prevalence, characterization, and associations. *Pediatrics*, *110*, 331–336.

Spielberger, C. D. (1988). *Manual for the state-trait anger expression inventory (STAXI)*. Odessa, FL: Psychological Assessment Resources.

Steinberg, T., Shmuel-Baruch, S., Horesh, N., & Apter, A. (2013). Life events and Tourette syndrome. *Comprehensive Psychiatry, 54*, 467–473.

Stephens, R. J., Bassel, C., & Sandor, P. (2004). Olanzapine in the treatment of aggression and tics in children with Tourette's syndrome—a pilot study. *Journal of Child and Adolescent Psychopharmacology, 14*, 255–266.

Storch, E. A., Jones, A. M., Lack, C. W., Ale, C. M., Sulkowski, M. L., Lewin, A. B., ... Murphy, T. K. (2012). Rage attacks in pediatric obsessive-compulsive disorder: Phenomenology and clinical correlates. *Journal of the American Academy of Child & Adolescent Psychiatry, 51*, 582–592.

Sukhodolsky, D., & Scahill, L. (2012). *Cognitive-behavioral therapy for anger and aggression in children*. New York, NY: The Guilford Press.

Sukhodolsky, D. G., Scahill, L., Zhang, H., Peterson, B. S., King, R. A., Lombroso, P. J., ... Leckman, J. F. (2003). Disruptive behavior in children with Tourette's syndrome: Association with ADHD comorbidity, tic severity, and functional impairment. *Journal of the American Academy of Child & Adolescent Psychiatry, 42*, 98–105.

Sukhodolsky, D. G., Smith, S. D., Mccauley, S. A., Ibrahim, K., & Piasecka, J. B. (2016a). Behavioral interventions for anger, irritability, and aggression in children and adolescents. *Journal of Child and Adolescent Psychopharmacology, 26*, 58–64.

Sukhodolsky, D. G., Vander wyk, B. C., Eilbott, J. A., Mccauley, S. A., Ibrahim, K., Crowley, M. J., & Pelphrey, K. A. (2016b). Neural mechanisms of cognitive-behavioral therapy for aggression in children and adolescents: Design of a randomized controlled trial within the National Institute for Mental Health Research domain criteria construct of frustrative non-reward. *Journal of Child and Adolescent Psychopharmacology, 26*, 38–48.

Sukhodolsky, D. G., Vitulano, L. A., Carroll, D. H., Mcguire, J., Leckman, J. F., & Scahill, L. (2009). Randomized trial of anger control training for adolescents with Tourette's syndrome and disruptive behavior. *Journal of the American Academy of Child & Adolescent Psychiatry, 48*, 413–421.

Sukhodolsky, D. G., Woods, D. W., Piacentini, J., Wilhelm, S., Peterson, A. L., Katsovich, L., ... Scahill, L. (2017). Moderators and predictors of response to behavior therapy for tics in Tourette syndrome. *Neurology, 88*, 1029–1036.

Wood, J. J., Piacentini, J. C., Southam-Gerow, M., Chu, B. C., & Sigman, M. (2006). Family cognitive behavioral therapy for child anxiety disorders. *Journal of the American Academy of Child & Adolescent Psychiatry, 45*, 314–321.

Yudofsky, S. C., Silver, J. M., Jackson, W., Endicott, J., & Williams, D. (1986). The Overt Aggression Scale for the objective rating of verbal and physical aggression. *American Journal of Psychiatry, 143*, 35–39.

FURTHER READING

Scahill, L., Sukhodolsky, D. G., Bearss, K., Findley, D., Hamrin, V., Carroll, D. H., & Rains, A. L. (2006b). Randomized trial of parent management training in children with tic disorders and disruptive behavior. *Journal of Child Neurology, 21*, 650–656.

Sukhodolsky, D. G., Eicher, G., & Leckman, J. F. (2013). Social and adaptive functioning in Tourette syndrome. In D. Martino, & J. F. Leckman (Eds.), *Tourette syndrome* (pp. 468–486). New York: Oxford University Press.

Chapter 13

Mindfulness for Tics

Hannah E. Reese, PhD
Department of Psychology, Bowdoin College, Brunswick, ME, United States

Mindfulness has been defined as, "paying attention in a particular way: on purpose, in the present moment, and nonjudgmentally" (Kabat-Zinn, 1994, p. 4). Although the concept of mindfulness originated in ancient Buddhist traditions, it has become the focus of western psychological study in the past 50 years. And in recent years, mindfulness has been increasingly integrated into contemporary psychological interventions for a wide range of disorders, such as borderline personality disorder (dialectical behavior therapy, Linehan, 1993), generalized anxiety disorder (Orsillo & Roemer, 2011), and major depression (Williams, Teasdale, Segal, & Kabat-Zinn, 2007).

Mindfulness can be cultivated in brief, informal practices (e.g., paying close, nonjudgmental attention to everyday activities such as brushing one's teeth, doing the dishes, taking a sip of coffee, taking a breath) and in formal meditative practices (e.g., sitting meditation, the body scan). Most mindfulness-based psychological interventions make some use of both types of practices. Among other things, the formal meditative practices are thought to build one's capacity for sustained mindfulness, and the informal practices allow one to integrate mindfulness into the moment-to-moment experience of one's life.

There are a number of reasons to believe that a mindfulness-based approach might be helpful for an individual with tics.

INCREASED ATTENTIONAL CONTROL

Mindfulness exercises are fundamentally exercises in attentional control. Individuals are asked to direct their attention to a focal point (an object, the breath, the body) and when their attention wanders, they are encouraged to gently and firmly bring their attention back to the focal point. This practice of repeatedly focusing one's attention, monitoring its focus, and redirecting the focus when needed has been shown to increase attentional control (Lutz, Slagter, Dunne, & Davidson, 2008). For individuals with tics, this increased

The Clinician's Guide to Treatment and Management of Youth with Tourette Syndrome and Tic Disorders.
DOI: https://doi.org/10.1016/B978-0-12-811980-8.00013-3

attentional control may enable them to more readily detect and attend to urges to tic, tics, and factors that make the tics more or less likely to occur. This awareness is essential in enabling the individual to enact behavioral changes.

INTEROCEPTIVE AWARENESS

A number of formal mindfulness practices, such as the body scan and mindful movement or yoga, are designed to increase awareness of one's body. Clinical experience suggests that many individuals with tics have learned to ignore their bodies because they are not cooperating. Although this is a perfectly reasonable response, the tendency to ignore one's body may make individuals less likely to notice urges to tic, tics, and internal physical states (e.g., tension, fatigue, physiological arousal) that may make the tics more likely to occur. Indeed, in a recent experimental study, Ganos et al. (2015) found that individuals with Tourette syndrome (TS) possess lower levels of interoceptive awareness relative to control subjects. Learning to attend to one's body, in a gentle, curious manner through mindfulness exercises may increase interoceptive awareness. This enhanced interoceptive awareness may, in turn, enable individuals to notice premonitory urges to tic, tics, and the internal states that make tics more likely to occur. Indeed, Ganos et al. found that among adults with TS, greater interoceptive awareness was associated with more premonitory urges. Once the individual notices a premonitory urge or another physical state associated with tic onset, the individual may use this information as a cue to respond differently to the urge to tic (e.g., allowing it to subside without ticcing) or to engage in self-care (e.g., rest, stretching, relaxation) to alleviate the physical state(s).

DISTRESS TOLERANCE

Mindfulness-based approaches emphasize *being with* uncomfortable thoughts, emotions, and bodily sensations rather than immediately trying to change or escape them. Through meditation, individuals are encouraged to sit with discomfort, to explore it, and to notice one's automatic cognitive or behavioral responses to these experiences. For example, it is very common to experience an itch somewhere on one's body while meditating. However, it is also very common to not become aware of an itch until one is already scratching it. That is, the individual has habitually done something to alleviate an uncomfortable sensation (i.e., the itch) prior to even becoming consciously aware of the sensation. In these moments, the individual may realize just how automatic many of our responses to discomfort are and that without awareness of our experience (e.g., the itch), we do not have a choice as to how to respond to it. With awareness, however, we can choose whether we would like to scratch the itch or tolerate it without trying to change it or escape it. This practice directly translates to tics and the urges to tic. Current behavioral models (Woods et al., 2008), suggest that individuals often perform tics in order to alleviate the discomfort associated with premonitory sensations. This conceptualization fits with many patients' understanding of their symptoms. For example, Kwak, Dat Vuong, and Jankovic (2003) reported that 71% of individuals with TS believed their tics would no longer occur if the premonitory sensations were eliminated. Similarly, Lang (1991) found that two-thirds of individuals with tics described *all* of their tics as voluntary responses to involuntary urges. Unfortunately, every time an individual eliminates the urge to tic by ticcing, he or she is unwittingly negatively reinforcing the tic itself (see Chapter 2, Psychoeducation About Tic Disorders and Treatment, for further discussion of current behavioral models). These attempts to escape or avoid distress are thus paradoxically creating more distress. Through mindfulness practice, individuals may be able to identify or create a space between the urge to tic and the tic itself. They may then be able to explore whether they could tolerate the distress associated with the urge, and to allow the urge to subside on its own without engaging in the tic. If needed, they can focus their attention on their breath while the urge subsides independently. In this way, the breath is functioning as a competing response, although it is typically not physically incompatible with the tic (except in the case of a vocal tic). By engaging in this practice, individuals may learn that they can tolerate the discomfort associated with the urge to tic and that the discomfort will not last forever. Indeed, in a recent study of a mindfulness-based treatment for tics (Reese, Vallejo, Rasmussen, Crowe, Rosenfield, & Wilhelm, 2015; p. 296) one participant reported, "I liked. . .being aware, and learning how to live with/hold the discomfort—that gets to the heart of what triggers most of my tics—discomfort over something."

DECREASED PHYSIOLOGICAL AROUSAL AND EMOTIONAL REACTIVITY

Mindfulness has also been shown to reduce physiological arousal and emotional reactivity (see Rubia, 2009 for a review). Given the body of research linking tic occurrence and exacerbation to arousal and emotion (e.g., Conelea & Woods, 2008), reduced physiological arousal and emotional reactivity may make tics less likely to occur. Additionally, many individuals with tic disorders experience comorbid emotional disorders or symptoms (e.g., anger outbursts, irritability, anxiety; Freeman et al., 2000; Groth, Debes, Rask, Lange, & Skov, 2017). By reducing overall levels of emotional reactivity, mindfulness may provide individuals with relief from some of these comorbid symptoms.

KINDNESS AND ACCEPTANCE

And finally, mindfulness practices, generally encourage a kind, accepting, and gentle stance toward oneself. This is a departure from how many people with tics have learned to treat themselves. Many have, unfortunately, grown up believing that they are defective, lack self-control, and need to "try harder." This attitude toward oneself can lead to frustration, sadness, and self-blame (see Chapter 5, Cognitive Restructuring About Tics, and Chapter 6, Improving Self-Esteem for Youth with Tourette Syndrome and Tic Disorders, for further discussion of tics and self-esteem). Thus, practice may help individuals extend kindness and compassion to themselves and to others in their life. Thus attitudinal shift could potentially improve an individual's well-being regardless of tic severity.

Evidence-Base

It is only in the past several years that researchers have begun to empirically test whether a mindfulness-based approach might be helpful for individuals with tics. Franklin, Best, Wilson, Loew, and Compton (2011) conducted an early pilot study in which they compared habit reversal therapy (HRT), the standard behavioral intervention for tics, to HRT plus acceptance and commitment therapy (ACT). ACT is a transdiagnostic intervention that focuses on increasing psychological flexibility by promoting mindfulness, acceptance, cognitive defusion, and valued action (Hayes, Strosahl, & Wilson, 1999). ACT teaches patients that attempts to control or avoid aversive private events are futile and often lead to an exacerbation of the aversive event. Franklin et al. hypothesized that this aspect of ACT might be particularly useful in addressing tic-related urges and associated negative emotional states. Thirteen adolescents received either HRT or HRT plus ACT over 10 weeks. Both treatments were associated with significant reductions in tic severity and improvements in global functioning from baseline to posttreatment, and 3-month follow-up. At one-month follow-up, both groups were classified as mild based on their symptom severity scores. However, HRT plus ACT did not outperform HRT alone at any time point. Indeed, visual inspection of the data suggests that HRT was associated with a more rapid decline in symptoms. The authors suggest that the relatively delayed response to the HRT plus ACT intervention may have occurred because ACT is arguably more abstract and challenging to employ. Thus, clinicians and patients may have needed more time to effectively implement the approach. Additionally, the authors noted that the five study clinicians, with one exception, were more familiar with HRT than ACT at the start of the study. Interestingly, the one clinician who was more familiar with ACT achieved better outcomes relative to those who were less familiar with the intervention. These observations point to the importance of adequate training in mindfulness-based interventions, and future studies should ensure that providers are equally familiar with all interventions. The authors also argue that future larger studies are necessary to determine whether HRT plus ACT is more helpful for individuals with comorbid conditions, as they would hypothesize.

In a more recent study, Reese et al. (2015) conducted an open pilot study of a modified version of mindfulness-based stress reduction (MBSR) for adults with TS or chronic tic disorder. MBSR is an 8-week program, originally developed in 1979 by Jon Kabat-Zinn at the University of Massachusetts (Kabat-Zinn, 1990). Through direct practice in meditation, MBSR promotes the development of nonjudgmental moment-to-moment awareness of one's bodily sensations, thoughts, emotions, and perceptions. Participation is highly experiential and centers around four primary meditative practices: the body scan, mindful movement (gentle stretching and yoga), sitting meditation, and walking meditation. In each of these practices, participants gain experience in directing their attention to the content of their moment-to-moment experience while refraining from any efforts to change their experience. Participants are encouraged to adopt a curious, patient, accepting, nonstriving, and nonjudgmental attitude toward themselves and their inner experience. To adapt the course for individuals with tics, the intervention provided psychoeducation regarding tics and the theory motivating the approach, included a tic-specific sitting meditation, and practices for promoting mindfulness of the factors that make tics better or worse. The tic-specific sitting meditation became a cornerstone of the experiential practice. Briefly, the meditation encouraged participants to mindfully notice any urges to tic. When urges were noticed, participants were instructed to ride the urge to tic like a wave, while anchoring one's attention to the breath, until the urge subsided on its own without engaging in a tic. The intervention also included group discussion regarding the informal, day-to-day implementation of a mindful approach to the tics and urges to tic. The intervention was cotaught by an expert MBSR teacher and a psychologist with expertise in tic disorders. Eighteen individuals (ages 16–67) completed 8 weekly 2-hour group sessions of MBSR-tics and a 4-hour retreat during the fifth or sixth week of the program. The intervention was associated with significant reductions in tic severity and tic-related impairment from baseline to posttreatment. Ten of the eighteen participants (58.8%) were deemed treatment responders by an independent evaluator. Gains were maintained at one-month follow-up. Symptomatic improvements were also significantly and positively associated with increases in mindfulness. The lack of a control condition does limit the conclusions that can be drawn from this study. However, the improvements observed were comparable to those achieved in the most recent multicenter trial of comprehensive behavioral intervention for tics (CBIT) for adults (Wilhelm, Peterson, Piacentini, Woods, Deckersbach, Sukhodolsky, et al., 2012) suggesting that mindfulness may be a promising treatment approach for individuals with tics.

Clearly, knowledge regarding the efficacy of mindfulness-based strategies for tics is limited. It is hoped that future research will allow clinicians and researchers to better understand the potential benefits of mindfulness for individuals with tics. Given the limited evidence-base, traditional behavioral approaches, such as habit reversal training (see Chapter 3, Habit Reversal Training for Tics) and CBIT (Woods et al., 2008) should be offered as a first-line psychosocial approach. Mindfulness-based strategies may be considered, however, as a means of augmenting traditional approaches and/or may be considered as a stand-alone intervention for individuals who are not willing to try traditional approaches or who have not responded to such approaches. Importantly, in the two studies mentioned above (Franklin et al., 2011; Reese et al., 2015), mindfulness-based approaches were not associated with adverse effects. It is recommend, however, that anyone wishing to integrate mindfulness practices into their work with individuals with tics, monitor their patients for progress and any adverse effects (e.g., tic worsening, increased anxiety) on an ongoing basis (see Lustyk, Chawla, Nolan, & Marlatt, 2009 for a discussion of adverse events associated with mindfulness and best practices in mindfulness meditation).

In the following section, a guide for adopting a mindfulness-based approach with individuals with tics is presented.

Integrating Mindfulness Into the Treatment of Individuals With Tics

Mindfulness is not only taught explicitly, through direct practice, but also embodied implicitly, by the teacher. In the session, the mindful clinician adopts an open, curious, and nonjudgmental approach to whatever experiences the individual brings to the session. In doing this, the clinician is modeling for the individual how one might approach one's own experiences. Therefore, it is strongly recommended that any clinician interested in integrating mindfulness into their clinical work with others, first practice mindfulness themselves. By developing one's own mindfulness, the clinician will develop a much deeper and richer understanding of the practices and their associated challenges. The clinician will also have a much greater capacity for mindfully responding to whatever arises in session.

The mindfulness exercises described below are largely drawn from prior work adapting MBSR (Kabat-Zinn, 1990) for individuals with tics (Reese et al., 2015). Although MBSR was developed for adults, mindfulness-based approaches have been successfully adapted for use with children (see Greco & Hayes, 2008 for an overview). Amy Saltzman and Philippe Goldin have been particularly influential in the development of an MBSR curriculum for children 8 years of age and older with or without their parents (Saltzman & Goldin, 2008; http://www.stillquietplace.com). Although this pediatric version of MBSR has not been empirically evaluated with children with tics, it serves as an example of a successful adaptation of an adult program to children. In their writings, Saltzman and Goldin emphasize the importance of using age-appropriate language, and making the practices fun and engaging. They have also substantially reduced the length of formal meditative practices, estimating approximately one minute of sustained practice for each year of age (Saltzman & Goldin, 2008). For example, they estimate that an 8-year-old child could be reasonably expected to engage in a practice for approximately 8 minutes. Eline Snel (2013) has also published some very accessible mindfulness exercises for kids aged 5 years and older, and their parents. Similar to those exercises described by Saltzman and Goldin, Snel's exercises are brief, employ simple language, and use metaphors to aid in comprehension and communication of relatively abstract concepts. Whenever engaging children in mindfulness exercises, clinicians should be cautious about forcing the practices upon children as a means of "fixing" whatever ails them. Doing so would be antithetical to the tenets of mindfulness and would likely not inspire the openness and curiosity necessary for engagement with the practice. As parents are often involved in the treatment of youth with tics, it is important that parents allow their child to engage with the mindfulness practices at their own pace and in their own way. While it is hoped that a mindful approach will result in fewer tics or a greater sense of well-being, it is important to consider that focusing too much on any single desired outcome will likely undermine the practices.

INTRODUCING MINDFULNESS

Mindfulness is an abstract concept and is best introduced experientially. A common way to introduce mindfulness is through the raisin exercise. In the raisin exercise, participants are provided with a raisin, although any other small item of food could serve as a substitute. When presenting the small food item, the clinician does not name the object. Instead, the clinician asks the individual to investigate the object (the raisin) as if it is the first time that he or she is encountering it. For example, the clinician might say:

> *In a moment, I will give you an object. I want you to imagine that you have just landed on earth from a far away land and you have never encountered this object before. Explore the object as if it is the first time you are seeing it.*

In mindfulness, this act of approaching something without expectations or preexisting knowledge is referred to as *beginner's mind*. The individual is then given the raisin and guided in silently exploring the raisin with all of their senses: sight, touch, smell, hearing, and finally taste. Throughout, the participant is encouraged to notice any thoughts or emotions that may arise in response to the object. After eating the raisin, the participant is asked, "*What did you notice?*" Often, in doing this exercise, participants notice a great deal. They notice the way in which the light bounces off the raisin.

They notice the variations in color and texture. They notice the juiciness of the raisin and the changing flavors as it enters their mouth. They may also notice thoughts that arise about the past (memories of past encounters with raisins), the present (commentary about this experience, "What am I doing? What is the point of this?"), or the future (e.g., "What will I say about this experience?"). They may also notice emotions or behavioral urges that arise in response to the raisin—liking it or not liking it, wanting or not wanting to eat it. They also often notice how much this encounter with a raisin differed from their previous encounters with raisins. In noticing all of this, the individual is being mindful. They are noticing the stream of perceptions, thoughts, and emotions that are occurring in the present moment. And they are also beginning to appreciate how mindful attention differs from our ordinary way of paying attention. This can be a very rich experience for participants in that they may start to question what they are not noticing in their daily lives. Some may even begin to understand that our views of the world and what is possible are constrained by what we notice. After completing this exercise, participants generally have a much better understanding of what we mean when we say mindfulness. However, if the clinician suspects that the participant is having difficulty connecting the exercise to the concept of mindfulness, the clinician might explicitly connect it. For instance, a clinician could say something like, "*What you just did, noticing the details of the raisin, the thoughts, emotions, and bodily sensations that you were having, that was mindfulness.*" Most people, however, do not struggle with making this connection. Indeed, this exercise generally serves as a very concrete, nonthreatening, and accessible introduction to mindfulness.

FOUNDATIONAL PRACTICES

The following practices are standard mindfulness-based meditative practices. They are practiced in MBSR (Kabat-Zinn, 1990) and many other mindfulness-based interventions. Although they are not tic-specific, these practices can teach individuals the skills (e.g., attentional control, interoceptive awareness, distress tolerance, acceptance, and kindness) that are necessary for working mindfully with urges to tic and tics. It is recommended that individuals gain some experience with these practices before trying to work mindfully with the tics or urges to tic directly. For example, in the Reese et al. (2015) study described above, participants engaged in these general practices for 2 weeks prior to the introduction of a tic-related practice. They then continued to do these foundational practices as they simultaneously built their capacity for working directly with the tics. A description of each practice is below. More detailed information can be found in Kabat-Zinn (1990) and links to audio recordings of the body scan, mindful movement, and sitting meditations can be found in the Appendix. As with the raisin exercise, after the participant has completed any of these exercises, the clinician should guide the participant in reflecting on what they noticed during the practice. This process is called *inquiry*. Inquiry may help the individual recall and explore what they are noticing in the practice, connect these observations to the more general themes of mindfulness (e.g., acceptance, impermanence, beginners mind), and consolidate their learning. To guide inquiry, clinicians often start out by simply asking, "*What did you notice?*" The participant can then describe what they noticed and will often spontaneously connect their observations to more general concepts or patterns that they are noticing. If they do not, the clinician may be able to facilitate this learning by asking follow-up questions such as, "*How was the way in which you paid attention in this practice different from how you normally pay attention?*" or "*How was observing your urges/tics in this way different from how you normally attend to your tics?*" or "*How might this practice be relevant to your tics?*" For a more in-depth discussion of inquiry and its role in facilitating the development of mindfulness see Crane et al. (2015), Felder, Dimidjian, and Segal (2012), McCown, Reibel, and Micozzi (2010) and Woods, Rockman, and Collins (2016).

Some individuals with tics may have tried meditation or yoga previously. It is not uncommon for these individuals to express some frustration with the practice of mindfulness. This is often because individuals with tics often feel an intense pressure to be still and quiet during the exercises. To reduce this pressure, it is recommended that the clinician explicitly state that there is no expectation of stillness or quiet during these practices. Similarly, there is no expectation of tic suppression. If the individual experiences a tic and/or urge to tic, he or she should notice those behaviors and urges. Similarly, the individual may also notice any thoughts or emotions that arise in response to the urges and/or the tics. However, the participant should not feel the need to maintain a perfect posture, be perfectly still, or tic free during the exercises. They should simply observe what is arising in the present moment, as impartially, and nonjudgmentally as possible.

BODY SCAN

The body scan was developed by Kabat-Zinn (1990) as a tool for establishing bodily awareness. As mentioned above, many individuals with tics will state that they intentionally ignore their bodies because their bodies are not "cooperative". In the body scan, individuals are guided by systematically directing their attention to their entire body, one part at a time. The intention of this practice is to pay careful, kind attention to the physical sensations present in the body without trying to change anything. In doing this, individuals can become better acquainted with the physical state of their body (tense, in pain, at ease) and practice simply allowing things to be without reflexively trying to fix or change them. In doing this, participants begin to develop greater attentional control, interoceptive awareness, and distress tolerance. Many individuals also find the body scan to be relaxing, although this is not the intent.

The body scan begins by having the individual adopt a comfortable position that he or she can maintain for the duration of the practice. Although it can be practiced in any position, many choose to lay flat on their back with their arms along their side, palms facing up, and their feet loosely falling away from one another. Once comfortable, the individual is given a series of instructions. For example, the clinician may say:

> *Please follow along with instructions as best you can. Take care of yourself, do your best to stay awake, and be present to what is here in each moment.*
>
> *It may be helpful to see this as a time that is totally set aside for you. There is nowhere else that you need to be, nothing else that you need to be doing. You may even see it as a nourishing time, a time in which you give yourself your complete attention.*
>
> *Some of the sensations that you observe in this exercise may be pleasant or unpleasant, mild or intense. In some areas of your body you may notice the absence of sensation. All of this is fine. Just do your best to stay with each sensation as it arises, noticing what each feels like. Perhaps seeing if you can let go of the very normal tendency to like or dislike any of the sensations, or want them to be different, but instead practice allowing the sensations to be, however they are. . .allowing the sensations to be exactly as you find them.*
>
> *And as best you can, be gentle with yourself, bringing a sense of kind curiosity, and compassion to whatever you may notice in the practice.*
>
> *It is also important to resist the temptation to try to relax in this practice. Striving to be anything other than what you are will only create tension. Instead, allow yourself to simply be aware of each moment, and each sensation you observe.*
>
> *Now, gently allow your eyes to close if that feels comfortable for you. If not, allow them to be slightly open with a soft, unfocused gaze.*

Following these introductory instructions, the clinician then leads the individual in directing their attention to various areas of their body. Typically, this begins by bringing attention to the points of contact that the body makes with the floor or chair, then the entire body, the breath, and then to particular parts of the body. The focus on specific parts of the body often begins with the toes on the left foot, and continues up the left leg, then to the toes on the right foot, up the right leg to the pelvic area, abdomen, chest, shoulders, arms (beginning with the fingers and traveling up), the neck, mouth, face, head, and then the entire body. Although a typical body scan lasts 35–40 minutes, the length of time can and should be modified to suit an individual's needs as previously discussed (e.g., a 15-year old might only be able to complete a 15-minute body scan). Tailoring of the exercise can be accomplished by reducing the number of body parts covered and/or shortening the length of time that each is focused on. Online audio recordings of the body scan can be found in Appendix.

MINDFUL MOVEMENT

Mindful movement is an opportunity to practice mindfulness of the body in motion. To do this, the clinician guides the individual in a series of gentle stretches and yoga postures. Kabat-Zinn (2009) provides a series of drawings of gentle stretches and postures that can be used for mindful movement (pp. 106–113). Additionally, links to audio and video recordings of yoga and other mindful movements can be found in Appendix. The clinician can and should modify these movements based on patient needs and physical ability. The movements that the clinician selects are not as important as the way in which the clinician encourages the participant to pay attention during the movements. As in the body scan, the individual is instructed to attend to the physical sensations present in their body with a sense of curiosity and kindness. The intention is to be fully present with the body in each moment without rushing through the movements to get to the end or to attain some outcome. The most important consideration is that the clinician should present these exercises as an opportunity to practice being aware of the body in motion. This practice may help individuals with tics by developing and maintaining their physical awareness, even when engaged in other activities. This may enable them to be more aware of the urges to tic, and also moments of heightened physiological tension or arousal that may make the tics more likely to occur throughout their day. Clinical experience suggests that individuals with tics often find mindful movement to be a more accessible practice because they do not feel pressure to be still and quiet.

SITTING MEDITATION

The most basic sitting meditation is a mindfulness of the breath meditation. This practice is generally done sitting on a cushion on the floor, but can be easily adapted to a chair. It can be of any length and should be adapted to the individual's needs based on developmental level and experience practicing mindfulness. After settling into a comfortable, dignified posture, the individual is guided in attending to the breath wherever the individual finds it to be most vivid: the belly, the chest, the throat, the nostrils. The individual is then instructed to attend to the direct sensations of each in-breath and each out-breath, for the duration of the meditation. Typically, in very little time, the individual will notice that his or her mind has wandered. This is normal and part of the practice. Upon noticing that the mind has wandered, the individual is instructed to note where it wandered to (e.g., daydreaming, memories, planning), and then gently and firmly return the attention to the breath.

This practice in sustaining one's attention, monitoring its focus, and reorienting attention, is the heart of the practice. Over time, many individuals experience greater ability to sustain attention on the breath. Often, with this enhanced attentional control, individuals can experience a greater sense of calm and stability. Of course, this is not always the case. In moments of greater mental volatility, the practice can be one in which the individual comes to learn how their mind tends to behave. For example, some individuals may note that their mind tends to go to the future. They may start making plans, creating lists, or worrying. Meanwhile, others may find that their mind tends to go to the past and ruminations on past events. This practice, in viewing the contents of one's mind from an objective, detached sense, can help individuals come to appreciate their thoughts, emotions, and bodily sensations as mental events that do not necessarily require a response. This practice also sets the stage for later practice in which patients are encouraged to witness their urges to tic with the same detachment and nonreactivity.

WORKING MINDFULLY WITH TICS AND URGES TO TIC

After having gained some experience with the foundational exercises, patients may be ready to work mindfully with the urges to tic and the tics themselves. Reese et al. (2015) introduce this practice with a "Riding the Wave" sitting meditation. The "Riding the Wave Meditation" is detailed in Box 13.1 and also available for download under the resources tab at: https://www.bowdoin.edu/faculty/h/hreese/. The intention of the meditation is to help individuals become as intimately familiar with the internal experience of ticcing. Individuals are guided in exploring the earliest premonitory signs with a sense of curiosity and compassion. And upon noticing these early signs, the individual is encouraged to explore the sensations with a sense of curiosity and kindness, and to practice allowing the urge to tic to subside independently, without trying to eliminate it by ticcing. In doing this, the individual is practicing distress tolerance. And consistent with the behavioral model of tics, every time the individual allows the urge to subside without expressing the tic, they are weakening the association between the urge to tic and the tic itself.

In Reese et al. (2015) individuals were encouraged to practice this formal sitting meditation daily from the third week of the program. They were also encouraged to mindfully attend to urges to tic informally and practice allowing the urge to subside independently, as possible, throughout the day.

MINDFULLY OBSERVING ANTECEDENTS AND CONSEQUENCES TO TICS

Mindfulness can also be used to informally observe the internal (e.g., thoughts, emotions, sensations) and external (e.g., people, places, things)

BOX 13.1 Riding the Wave

Transcript of "Riding the Wave" meditation

As we have discussed, tics are often preceded by what we call a premonitory urge—an itch, tension, or pressure, that pushes you to tic to get rid of the urge. Our hope is that the following practice will guide you in becoming more aware of these urges—what they feel like in your body, where they are, how long they last—and the connection between these urges and your tics. And in time, you may be able to practice observing these urges, allowing them to go away on their own. It might be helpful to think of this practice like riding a wave—seeing the approaching water from a distance, watching it rise, and allowing it to pass through you and collapse, without needing to do anything to get rid of it, or push it away, but allowing it to go away on its own, without engaging in the tic—all the while using your breath as an anchor to steady yourself. Over time, with practice, you may see that the waves become smaller, less intense, and occur less frequently.

When you are first doing this practice, we recommend that you select one tic and its associated urge to focus your attention on. As you practice more, you may be able to expand your attention to include several or all of your tics and urges to tic at the same time.

As you complete the practice, try as best you can to not judge yourself or your experience. This is very difficult work. The practice is asking you to respond differently to processes that have been in place for years. This isn't something that can be learned overnight. Above all, we ask that you practice patience and kindness with yourself. Every new urge presents another opportunity for practice. And every response, presents an opportunity for learning.

Now, let's begin by adopting an upright, comfortable, dignified posture. If you are sitting in a chair, trying to sit away from the back of the chair so that your back is supporting itself. If you feel comfortable, closing your eyes or fixing your gaze gently on a spot in front of you. Closing your lips gently together and beginning to breathe through your nose.

And now bringing your attention to your breath, wherever you notice it in your body. It may be in your nose, your chest, or your belly. Wherever you notice the breath, try to notice the sensations present in that spot. Perhaps the rise of your belly with each in-breath, and the fall of your belly with each out-breath. Perhaps the sensation of air entering your nose with each in-breath and escaping with each out-breath. There's no right or wrong place to notice the breath. Just choose one location for this practice, perhaps where you feel it most strongly, and practice focusing your attention on the breath in that spot. There's no need to control your breath—making it slower or deeper. Just letting the body breathe itself and noticing the sensations associated with each in-breath and each out-breath for the next few minutes.

PAUSE (~2 minutes)

By now, you may have noticed some tics or urges to tic. When you notice the urge to tic, or a tic itself, with great kindness, patience, and compassion for yourself, see if you can remain curious and present to what is happening moment-by-moment-by-moment in your body and in your mind. The intention is to become as familiar as possible with what it feels like to experience an urge and a tic. Shifting your attention, if you care to, away from the breath and to the sensations that are present in this moment. What does it feel like? Where is it in your body? What are the earliest

(Continued)

BOX 13.1 (Continued)

sensations that you experience? A tingling, an itch, a pressure? How strong is the urge? And what happens to it over time? Does it come and go? Is there any space between the urge to tic and the tic itself? Some space, even the tiniest one, in which you could choose to respond rather than react to the urge—choose to allow the urge to subside on its own, rather than getting rid of it by doing the tic?

For the next few minutes, practice attending to your breath, focusing on each in-breath and each out-breath. And if you should notice an urge to tic or a tic itself, expand your attention to include the urge and/or the tic itself. In time, you may also practice exploring what happens if you allow the urge to come and go on its own—all the while anchoring yourself to your breath.

PAUSE (~4 minutes)

You may have noticed that your mind has started to wander. This is natural, normal, and part of being human. What is important is that once you notice your mind is elsewhere, you gently bring it back to your breath—focusing on each in-breath and each out-breath. You may do this 100 times or more before the practice is over and that is fine. It is the act of bringing your attention back to the sensations that are present in this moment that is important.

PAUSE (~1–2 minutes)

If you have been finding this difficult, or frustrating, that is natural too. If you find yourself getting frustrated or angry, or you notice judgmental thoughts like, "I'm not doing this right", try to note those feelings and thoughts, as they happen, with gentle curiosity—taking a step back, and perhaps saying, "hmph—look at that emotion" or "look at that thought." Perhaps also taking a moment to note how these thoughts or emotions might be affecting your body. Have your shoulders tightened? Has your jaw clenched? Once you have noted these things, you can then return to the practice of attending to the breath while remaining open to urges and tics.

PAUSE (~1–2 minutes)

Continue this practice for a few more minutes. When you hear the sound of a bell, you can gently open your eyes.

PAUSE (~2–3 minutes)

BELLS

antecedents and consequences that are associated with tic worsening. In Reese et al. (2015), clinicians assigned this informal exercise as home practice. Individuals were instructed to pause several times throughout each day, upon noticing a tic, to make note of their internal environment and external environment. With repeated observations, individuals could start to observe patterns associated with tic worsening. Then, if appropriate, they could devise behavioral strategies for reducing the impact of these factors. This is very similar to the functional analysis conducted in CBIT (Woods et al., 2008), although participants were encouraged to monitor the factors associated with tic occurrence on an ongoing basis, rather than to reflect on them retrospectively. Example monitoring forms can be found in the Appendix. Individuals could use paper forms or their smartphone or other digital devices to record their observations.

Challenging or Complex Issues

What if My Patient Struggles to Understand the Principles of Mindfulness?

Mindfulness can be an abstract concept to grasp. If your patient is struggling to understand the intention of the practices, it is recommended that the clinician reexamine the instructions that have been provided to the patient. Is the language simple and straight-forward? Are enough instructions provided. . .or perhaps too many? The practices that have been developed for children (e.g., Saltzman et al., 2008; Snel, 2013) are often the easiest to understand and may serve as an excellent reference.

How Should I Involve Parents or Other Caregivers in Treatment?

Whenever possible, it is important to actively involve parents or other caregivers in mindfulness-based interventions. This will enable the caregivers to understand what the child is doing in treatment, understand mindfulness, and perhaps better support the child in his or her practice. Indeed, as Greco and Hayes (2008) point out, if the child is being taught mindfulness in the clinic, but is living in an environment or culture that is unsupportive of its tenets (i.e., nonjudgmental acceptance of one's moment-to-moment experience), the child may be confronted with very mixed messages. For this reason, it is important that parents be aware of and supportive of the mindfulness-based approach to working with tics. To do this, the clinician can invite the caregiver(s) to practice the mindfulness exercises right alongside the child in session and at home. This may foster discussion between the caregiver and child about the practices and their effect on the caregiver and child, and promote a culture of mindfulness in the household.

Should I Apply Mindfulness During a "Tic Attack?"

Mindfulness is a skill that must be developed over time. Given its complexities, it is not recommended that patients try to learn mindfulness as a "quick fix" to reduce tics during a "tic attack." If, however, a patient has been practicing mindfulness for some time, and feels that he or she can bring his or her mindfulness to the moment, there is no reason to believe that mindfulness might not be helpful. Adopting an impartial, nonjudgmental stance on the moment may reduce one's emotional response to a bout of tics, which are typically very frustrating and upsetting for the individual. In mindfulness, one learns to accept the past. Thus, when one has just ticced, it is not something to be fought against or to hate, but to simply note because nothing more can be done about it. This approach could help individuals not beat themselves up for having just ticced (it already happened so no amount of disappointment will change that) and move on to the present moment.

Attention-Deficit Hyperactivity Disorder (ADHD) is Commonly Comorbid With Tics. Will Mindfulness be Helpful if my Patient Already has Trouble Paying Attention?

Although this has not been empirically tested, there is reason to believe that mindfulness-based approaches might actually be a good fit for individuals with tics and comorbid ADHD. Indeed, there is a growing literature to support the use of mindfulness-based strategies for children and adults with ADHD, many of whom were not concurrently taking ADHD medications (Bögels, Hoogstad, van Dun, de Schutter, & Restifo, 2008; Van der Oord, Bögels, & Peijnenburg, 2012; Van de Weijer-Bergsma, Formsma, de Bruin, & Bögels, 2012; Zylowska et al., 2008). For example, Van de Weijer-Bergsma et al. (2012) tested an 8-week mindfulness-based training for adolescents aged 11–15 and their parents. After treatment, the adolescents reported decreased attentional and behavioral problems and improved executive functioning. The authors incorporated many of the traditional mindfulness-based strategies in their intervention, but also developed mindfulness exercises specific to the challenges faced by youth with ADHD (e.g., distractibility). They also stated that the training was conducted in a stimulus-free environment with additional structural supports (e.g., a predictable routine, and a clearly outlined class schedule that was visible to all participants). Compliance with the exercises was also monitored and rewarded. Thus, it may be necessary for the clinician to modify the delivery of the exercises to help patients engage with them, but there is reason to believe that these interventions can be effective with this population.

CONCLUSION

In conclusion, there is recent evidence to suggest that a mindfulness-based approach may be helpful for individuals with tics. Given their strong empirical support, traditional behavioral approaches, such as habit reversal training (see Chapter 3, Habit Reversal Training for Tics) and CBIT (Woods et al., 2008) should be offered as first-line psychosocial treatment. However, mindfulness-based strategies may be considered as a means of augmenting traditional therapy and/or as a stand-alone intervention for individuals who are unwilling to try or unresponsive to traditional behavioral approaches. Future research will hopefully allow clinicians, researchers, and patients to more fully understand the potential benefits of this promising approach.

REFERENCES

Bögels, S. M., Hoogstad, B., van Dun, L., de Schutter, S., & Restifo, K. (2008). Mindfulness training for adolescents with externalizing disorders and their parents. *Behavioral and Cognitive Psychotherapy, 36*, 193–209.

Conelea, C. A., & Woods, D. W. (2008). The influence of contextual factors on tic expression in Tourette's syndrome: A review. *Journal of Psychosomatic Research, 65*, 487–496.

Crane, R. S., Stanley, S., Rooney, M., Bartley, T., Cooper, L., & Mardula, J. (2015). Disciplined improvisation: Characteristics of inquiry in mindfulness-based teaching. *Mindfulness, 6*(5), 1104–1114.

Felder, J. N., Dimidjian, S., & Segal, Z. (2012). Collaboration in mindfulness-based cognitive therapy. *Journal of Clinical Psychology, 68*(2), 179–186.

Franklin, M. E., Best, S. H., Wilson, M. A., Loew, B., & Compton, S. N. (2011). Habit reversal training and acceptance and commitment therapy for Tourette syndrome: A pilot project. *Journal of Developmental and Physical Disabilities, 23*(1), 49–60.

Freeman, R. D., Fast, D. K., Burd, L., Kerbeshian, J., Robertson, M. M., & Sandor, P. (2000). An international perspective on Tourette syndrome: selected findings from 3500 individuals in 22 countries. *Developmental Medicine & Child Neurology, 42*(7), 436–447.

Ganos, C., Garrido, A., Navalpotro-Gómez, I., Ricciardi, L., Martino, D., Edwards, M. J., … Bhatia, K. P. (2015). Premonitory urge to tic in Tourette's is associated with interoceptive awareness. *Movement Disorders, 30*, 1198–1202.

Greco, L. A., & Hayes, S. C. (2008). *Acceptance & mindfulness treatments for children & adolescents: A practitioner's guide*. New Harbinger Publications.

Groth, C., Debes, N. M., Rask, C. U., Lange, T., & Skov, L. (2017). Course of Tourette syndrome and comorbidities in a large prospective clinical study. *Journal of the American Academy of Child & Adolescent Psychiatry, 56*(4), 304–312.

Hayes, S. C., Strosahl, K., & Wilson, K. G. (1999). *Acceptance and commitment therapy: Understanding and treating human suffering. New York*: Guilford.

Kabat-Zinn, J. (1990). *Full catastrophe living: Using the wisdom of your body and mind to face stress, pain, and illness*. New York: Dell Publishing.

Kabat-Zinn, J. (1994). *Wherever you go, there you are: Mindfulness meditation in everyday life*. New York: Hyperion.

Kabat-Zinn, J. (2009). *Full catastrophe living: Using the wisdom of your body and mind to face stress, pain, and illness (15th Anniversary Edition)*. New York: Bantam.

Kwak, C., Dat Vuong, K., & Jankovic, J. (2003). Premonitory sensory phenomenon in Tourette's Syndrome. *Movement Disorders, 18*(12), 1530–1533. Available from http://dx.doi.org/10.1002/mds.10618.

Lang, A. (1991). Patient perception of tics and other movement disorders. *Neurology, 41*(2, Pt 1), 223–228.

Linehan, M. (1993). *Cognitive-behavioral treatment of borderline personality disorder*. Guilford Press.

Lustyk, M. K., Chawla, N., Nolan, R., & Marlatt, G. A. (2009). Mindfulness meditation research: Issues of participant screening, safety procedures, and researcher training. *Advances in Mind-Body Medicine, 24*(1), 20–30.

Lutz, A., Slagter, H. A., Dunne, J. D., & Davidson, R. J. (2008). Attention regulation and monitoring in meditation. *Trends in cognitive sciences, 12*(4), 163–169.

McCown, D., Reibel, D., & Micozzi, M. S. (2010). *Teaching mindfulness. A practical guide for clinicians and educators*. US: Springer.

Orsillo, S. M., & Roemer, L. (2011). *The mindful way through anxiety: Break free from chronic worry and reclaim your life*. Guilford Press.

Reese, H. E., Vallejo, Z., Rasmussen, J., Crowe, K., Rosenfield, E., & Wilhelm, S. (2015). Mindfulness-based stress reduction for Tourette syndrome and chronic tic disorder: a pilot study. *Journal of Psychosomatic Research, 78*(3), 293–298.

Rubia, K. (2009). The neurobiology of meditation and its clinical effectiveness in psychiatric disorders. *Biological Psychology, 82*(1), 1–11. PubMed PMID: 19393712.

Saltzman, A., & Goldin, P. (2008). Mindfulness-based stress reduction for school-age children. In L. A. Greco, S. C. Hayes, L. A. Greco, & S. C. Hayes (Eds.), *Acceptance and mindfulness treatments for children and adolescents: A practitioner's guide* (pp. 139–161). Oakland, CA, USA: New Harbinger Publications.

Snel, E. (2013). *Sitting still like a frog: Mindfulness exercises for kids (and their parents)*. Shambhala Publications.

Van der Oord, S., Bögels, S. M., & Peijnenburg, D. (2012). The effectiveness of mindfulness training for children with ADHD and mindful parenting for their parents. *Journal of Child and Family Studies, 21*(1), 139–147.

Van de Weijer-Bergsma, E., Formsma, A. R., de Bruin, E. I., & Bögels, S. M. (2012). The effectiveness of mindfulness training on behavioral problems and attentional functioning in adolescents with ADHD. *Journal of Child and Family Studies, 21*(5), 775–787.

Wilhelm, S., Peterson, A. L., Piacentini, J., Woods, D. W., Deckersbach, T., Sukhodolsky, D. G., et al. (2012). Randomized trial of behavior therapy for adults with Tourette syndrome. *Archives of General Psychiatry, 69*(8), 795–803.

Williams, M., Teasdale, J. D., Segal, Z. V., & Kabat-Zinn, J. (2007). *The mindful way through depression: Freeing yourself from chronic unhappiness*. Guilford Press.

Woods, D. W., Piacentini, J. C., Chang, S., Deckersbach, T., Ginsburg, G. S., Peterson, A. L., ... Wilhelm, S. (2008). *Managing Tourette syndrome: A behavioral intervention for children and adults*. New York, NY: Oxford University Press.

Woods, S.L., Rockman, P., & Collins, E. (2016). A contemplative dialogue: The inquiry process in mindfulness-based interventions. Retrieved from <http://www.mindfulnessstudies.com/wp-content/uploads/2016/02/Woods-S.-L.-Rockman-P. Collins-E.-2016-A-Complentative-Dialogue.pdf>.

Zylowska, L., et al. (2008). Mindfulness meditation training in adults and adolescents with ADHD a feasibility study. *Journal of Attention Disorders, 11*(6), 737–746.

FURTHER READING

Abramovitch, A., Reese, H., Woods, D. W., Peterson, A., Deckersbach, T., Piacentini, J., ... Wilhelm, S. (2015). Psychometric properties of a self-report instrument for the assessment of tic severity in adults with tic disorders. *Behavior Therapy, 46*(6), 786–796.

Chang, S., Himle, M. B., Tucker, B. T., Woods, D. W., & Piacentini, J. (2009). Initial psychometric properties of a brief parent-report instrument for assessing tic severity in children with chronic tic disorders. *Child & Family Behavior Therapy, 31*(3), 181–191.

Gaffney, G. R., Sieg, K., & Hellings, J. (1994). The MOVES: A self-rating scale for Tourette's syndrome. *Journal of Child and Adolescent Psychopharmacology, 4*(4), 269–280.

Mitchell, J. T., McIntyre, E. M., English, J. S., Dennis, M. F., Beckham, J. C., & Kollins, S. H. (2013). A pilot trial of mindfulness meditation training for ADHD in adulthood: Impact on core symptoms, executive functioning, and emotion dysregulation. *Journal of Attention Disorders*. Available from http://dx.doi.org/10.1177/1087054713513328.

APPENDIX

External Environment Monitoring Form

This form is designed to help you observe things outside of yourself, such as people (e.g., being around a certain person, being in a crowd), places (e.g., being in the car, in bed, in a movie theatre), and things/activities (e.g., a certain piece of clothing, a certain light or sound, talking on the phone, watching TV), that are associated with the tics.

Some things may set the stage for tics being more likely to occur (e.g., being in a movie theatre), whereas some may only occur after the tic (e.g., your spouse or parent asks you to stop). Just write down whatever you observe. The before column is for people, places, and things, that you observe before a tic or bout of tics. The after column is for observations that occur after the tic or bout of tics. The form is intended to guide your observations, but don't let it constrain you. If you also notice how these external events affect your internal environment, make note of that too. Try to make observations for at least one tic or bout of tics per day. The more observations you collect, the more likely it is that you will be able to see what patterns emerge.

Day/Time	Before	After

Internal Environment Monitoring Form

Use the following table to record your observations regarding your internal environment: your thoughts, emotions, and bodily sensations. Try to observe whatever arises immediately before or after a tic or bout of tics. You might not write something in every box--just write whatever you notice. Be curious—see if you can slow the process down enough to really notice what arises rather than writing down what you *know* to be true or *expect* to be true.

	Before	After
Thoughts Emotions Sensations		
Thoughts Emotions Sensations		
Thoughts Emotions Sensations		
Thoughts Emotions Sensations		
Thoughts Emotions Sensations		

Resource	Description	Access
https://www.bowdoin.edu/faculty/h/hreese/	A website maintained by the author which offers the tic-specific sitting meditation described above for download under the resources tab.	Free
http://www.mindfulnesscds.com/	A website through which CDs or digital files of guided meditations by Jon Kabat-Zinn, the creator of MBSR, can be purchased.	Available for purchase
http://marc.ucla.edu/mindful-meditations	A website maintained by the University of California Los Angeles Mindful Awareness Research Center that offers a range of brief (3–19 minute)	Free

(*Continued*)

(Continued)

Resource	Description	Access
	body scan and sitting meditations in English and Spanish.	
https://health.ucsd.edu/specialties/mindfulness/programs/mbsr/Pages/audio.aspx	A website maintained by the University of California San Diego Center for Mindfulness that offers a range of body scan, sitting meditation, and yoga audio and video recordings.	Free
Saltzman, A. (2014). *A still quiet place: A mindfulness program for teaching children and adolescents to ease stress and difficult emotions.* New Harbinger Publications.	A guide detailing the 8-week MBSR program that Amy Saltzman, M.D. created for children 8 years of age and older. Comes with downloadable exercises.	Available for purchase.
http://www.stillquietplace.com/practice-videos/	A website maintained by Amy Saltzman, M.D. that offers two sitting mediation and one mindful stretching video.	Free
Snel, E. (2013). *Sitting still like a frog: Mindfulness exercises for kids (and their parents).* Shambhala Publications.	A guide for parents who want to practice mindfulness with their children. Comes with a CD of 11 guided meditations.	Available for purchase.
Wolf, C., & Serpa, J. G. (2015). *A clinician's guide to teaching mindfulness: The comprehensive session-by-session program for mental health professionals and health care providers.* New Harbinger Publications.	A detailed reference for clinicians wishing to teach mindfulness to their patients. Example meditation scripts are included.	Available for purchase.
https://soundcloud.com/mindfulmagazine/body-scan-meditation-for-kids	A 12-minute body scan meditation for kids.	Free
https://www.headspace.com/	A popular mindfulness app that offers brief, accessible meditations.	Some basic meditations available for free, others available for purchase.
http://www.freemindfulness.org/download	A website maintained by Peter Morgan, a clinical psychologist, offering audio recordings of meditations that are commonly done in MBSR and/or Mindfulness-based Cognitive Therapy.	Free

Chapter 14

Family Issues Associated With Tics

Michael B. Himle, Brianna C.M. Wellen and Loran P. Hayes
Department of Psychology, University of Utah, Salt Lake, UT, United States

INTRODUCTION

The past quarter-century has witnessed substantial progress in treating persistent tic disorders (PTDs, including Tourette disorder, TD) using both medical and behavioral approaches (Himle & Capriotti, 2016; Scahill et al., 2006a). While these advancements are encouraging, most existing treatments for youth with PTD focus exclusively on reducing the child's tic symptoms and assume that tic reduction will be sufficient to ameliorate PTD-related sequelae and improve functioning (Ginsburg & Kingery, 2007). However, there is a growing literature showing that the impact of PTD often extends beyond the affected child. Numerous studies have shown that parenting a child with PTD is stressful on caregivers and can negatively impact the entire family system (Conelea et al., 2011; Ramanujam et al., 2015; Storch et al., 2007). The aim of this chapter is to help clinicians appreciate the importance of providing comprehensive, family-based clinical care when working with a child with PTD. The chapter begins with a brief review of how PTD and comorbid symptoms can negatively affect family functioning. It then discusses specific factors that are important for clinicians to consider when working with a family of a child with PTD and provides practical recommendations for how providers can intervene to reduce stress and burden on the family, improve resilience and family functioning, and increase treatment engagement.

THE IMPACT OF TICS AND COMORBID SYMPTOMS ON FAMILY FUNCTIONING

Understanding how PTD affects family functioning begins by appreciating the impact of PTD on the affected child, as social-emotional and behavioral problems in children have a reciprocal relationship to the well-being of

The Clinician's Guide to Treatment and Management of Youth with Tourette Syndrome and Tic Disorders.
DOI: https://doi.org/10.1016/B978-0-12-811980-8.00014-5

caregivers and siblings (Angold et al., 1998). Although some children with PTD are quite resilient and are not particularly bothered by their tics, many youths with PTD experience substantial tic-related functional impairment. In one of the largest studies to date, Conelea et al. (2011) conducted an online survey with 740 parents of children with PTD and found that both parents and children generally agreed that tics had an overall negative impact on the child's social, academic, and psychological functioning. Similarly, Storch et al. (2007) found that 36% of children reported at least one significant tic-related problem at school (e.g., difficulty writing, doing homework, or concentrating) and 25% reported that tics affected them socially (e.g., being teased, having trouble making friends). In addition to directly impacting the affected child, PTD has been shown to negatively affect caregivers and disrupt family functioning. For example, studies have shown that parents of children with PTD report considerable levels of objective burden (e.g., financial cost, disruption to daily routines, and interruption of personal time) and subjective strain (social isolation, worry, anger, stigma, and guilt; Conelea et al., 2011; Ramanujam et al., 2015). Likewise, studies have shown that tics often interfere with home activities, such as completing chores, disrupt morning, or bedtime routines, cause friction with siblings and parents, or make it difficult to go on family outings (e.g., vacation, church; Storch et al., 2007). A summary of some of the ways having a child with PTD can negatively impact the family is provided in Table 14.1.

In addition to the tics, psychiatric comorbidity is common in PTD and can cause or exacerbate functional impairment. Large international samples have found that as many as 90% of individuals with PTD (in clinical samples) experience at least one comorbid psychiatric condition, with most meeting criteria for at least two comorbid diagnoses in addition to PTD (referred to as PTD + ; Freeman et al., 2000). Studies have also shown that both internalizing and externalizing comorbidity are associated with decreased self-esteem, relationship problems, and functional impairment across most psychosocial domains, including family functioning (O'Hare, Helmes, Reece, Eapen, & McBain, 2016; Storch et al., 2007). For example, children with comorbid attention deficit hyperactivity disorder (ADHD), which is particularly common in PTD + , often need close monitoring and frequent reminders to complete simple tasks, take longer to complete homework, act impulsively, defy requests and commands, and misplace or lose important items. Likewise, children with comorbid obsessive-compulsive disorder (OCD), another common comorbidity in PTD + , often get "stuck" on tasks, get upset when rituals are interrupted, seek constant reassurance, involve family members in their rituals, and shape parents to commit time, energy, and resources to accommodate their symptoms in order to avoid a meltdown. In addition to being a significant source of familial distress, tics and comorbidity can also negatively impact the child's functioning at school, resulting in parents spending considerable time and energy working with (sometimes

TABLE 14.1 Examples of How Tics Can Affect Family Functioning

Tics can...
• Be distracting, making it hard for the child to focus on tasks • Directly interfere with homework (e.g., writing tics, eye-tics, head jerking) • Disrupt morning or bedtime routines • Interfere with leisure activities (e.g., hobbies) • Interfere with the child's activities of daily living (e.g., bathing, dressing, eating, toileting) • Limit the child's activities due to muscle fatigue and pain, eyestrain, and/or headaches • Cause injury to the child in severe cases • Disrupt the child's sleep • Lead to teasing from siblings (and sometimes even parents) • Become the focus of parental attention • Lead to avoidance of social activities (e.g., vacations, church) • Be a source of worry, confusion, frustration, and tension for parents • Be difficult to distinguish from comorbid symptoms and developmentally normal behavior, making it difficult for parents to know how (or not) to respond to the child's behavior. • Be a source of financial strain (medical bills) • Be time demanding for caregivers (doctors' visits, seeking school accommodations, etc.) • Cause the family to spend more time with, or give more attention to, the affected child than his/her siblings • Result in the child being excluded from family activities (e.g., going to movies, eating meals with the family) • Cause conflict with extended family • Be embarrassing and/or stigmatizing for the child and his/her parents • Cause the parents to inappropriately reduce their expectations for the child. • Lead to parent-school conflict

battling) the school to ensure that the child is receiving appropriate academic accommodations (see Chapter 8: Tourette's in the Classroom: Support and Guidance on Education Issues for Clinicians). Many children with PTD also experience nondiagnostic problems including sleep disruption, sensory sensitivities, somatic complaints, perfectionism, and fine motor delays. Because these symptoms are not specific to PTD (or any particular comorbid diagnosis), they are often overlooked, but can place additional burden on caregivers and the family system (Freeman et al., 2000; Houghton, Capriotti, Conelea, & Woods, 2014).

Based on the extant literature and the authors' clinical experience, two important aspects should be considered by clinicians when working with PTD. First, it is important to be mindful of the fact that the impact of PTD often extends well beyond the affected child. Thus in addition to assessing the functional impact of PTD on the affected child, clinicians should also carefully assess how the child's tics and comorbid symptoms are affecting caregivers and siblings. Second, clinicians should not assume that successfully treating a child's tics will sufficiently ameliorate the negative impact of PTD or comorbidity on other members of the family. In fact, secondary analyses from a large randomized controlled trial of behavior therapy focused on reducing tics (i.e., Comprehensive Behavioral Intervention for Tics, CBIT) showed that, even among treatment responders, parents reported only modest improvements in caregiver strain, family functioning, and comorbid symptoms (Woods et al., 2011).

IMPROVING FAMILY FUNCTIONING IN PERSISTENT TIC DISORDERS

While much more empirical work is needed to better understand how to optimally support families affected by PTD, clinical experience suggests that taking a comprehensive approach that incorporates tic-specific interventions (e.g., HRT, CBIT) into a broader framework of providing psychosocial support and family-based therapy can reduce caregiver burden, improve family functioning, and increase treatment adherence. Specifically, the comprehensive approach outlined in this chapter emphasizes the importance of (1) helping the family to prioritize treatment targets and goals (see Chapter 1: Introduction to Treatment and Management of Youth With Tourette Disorders and Tic Disorders), (2) providing thorough psychoeducation (see Chapter 2: Psychoeducation About Tic Disorders and Treatment), (3) identifying and fostering the child's strengths (see Chapter 6: Improving Self-Esteem for Youth With Tourette Syndrome and Tic Disorders), and (4) teaching the family healthy ways to talk about tics with other (see Chapter 7: Talking About Tics With Peers and Coping in Social Interactions). Because these topics are discussed in detail in other chapters, this chapter will provide only a brief review of each in order to highlight particular points of relevance for improving family functioning. We will then more thoroughly examine several additional factors that clinicians should consider when working with families with PTD, including: (1) assessing and understanding the family's early experiences with PTD and the health care system, (2) helping the family to differentiate tics from nontic behaviors and managing comorbidity, (3) teaching families effective ways to respond to the child's tics using a function-based approach, (4) increasing support for the patient, parent, and family, and (5) coordinating care.

Helping the Family to Prioritize Treatment Targets and Goals

Prior to entering treatment, parents often lump their child's tics and comorbid symptoms together under the "Tourette's" diagnostic label. In doing so, clinicians may be left with the impression that the child's tics are the primary problem (as clinicians understand that the diagnosis refers only to tics) and the reason that the family is seeking treatment. Such assumptions can lead to confusion and dissatisfaction if the clinician, child, and parents are in disagreement about treatment goals and priorities. As discussed in Chapter 1, Introduction to Treatment and Management of Youth With Tourette Disorders and Tic Disorders, it is essential for clinicians to carefully explore which specific symptoms are impacting whom and why, and then determine which symptoms are contributing the greatest burden on the family and child. Prior to beginning treatment, it can be helpful to have the child and his or her parents independently create lists of the 5–10 most bothersome things about PTD and then to rank them from most to least bothersome. Similarly, parents and the child can be asked to list and rank order the five most important outcomes they would like to see from treatment. In doing this, a clinician can discover whether parents and children have similar views of which symptoms are the most bothersome and why, as well as clarify disagreements about treatment expectations. Gathering parent and child input regarding their experiences and perception of the problem can also help to establish a collaborative working alliance, inform the clinician's case formulation and treatment plan, clarify treatment expectations, and increase treatment engagement.

Providing thorough Psychoeducation

How a family is affected by PTD can be heavily influenced by the timing, amount, and quality of psychoeducation they receive and the advice they are given regarding how to manage their child's symptoms. Unfortunately, many parents report that they receive little helpful guidance and remain confused about diagnostic terms and treatment options. For example, it is not uncommon for parents to assume (or to be told) that their child does not have TD because he/she does not have comorbidity (which is in fact *not* required for a TD diagnosis) or that their child's comorbid symptoms (e.g., noncompliance, compulsions, swearing) are tics. This can leave parents confused about which behaviors their child can, and cannot, control. Likewise, some parents have been told that medication for tics should unequivocally be avoided due to serious side effects or that behavioral interventions, such as CBIT, will make tics worse (e.g., cause a tic rebound, cause new tics to start, make the child self-conscious), despite a wealth of research showing this to be rare (e.g., Peterson et al., 2016). Lack of information about PTD and its treatment can leave families feeling helpless or pessimistic about available treatment options and decrease the likelihood that they will seek and utilize effective interventions. As discussed in Chapter 2: Psychoeducation About Tic Disorders and Treatment, thorough psychoeducation can, among other things, promote positive attitudes and healthy interactions toward youth with PTD, increase treatment engagement and adherence, help to reduce guilt and stigma surrounding the PTD diagnosis, restore trust in health care providers, and create optimism for the future by helping parents understand that PTD is a manageable condition.

Identifying and Fostering the Child's Strengths

In working with children with PTD, especially those with complex comorbidity, it can be easy for the parents (and even clinicians) to focus exclusively on the child's struggles. It is equally important, however, to identify and highlight the child's strengths (see Chapter 6: Improving Self-Esteem for Youth With Tourette Syndrome and Tic Disorders on improving self-esteem). In one interesting study, Steinberg, Shmuel-Baruch, Horesh, and Apter (2013) found that positive life events, such as academic success and compliments from teachers, were associated with decreased tic severity, suggesting that focusing on the child's strengths and promoting success in other areas might confer some clinical benefit. It is recommended that, for most children, at least one of the goals for treatment focus on fostering or developing the child's strengths and/or increasing time spent in preferred activities. These might include joining a sports team, pursuing a new hobby, learning to play an instrument, joining a club at school, or volunteer work, to name just a few. When appropriate, clinicians should place particular emphasis on increasing time spent in any activities that the child and family enjoy doing together (or had enjoyed in the past), but have been avoiding due to tics. In addition, it may be useful to assign tasks at home that the child can easily master, such as completing chores (along with contingent reinforcement and ample praise from the parents), helping prepare meals, or taking responsibility for his/her morning or bedtime routine. Focusing at least part of treatment on fostering the child's strengths and self-efficacy can help to create a sense of resilience and accomplishment in the child, improve parent–child relationships, and decrease parental distress.

Teaching the Family Healthy Ways to Talk About Tics and Comorbidity with Others

As noted in Chapter 7, Talking About Tics With Peers and Coping in Social Interactions the importance of teaching children to effectively talk about PTD with others is highlighted by several studies showing peer education and self-disclosure have been shown to increase positive attitudes toward, and social acceptability of, individuals with PTD (Nussey, Pistrang, & Murphy, 2013; Olufs, Himle, & Bradley, 2013; see Chapter 7: Talking About Tics With Peers and Coping in Social Interactions for specific strategies for helping children learn to talk about their tics with peers). It is important to note, however, that parents can also struggle to know how and when to disclose that their child has PTD. For example, parents often worry that telling teachers that their child has been diagnosed with PTD (or a comorbid psychiatric condition) will result in the child being treated differently by his or her teacher, reduced academic expectations, or will create conflict with the school (see Chapter 8: Tourette's in the Classroom: Support and Guidance on Education Issues for Clinicians for strategies for managing tics at school). Some parents even avoid talking with their child about his/her diagnosis and symptoms out of fear that doing so will be stigmatizing or damage the child's self-esteem. Socially noticeable and/or inappropriate tics can be particularly stressful for parents because they are often misunderstood by the general public and draw attention to the child and/or parent, which can be embarrassing. When this happens, some parents resort to making excuses or even lying about their child's tics, apologizing for their child's behavior, or avoiding public places. In addition to being upsetting to parents, if observed by the affected child, this can lead to shaming and contribute to self-esteem problems. As such, it can be helpful for clinicians to use the same strategies they use with children (see Chapter 7: Talking About Tics With Peers and Coping in Social Interactions) to help parents learn to appropriately talk about their child's tics and comorbid symptoms with others (e.g., making and practicing sample scripts for different social situations in which tics or comorbid symptoms might cause problems).

Clinicians should also emphasize to parents that it is important that they lead by example and model the behaviors they want to see in their child. For example, if a parent models social avoidance, makes excuses, or apologizes for their child's tics in public, the child is likely to do the same. Rather, it is important for parents to model assertiveness, as well as how to provide brief, nonjudgmental education about PTD to others. Several resources for helping parents and children educate others about PTD are available online from the Tourette Association of America (www.tourette.org under the "Resources and Support" tab). Finally, it is important that the family learn how to effectively talk about tics and comorbid symptoms at home. Specifically, it is essential for the parents to provide a supportive environment in which their child feels comfortable expressing his/her thoughts, concerns, and experiences with tics without fear of being judged or dismissed, or that doing so will worry or inconvenience the parents. In addition, it is important that parent-initiated discussions about tics take place at a time when the parents and child are calm and can effectively communicate and that adult discussions about the child's tics (e.g., how they frustrate the parents, the parents' worries about tics) occur when the child is not nearby and cannot overhear.

Assess and Understand the Family's Early Experiences With Diagnosis and Care

How a family adjusts to having a child with a PTD is often rooted in their prior experiences with the health care system. Despite recent progress in recognizing, understanding, and treating PTD, research has shown that parents are often frustrated by delays in receiving a diagnosis, limited understanding of tics and PTD among general practitioners, and have received little information about PTD from health care providers following diagnosis (Cuenca et al., 2015). As a result, confidence in the health care system can be eroded. In addition, families may be left to struggle on their own to make sense of their child's behavior and many seek information from sources of questionable authority (e.g., friends, family members, or the internet). Since parents may not adequately understand their child's problems due to inadequate psychoeducation, many parents rely upon well-intentioned but ineffective parenting strategies to alter their child's behavior and express frustration when those strategies do not work (see Chapter 11: Brief Trans-diagnostic Parent Training : A Strengths-Based, Parent-Centered Treatment for Youth With Tourette Syndrome). Consider the following description provided by the mother of an 11-year-old girl with PTD during a recent clinical encounter with a clinician:

> *"She started having tics when she was three or four, right before she started kindergarten. She would blink all the time and make these funny looking faces. We laughed at them at first, but we also worried that she might get teased at school, so we would tell her to stop. I know now that she couldn't stop, and I can't tell you how much guilt I have about that. We took her to her pediatrician who told us not to worry about it, that it was normal and that she would grow out of it. Then she started clearing her throat. It seemed to come on overnight and would happen all the time. We took her back to the doctor, had her tested for allergies, and were told that she was allergic to dust mites. We tried antihistamines, but they didn't seem to help. Things got really bad about the time she started second grade. Suddenly we couldn't get her to go to school. I would have to drive her to school every day and walk her to the classroom. But when we got there, she would cry and cling to me as if the world was coming to an end. She couldn't tell me why she was so upset. I didn't know what to do. I tried to reason with her. I would bribe her. I would even sometimes yell at her. Nothing worked. Most days I would just leave her there, in the hallway or with her teacher, crying and ticcing like crazy. I can't tell you how embarrassing it was. I felt like such a failure as a parent. It just seemed like the parenting tricks we used with our other four children didn't work with her. We tried time out, we tried sticker charts, we even resorted to yelling and taking things away. But nothing seemed to work. Finally, we just gave up. And I know it affected my other kids because she was getting so much attention and always getting her way. We tried to get help. We took her to more doctors and therapists than I can count. We spent a lot of time and money trying to figure out what was wrong with her and what we had done wrong. Then one night my sister called me and told me she had seen a story on TV about Tourette's. I looked it up online and it seemed to describe everything she was dealing*

with—the sensitivities, the anxieties, the tics. We went back to our pediatrician and she said yes, it's Tourette's, like she knew this all along. She didn't really give us much advice for what to do about it, except to say we needed to learn to live with it and that if it got really bad, we could try medication, but the possible side effects were scary. She also told us not to overreact, that parents are usually more bothered than the kids. We were happy to finally know it was Tourette's, but the advice we got wasn't very helpful. To tell us to just live with it—what did she think we were doing? That's an easy thing to say. After that, we pretty much gave up on the doctors and decided we were going to have to figure this out on our own."

For clinicians who work with PTD, such accounts are quite common. Parents of children with PTD often recognize symptoms early and appropriately seek (and rely upon) help from medical professionals to understand their child's problems. While some families are fortunate to find a knowledgeable and experienced provider who confirms a diagnosis and makes helpful treatment recommendations, many parents are left to make sense of, and deal with, the symptoms on their own. In fact, a study of 314 parents of children with PTD (Mol Debes, Hjalgrim, & Skov, 2008) found that the median delay between the onset of symptoms (tics or comorbid symptoms) and diagnosis of PTD was 5.3 years and the median delay between onset of tics and diagnosis of PTD was 2.8 years. Furthermore, on average, families had consulted 2–3 professionals before a PTD diagnosis was conferred.

Early interactions with health care providers can also influence how parents (and their child) reacts to, and copes with, a PTD diagnosis. For many parents, the initial reaction to receiving a diagnosis is one of relief at finally having a medical explanation for their child's symptoms. Some parents, however, report feelings of anger and resentment that the diagnosis was not conferred earlier, fear and uncertainty about their child's future, and confusion and misunderstanding regarding medical and diagnostic terms. Some parents also react to a PTD diagnosis with blame (of themselves or another caregiver), denial, confusion, fear about the child's future, and/or guilt (Ginsburg & Kingery, 2007). To illustrate, consider the following summary of a clinical conversation between a clinician and the mother of a 10-year-old boy (Billy) during an initial clinical visit after the child was diagnosed with TD by his pediatrician:

"After we left Dr. Winston's office, I went home and tried to understand what he said about Billy and Tourette's. I went on the internet, just like he said, and I got really freaked out. I don't mean to question Dr. Winston, but are you sure he has Tourette's? I saw all of these videos of kids and adults with Tourette's on the internet, and they all seem so much worse than Billy. I thought Tourette's was swearing, and Billy doesn't swear. And I was reading this blog about Tourette's, and everyone there talked about how their kids have ADD and OCD and how they are always mad and get aggressive. But

Billy doesn't have any of those problems. Are you sure he doesn't just have tics? After watching the videos, I kept thinking, is that what's going to happen to Billy? And I talked with Billy's dad last night [the parents are divorced]. Dr. Winston told us that Tourette's is genetic. I know that he [Billy's father] had some OCD when he was a kid, but I think he had tics too, he was just calling them OCD. I got so mad at [Billy's father], why didn't he tell me that? I feel like this is his fault and now he's out of the picture and I am left cleaning up his mess. And now that I know that Billy can't stop the tics, I'm mad at myself for the way I treated him, especially for punishing him when he was having tics. How was I supposed to know that he couldn't control them? So now what? I really don't want to bring Billy back to see any doctors because I don't want him to know he has Tourette's. I don't want him to know the stuff I know."

The above clinical encounter highlights the confusion, blame, frustration, and myriad of emotions that parents can experience when their child receives a diagnosis of PTD. Unfortunately, many medical professionals overlook or underestimate the impact that a PTD diagnosis has on the family (Rivera-Navarro, Cubo, & Almazan, 2009). While it is not possible to go back in time, understanding a family's journey to diagnosis and assessing their current understanding of PTD is important because it can provide a wealth of clinically useful information. For example, the time between symptom onset and diagnosis is often characterized by an increasing level of family strain, feelings of confusion, fear, and exasperation among caregivers, and, in some cases, ineffective and coercive parent–child interactions that need to be targeted in treatment. It is also important to understand how the parents conceptualize their child's tics and comorbid symptoms (involuntary vs voluntary, planned vs reactive) and how they have reacted to them in the past (ignored vs punished, etc.). Based on this information, the clinician can begin to better advise the parents on how to respond to their child's tics in a healthier and more effective way. Finally, listening to the family's history can help to lay the foundation for a collaborative therapeutic relationship and identify potential barriers to treatment.

Differentiating Tics From NonTic Behavior and Managing Comorbidity

Among the most difficult and frustrating tasks facing parents of children with PTD are differentiating tics from comorbid symptoms (and developmentally normal behavior) and knowing how to appropriately respond (or not respond) based on whether the behavior is, or is not, a tic. Inappropriately responding to a child's tics or comorbid symptoms can exacerbate PTD, reinforce problematic behavior, and/or negatively affect the parent–child relationship.

Even prior to a formal diagnosis of PTD, some parents realize that their child cannot control his/her symptoms, even if they do not recognize them to be tics. However, tics that more closely resemble purposeful behaviors (e.g., contorted facial expressions, eye-rolling, shoulder shrugging, squeaking, spitting) are often more difficult for parents to understand, explain, and separate from the social evaluation they might give a purposeful behavior. As a result, some parents assume that their child can control his/her tics and use well-intentioned, but ineffective parenting strategies in an attempt to reduce the behavior (see Chapter 11: Brief Trans-diagnostic Parent Training: A Strengths-Based, Parent-Centered Treatment for Youth With Tourette Syndrome). In such cases, it is common for parents to tell their child to stop their tics and issue reprimands when the child does not comply. When this does not work, some parents resort to coercive and punitive techniques that are ineffective and can strain the parent–child relationship. For example, consider the case of a child who developed a spitting tic early in the course of PTD. His parents disclosed that they assumed he had learned this from friends on the baseball team and repeatedly told him to stop because it was disrespectful and socially inappropriate. When their directives failed to eliminate the spitting (i.e., "he did not listen"), they attempted to use time-out strategies when they caught him spitting at home. However, the tic increased in frequency over the course of several months (a common phenomenon in the clinical course of PTD), and as a result, his parents removed him from the baseball team as punishment for failure to discontinue spitting. This punishment also failed to decrease the spitting tic and further strained the parent–child relationship.

One of the most important tasks for a clinician working with a family with PTD is helping the parents to understand, which behaviors the child can and cannot control, so that they can respond appropriately and effectively. This is especially important when comorbidity is present. For example, it is not uncommon for parents to mistake comorbid symptoms (e.g., shouting, swearing, hitting, engaging in compulsions) for tics. Because of this, parents might hesitate to implement appropriate consequences, become overly permissive, allow escape or avoidance from tasks and expectations, and/or generally fail to respond to the behavior appropriately, which can reinforce and exacerbate nontic problem behaviors.

In all fairness to parents, differentiating tics from comorbid symptoms is an often difficult task, even for experienced clinicians. While simple motor and vocal tics are relatively easy to identify, differentiating complex tics from comorbid symptoms can be challenging. For example, complex tics, such as touching, tapping, and rewriting can be difficult to distinguish from compulsions associated with OCD, coprolalia (obscene vocal tics) can be difficult to distinguish from nontic swearing, normative repetitive behaviors, such as knee bouncing, knuckle cracking. can easily be confused with motor tics, and frequent motor tics can mimic the symptoms of ADHD because they make it difficult for the child to concentrate or make the child fidget. Clinical experience suggests that the following considerations can be helpful for distinguishing between complex tics and nontic behavior: (a) it is relatively rare for complex tics to be the first tics to emerge, so assessing the timing of symptom onset can be informative, (b) complex tics are often performed to alleviate a sensory urge rather than to neutralize an obsessive thought or anxiety, (c) although tics often fluctuate in response to contextual cues, they are rarely completely constrained to particular settings, activities, or mood states, and (d) most children (especially older ones) are able to differentiate their tics from purposeful behavior and, if explored in a nonjudgmental manner, will disclose whether or not the behavior in question is a tic.

Teaching Families Effective Ways to Respond to Tics Using a Function-Based Approach

One of the primary components of our comprehensive approach to PTD management is using a function-based assessment and intervention (FBAI) approach to decrease tic-related functional impairment and situational exacerbations (see Himle et al., 2014; Woods et al., 2008). The FBAI approach is based on behavior-analytic research showing that tics, even though they are involuntary, can be influenced by contextual factors (i.e., antecedents) and social reactions (i.e., consequences or reactions that follow the tics; Himle et al., 2014). For example, it is not uncommon for tics to occur at higher frequency or intensity in specific settings (e.g., quiet places, home vs school), during certain activities (e.g., in the car, during mealtime, during homework), or around specific people (e.g., one parent vs the other; Conelea & Woods, 2008). Internal antecedents, such as mood states (e.g., anxiety, stress, excitement, boredom), have also been shown to worsen tics (Conelea & Woods, 2008). Finally, tic-contingent reactions, such as talking about tics, telling the child to stop ticcing, teasing, mimicking, attention, and escape or avoidance of nonpreferred tasks (e.g., homework, chores,), can also serve to increase tic severity (Himle et al., 2014). This is not to say that these factors *cause* tics, but rather that tics, like all behaviors, are influenced by specific contexts, as well as consequences that occur contingent upon tic performance.

The goal of the FBAI approach to tic management is to use an individualized, systematic approach to help the parent(s) and child to identify settings and reactions that are associated with *problematic* tic exacerbations. Once identified, the clinician can help the family to modify the situation (to the extent possible) or change the way they react to the tics with the goal of reducing tic-related interference and functional impairment. In other words, the goal is to help the family predict and appropriately respond to situations in which the tics might increase in severity and to help them problem-solving ways to reduce the impact of tics on the affected child and family.

Likewise, helping parents to understand that tic exacerbations might be a sign that their child is struggling to regulate his/her emotions can help to reduce parental frustration, increase tolerance of the tics, and signal that the parent should respond by helping the child to more effectively cope with and problem solving the tic-exacerbating situation.

To illustrate the FBAI approach to tic management, consider the case of Johnny, an 11-year-old boy with TD, OCD, and anxiety. Early in treatment, the clinician introduced the concept of FBAI to Johnny's parents and discovered that his vocal tics occurred with unusually high frequency and intensity at home after school. Below is an abbreviated transcript of the conversation between the clinician and Johnny's parents:

Clinician: We have talked a lot about how Johnny's tics are involuntary, meaning that although he can suppress them for a little bit, he can't control them completely and he certainly does not do them on purpose. But a lot of parents and children notice that all or some tics are worse in certain situations compared to others. Have you noticed any situations in which Johnny's tics are particularly frequent or noticeable?

Parent: Absolutely. His vocal tics are really bad when he gets home from school.

Clinician: That's a really interesting observation. We hear that a lot. And many parents attribute the worsening after school to suppressing tics during the day. We call that a tic rebound. And for a small subset of children, tics do get a little bit worse after they try to suppress their tics. But we have done a lot of research on this topic and we know that most children are not able to suppress their tics all day and suppression doesn't generally worsen tics. And in talking with Johnny and his teachers, it sounds like he is ticcing a quite a bit at school.

Parent: That's true, but he certainly tics more after school than he does in the classroom.

Clinician: That's really helpful information. Is it problematic that he tics more when he gets home?

Parent: For sure, it's a huge problem. He tics so much that he can't do anything else. We used to make him do his homework after school, like his brother does, but his tics are so severe that he can't concentrate. No one can concentrate on anything when he's in the room.

Clinician: That sounds really frustrating for everyone. How do you manage that on a daily basis?

Parent: We usually just let him go to his room to get his tics out while he watches TV.

Clinician: Does that seem to be working well for you? Do you feel like allowing him to watch TV until he gets his tics out has solved the problem?

Parent: In some ways, yes. We don't hear his tics as much. But I wish he was able to do his homework, he's really falling behind in school. And it creates a lot of conflict at home because his brother doesn't understand why he has to do homework when Johnny doesn't. So we end up in a power struggle with his brother. And sometimes Johnny ends up in his room for hours. He doesn't even come downstairs to eat dinner with the family and it's made it almost impossible to do anything as a family, like go to restaurants for dinner.

Clinician: Again, this is really helpful information, and it sounds like his tics are really getting in the way after school. And you are not alone, many families struggle in similar ways when tics are bad. I would like to talk with you a little bit about something we call a "function-based" approach to tic management.

This is a clinical term we use to describe that tics, although involuntary, can be made worse by certain settings, activities, and reactions. In other words, although he's not ticcing more on purpose after school, and he certainly isn't ticcing on purpose in order to get out of tasks or to get attention, those things can still make the tics worse. That's just how the brain works. When a behavior is rewarded, the brain tells the body to do that behavior again and again in certain situations. In most cases, how parents react to tics is meant to be helpful and it usually makes things better in the short term. But in some cases, those well-intentioned reactions can backfire and unintentionally make the tics worse in the long term. In Johnny's case, it doesn't sound like allowing him to go to his room and watch TV is making the tics better in the long term and it's causing other problems at home. It also isn't getting at the root of the problem because we don't know why his tics are getting worse after school. By using a function-based approach, we can try to figure out why his tics are worse after school and make some adjustments to his routine and your reactions so that we can reduce the after school tics and get him back to doing his homework and other after-school activities.

Parent: That makes sense. How should we respond to his tics?

Clinician: To figure that out, we have to gather some more information. The first step is trying to figure out what's making the tics worse in the first place. We call these the ABCs. That stands for Antecedents, Behaviors, and Consequences. In this case, the behavior, the B, is his vocal tic. Antecedents, the A's, are the situations in which the tic happens more often. You have already told me that his vocal tics are worse after school. But it would be helpful to have more information about what is leading up to his tics getting worse. For example, do the tics explode when he walks in the door, or do they get progressively worse as the day goes on? Consequences, the C's, are what happen as a result of the tics that might be making the tics worse. We already have some good information about consequences. We know that he is allowed to watch TV, which is rewarding, and he doesn't have to do his homework, which is also rewarding. But we need to cover all of our bases and really understand what is happening before and after he gets home from school that might be making his tics worse in the long run. To identify the ABCs, over the next week, I am going to ask you to pay particular attention to what situations make his vocal tics worse and how you and others respond to his tics. I will ask you to write down this information on a form that I will give you at the end of the session. If we can figure out what ABCs are making the tics worse, we can come up with a plan for how to reduce his tics after school so that they are not causing as much of a problem.

In using the FBAI approach to tic management, the clinician was able to determine that Johnny's tics were worse after school and that his parents were responding in ways that were potentially reinforcing (i.e., worsening) his tics (i.e., allowing him to go to his room and engage in a preferred activity while avoiding homework). Johnny's after school tic exacerbations had placed considerable strain on the family because he was falling behind in school, his younger brother was becoming disrespectful and noncompliant, and they had stopped engaging in after-school family activities (e.g., eating meals together, going to restaurants). Conceptualizing Johnny's case from an FBAI perspective and collecting ABC data between sessions revealed several additional factors related to after-school tic exacerbations. First, it was discovered that a peer on the school bus (a tic-exacerbating antecedent) was teasing Johnny about his tics (a tic-exacerbating consequence), which angered Johnny and made his tics worse. Second, Johnny's mother acknowledged that her conflicts with Johnny's younger sibling, which usually occurred after school, resulted in emotional "yelling matches," which made Johnny's tics even worse. Finally, it was apparent that Johnny was receiving a lot of attention from his mother (a tic-exacerbating consequence) when he arrived home from school (she would frequently express frustration about his tics, etc.). Based on this information, several intervention strategies were planned and implemented. First, the bus driver was notified of the teasing and Johnny and a friend began sitting in the front of the bus near the driver (an antecedent intervention), which eliminated the teasing. Second, Johnny's mother was instructed to ignore the tics after school (a consequence-based intervention). It was also clear that Johnny was escaping/avoiding homework contingent on tic exacerbations (a tic-exacerbating consequence) and gaining access to a preferred activity (television) when his tics were worse, so a reward program was implemented in which both Johnny and his brother could earn television time for completing their homework, and Johnny's homework time was scheduled in the morning when his tics were less severe. Finally, the family agreed to regularly engage in family activities, such as going to a park, in the afternoons and to attend these activities regardless of the severity of Johnny's tics after school. By modifying tic-exacerbating antecedents and consequences (along with other therapeutic activities such as habit reversal, anxiety management, and others), Johnny's tics decreased substantially (albeit slowly) after school, his brother's behavior improved, and his mother reported a significant reduction in stress.

Several caveats to the FBAI approach warrant mention. First, not all tic-exacerbating factors need to be addressed. For example, if a child's tics are transiently worse when the child is engaged in his/her favorite activity, but this is not causing any problems, it is not recommended that the activity is taken away (especially if you want the child to stay engaged in treatment). On the other hand, if the activity is exacerbating tics to the point that they are interfering with appropriate expectations or the child's normal routine (i.e., inability to complete schoolwork later that evening), then this should be addressed, for example, by scheduling the tic-exacerbating activity for after homework is complete. By focusing on problematic tic exacerbations (versus all tic exacerbations), the clinician can concentrate his/her efforts in a way that is more productive and beneficial. Second, although FBAI-based recommendations are often quite simple and straightforward, they require careful planning and need to be feasible. For example, if a child's tics are exacerbated by fatigue, simply recommending that the child "get more sleep" is not a recommendation that is likely to be followed. Rather, the therapist should carefully assess the child's sleep hygiene and make a detailed plan and specific recommendations for how to improve the child's sleep. Likewise, not all parents are able (or willing) to simply ignore tics. For example, even subtle, nonverbal tic-contingent reactions (e.g., eye-rolling, frustrated or concerning looks from the parent) are a form of attention. It is helpful to teach parents to engage in planned ignoring and have them practice how to ignore tics during sessions so that the clinician can provide corrective feedback. In addition, some tics (e.g., self-injurious tics) cannot always be completely ignored because of safety concerns, so it is important to generate a detailed plan for how the parents should respond to such tics if the FBAI reveals that they are potentially worsened by attention. Finally, tic-exacerbating patterns are usually established through extensive experience and can be resistant to change. Consider the following transcript from the case of Johnny described above:

Clinician: Last week we started working on ignoring Johnny's vocal tics after school. How has that been going?

Parent: Not very well. It's really hard because the tics are so loud. In fact, for the first few days, the tics actually seemed to be worse when we ignored them. It's really been a struggle.

Clinician: I'm sorry it's been so difficult. How often have you been successful in ignoring his tics after school?

Parent: I would say that I have been able to ignore them most of the time, may be 80% of the time. Sometimes they just get so loud that I have to say something. I know I shouldn't, but it doesn't seem to be working so I need to do something. What else can we do?

Clinician: I'm really pleased to hear that you have been successful 80% of the time. That's a good start. I want to hear more about the times when you have been successful and also the times that you have been unsuccessful. But first, it's important to understand a few things. First, it is not uncommon for tics to get worse when you start ignoring them, at least in the short term. We call this an extinction burst. Basically, whenever you stop rewarding a behavior, the brain increases the behavior in an attempt to get the response it's used to getting. It's actually a sign that the intervention is working. Over time, those short-term increases will get less and less. The key is to be consistent. If the brain learns that a response, in this case, attention will come every once in awhile, the behavior will continue. In fact, it will learn that the way to get attention from you is to get louder or more frequent. So in essence, it learns that increasing tics will pay off.

Parent: So giving attention once in awhile is the same as giving attention every time?

Clinician: In some ways, yes. It's important to remember that these patterns have been established over a very long period of time and will take time to correct. How many times do you think you gave his tic attention prior to starting treatment?

Parent: I couldn't even guess. Hundreds, may be more.

Clinician: Exactly. So the brain is used to getting attention for the tics. It's going to take time for it to learn that the tics will not be rewarded with attention. But again, consistency and patience is the key. But I know that is very difficult, so let's talk about those times when you have had a hard time ignoring and see if we can give you some strategies to make those easier. Can you give me an example of when you gave the tics attention, what was happening?

Parent: Yesterday. He came home and it had already been a stressful day. He came through the door and his tics were actually not that bad. So I asked him to help out with his brother's homework while I made a call for work. Then his tics got really loud and he stopped helping his brother, it was basically chaos. I had to go back into the den, where they were supposed to be doing homework, several times to tell them to quite down. I finally had to reschedule my call and hang up.

Clinician: You said several important things. First, you said his tics were actually better than usual. That could be a sign that ignoring is working. Second, you said that you had a stressful day and had a work call. Do you find it more difficult to ignore his tics when you are stressed or multitasking?

Parent: Of course.

Clinician: Okay, that gives us something to work with. You also said that when his tics flared up, you went back into the den several times and told them to quite down. Do you think that is consistent with ignoring his tics?

Parent: No, I suppose not.

Clinician: Okay. So we need to work a little bit on consistency in ignoring his tics, which is perfectly normal! This is more difficult than it sounds. We need to give you some strategies to help you to be better able to ignore his tics when you are stressed out.

Parent: In retrospect, I shouldn't have scheduled the call for that time. I should have just done it the next morning when the kids were at school so I could focus on our after-school plan.

Clinician: Don't beat yourself up about it. These interventions sound simple, but usually are more difficult than we think. We learned some important things from your experience yesterday and we can make some simple adjustments to improve the likelihood of success. So that is what we will focus on today, helping you to be more consistent in ignoring and giving you strategies to help you during those times when ignoring is really hard. I would also like to have you continue to record the ABCs, like we did before, so that we can be sure we are not missing anything. Finally, I think it would be helpful if we came up with a way to rate how bad the tics are after school so we can see if things are getting better in the long term. It's easy to pay attention to the short-term increases and assume that the intervention is not working, but the goal is to reduce the tics in the long term

The case of Johnny provides an example of how a systematic and individualized FBAI approach can be employed to identify and alter tic-exacerbating antecedents and consequences, which in turn can help to reduce tics and tic-related interference, help families respond to tics in a healthier way, and improve overall family functioning. In addition, the FBAI approach to tic management shares underlying conceptual and procedural similarities with other empirically-supported interventions for common comorbid symptoms (e.g., parent training for noncompliance, scaffolding to decrease parental accommodation for OCD) and thus provides a useful framework for addressing nontic symptoms later in treatment. A step-by-step guide for how to implement the FBAI approach is outlined in the CBIT treatment manual (Woods et al., 2008) and some illustrative examples of antecedent- and consequence-based intervention strategies are provided in Tables 14.2 and 14.3.

TABLE 14.2 Examples of Function-Based Antecedent Interventions

Tic-Exacerbating Antecedents	Examples of Function-Based Antecedent Interventions
Stress & Anxiety	• Teach relaxation strategies (e.g., progressive muscle relaxation, relaxed breathing, mindfulness) • Teach coping strategies (e.g., self-statements, thought challenging) • Minimizing unnecessary stressors
Fatigue	• Teach good sleep hygiene/routine • Scheduled breaks during demanding tasks (independent of tic exacerbation) • Break tasks down into manageable components
Transitions	• Activity scheduling (e.g., using daily and monthly visual planners) & advanced warning of major changes to daily routine or events • Countdown transition "alerts" (e.g., 10-minutes before transition between activities, then 5 minutes, then 1 minute)
Boredom	• Assign pleasurable activities/choice of activity from menu • Assign easily mastered tasks (e.g., chores) • Schedule activities for child throughout the week
After school	• 15 minute break before demanding tasks for which tics will interfere (e.g., homework, chores) • Have a planned after-school routine • Complete essential tasks at low-risk times (e.g., homework in the morning or later in the evening)
Television/Video Games	• Minimize screen time • Limit access to times in which tics will not interfere with subsequent activities (e.g., TV after homework)
In public	• Practice how to respond to others/discuss/disclose his or her tics • Explore expected outcomes versus realized outcomes (e.g., people comment vs fear that people will comment) • Increase/substitute social activities that are less likely to be impacted by tics (e.g., going to a park rather than the library)

Increasing Support for the Patient, Parent, and Family

Another source of stress for families managing PTD is a sense of social isolation. On a positive note, at least one study has found that caregivers' perceived social support partially mediated the association between caregiver strain and tic symptom severity, suggesting that increasing social support for caregivers might be therapeutic and serve as a protective factor against the

TABLE 14.3 Examples of Function-Based Consequence Intervention

Tic-Exacerbating Consequences	Examples of Function-Based Consequence Interventions
Parental/sibling attention	• Help parents understand that although attention can exacerbate tics, the child is not ticcing on purpose to get attention. • Teach parents to selectively ignore tics and tic exacerbations • Provide noncontingent attention • Talk about tics at a scheduled time each day/night or when tics are relatively mild. • Do not tease or mimic tics • Talk about tics when parents and child are calm • Allow child to initiate tic-related discussions. • Minimize tic-related gestures of comfort • Teach parents to prompt tic-management strategies rather than comment on tics per se (e.g., prompt use of relaxation strategies, habit reversal strategies) • Praise use of tic-management strategies • Parents should express their frustrations and concerns about tics when the child is not present and cannot overhear.
Escape or avoidance of tasks because of tics	• Parents should understand that escape/avoidance can serve to worsen tics in the long run, but that does not mean that the child is ticcing on purpose to get out of activities • Child should be supportively encouraged to "push through" to complete tasks during mild tic exacerbations • For more severe exacerbations, child should be allowed a break from the task, but should return to complete the task as soon as tics have subsided. Parent should prompt and encourage the child to use tic-management strategies (e.g., relaxation, habit reversal exercises) during the break • If child is allowed to leave a situation because of tics (e.g., leave the table during homework), he/she should still be asked to complete the task in a timely manner to the best of his/her abilities (e.g., do homework in his/her bedroom). • Parent should set realistic expectations for, and encourage, their child to engage in developmentally appropriate activities (e.g., sports, hobbies, academics, social gatherings). • For tasks in which the child struggles, he/she should be encouraged to attempt the task independently before providing support

(Continued)

TABLE 14.3 (Continued)

Tic-Exacerbating Consequences	Examples of Function-Based Consequence Interventions
	• Social outings should be planned in a way that minimizes the impact of tic exacerbations (e.g., going to outdoor movies rather than the movie theater). • Social activities that are less likely to be impacted by tics should be encouraged, especially if the family is avoiding other social activities because of tics.

burden of parenting a child with PTD (Schoeder & Remer, 2007). To increase social support, we encourage parents to attend local PTD support group meetings or connect them with other parents of children with PTD, encourage them to find time to engage in other social activities not related to tics or caregiving (e.g., joining a book club), and to schedule time each day or week to attend to their own needs (e.g., go on a weekly date with their spouse, having coffee with a friend, going to the gym). It is also important that families share in the responsibility of caring for the child with PTD. For example, if it is not possible for both parents to attend therapy sessions, clinicians might ask the parents to alternate which parent attends therapy with their child each week. This ensures that the parents are sharing the responsibility of caring for their child, gives the other parent time to attend to other matters (e.g., self-care, spending time with the other children), and also ensures that both parents are aware of what is taking place during treatment. When applicable, it is also important for parents to spend individual time with other children in the household. In fact, clinicians may routinely assign parents to spend an equal amount of one-on-one time with their nonaffected children as therapy homework. For example, if a clinician assigns 30 minutes of therapy homework between the parents and PTD affected child, they may consider assigning 30 minutes of a one-on-one activity with the sibling(s). This can help to prevent or remediate problems related to the attention that the affected child is receiving.

Another often overlooked contributor to family functioning, as well as treatment adherence, is the psychological well-being of parents. Numerous studies have shown that PTD, OCD, and ADHD are heritable (Santangelo et al., 1996). Not surprisingly, many parents, in addition to the burden of parenting a child with PTD, struggle with their own mental health issues. This can have a profound negative effect on family functioning and can create a stressful home environment, which has been shown to predict poorer prognosis for PTD/PTD + (Lin et al., 2007). Parental mental health problems can also decrease tolerability for the child's symptoms, result in inconsistent use of effective parenting strategies, lead to under involvement in the child's care, and hinder the appropriate utilization of treatment and educational services for their child. In addition, parenting more than one child with psychological or behavioral health issues can add significant caregiver burden for any parent regardless of their own mental health, emphasizing the importance of asking about the mental and behavioral health of siblings. These factors need to be carefully considered early in the course of treatment planning.

Finally, studies have shown that major stressful life events (e.g., divorce, significant illness, death of a relative or friend, relocation, job loss) can increase family strain and negatively affect family functioning (Lavee, McCubbin, & Olson, 1987). Although most such events are not planned and cannot be avoided, it is important to understand their potential impact on both the caregivers and the child with PTD. Consistent with clinical experience, several studies have shown that stress is associated with a transient (and possibly long term) worsening of tic symptoms. For example, Steinberg et al. (2013) analyzed the impact of both major (e.g., divorce) and minor negative life events (interpersonal interactions, such as arguments, academic failures) on the severity of tics and comorbid symptoms in children with PTD and found that the number of negative life events was positively associated with increased tic severity, depression, anxiety, and aggression. In fact, clinical experience suggests that symptom worsening due to life events (e.g., beginning of the school year) is often the impetus for families to bring their child to therapy. However, while in some cases life stressors can motivate positive change, such as the initiation of treatment, caregivers who are managing multiple stressors may often find it more difficult to tolerate and manage their child's symptoms, struggle to follow through with treatment recommendations, and be more likely to cancel sessions and terminate treatment prematurely. While not all life stressors can be predicted, avoided, or remediated, it is important for clinicians to assess family stressors, help them understand their potential impact on their child's symptoms, and work with parents to eliminate and minimize unnecessary sources of stress to the extent possible.

Coordination of Care

Another factor that can contribute to how a family copes with PTD is the availability (or lack thereof) of informed and coordinated interdisciplinary care. Bitsko et al. (2012) analyzed data from the 2007 to 2008 National Survey of Children's Health and found that 64% of parents of children with TD reported that their child needed or used more medical, mental health, and educational services than most same-aged children. Furthermore, only 44% of TD parents reported that their child receives effective care coordination. Given such high health care needs, it is not surprising that clinicians frequently encounter parents who express frustration because they unable to obtain appointments with recommended treatment providers, encounter long waitlists to see knowledgeable providers, complain of a lack of sharing of information between interdisciplinary providers, feel the need to constantly educate physicians and educators about their child's PTD, and receive an overwhelming number of referrals to various specialists. While some parents have the time, resources, and capability to manage their child's care effectively, many find this process overwhelming and prohibitively time-consuming. Furthermore, specialists tend to be concentrated in metro areas, and patients and their families living outside of metro areas experience the added burden of travel time to attend specialist appointments. For instance, consider a case in which a mother was diligently taking her child to PTD-related visits (occupational therapy, behavior therapy, biofeedback, and medication management visits) four afternoons per week, each at a different location. This schedule left her little time to attend to her own needs or to those of her family and she frequently canceled or no-showed for sessions. It is easy to see how such demands can negatively impact the well-being of the caregiver and the functioning of the entire family system. More often, however, parents may fail to take advantage of care options available to them because they are uncertain about which services are needed and/or where to go to receive them. In other words, simply recommending that a family "see a physician for medication management" is not a particularly helpful recommendation. Finally, some parents fail to seek, or actively resist, potentially helpful services (e.g., behavior therapy) for their child because they have prioritized services that they are hopeful will work but lack empirical support. For example, Woods, Conelea, and Himle (2010) surveyed 740 parents of children with PTD regarding treatment utilization and found that many families reported having sought a variety of interventions that lack empirical support, including dietary supplements and modifications, acupuncture, aromatherapy, chiropractic therapy, massage therapy, and sensory integration treatment. In some cases, these treatments consume considerable time and financial resources that could be spent on empirically-supported services (e.g., educational services, behavioral therapy).

One way that clinicians can help to reduce family strain and burden is to help them coordinate their clinical care. Specifically, clinicians are encouraged to (1) be aware of PTD experienced and knowledgeable providers in their area (the Tourette Association of America maintains a provider list that can be accessed at www.tourette.org) and, to the extent possible, stay abreast of their availability to take new patients, (2) assess which health and educational services would be beneficial for the family and child, which services they are and are not utilizing, and help them to prioritize those services that will be most helpful based on their child's difficulties, (3) identify and problem solve logistical barriers to receiving care-related services (e.g., transportation availability, financial resources, child-care options for siblings), and (4) help families organize information that they can share across service providers. Clinical experience suggests that these relatively simple activities are often overlooked by clinicians, but can significantly reduce caregiver burden, improve optimism, and improve service utilization and treatment adherence.

SUMMARY AND CONCLUSIONS

The aim of this chapter was to help clinicians appreciate the importance of providing comprehensive, family-based clinical care when working with a child with PTD. Although efficacious interventions for reducing tics are available and are highly recommended when tics are problematic, interventions focused purely on reducing tic severity do not always fully address PTD-related problems in family functioning. Research and clinical experience remind clinicians that the effects of PTD and PTD + can be particularly disruptive to the family system and can lead to patterns of behavior and interaction amongst family members that increase caregiver stress and burden, worsen PTD symptoms, and interfere with treatment compliance. Thus a comprehensive family-based approach to caring for and treating PTD/PTD + is recommended that takes into account and balances the needs of the affected child along with other family members. While this comprehensive approach is guided by the current empirical literature and clinical experience, it is important to note that such an approach has not yet been thoroughly tested in treatment outcome studies. Future research is needed to better understand the impact of PTD on caregivers and siblings and to evaluate comprehensive approaches to treating PTD/PTD + to produce outcomes beyond reductions in tic severity.

REFERENCES

Angold, A., Messer, S. C., Stangl, D., Farmer, E., Costello, E. J., & Burns, B. J. (1998). Perceived parental burden and service use for child and adolescent psychiatric disorders. *American Journal of Public Health, 88*, 75–80.

Bitsko, R. H., Danielson, M., King, M., Visser, S. N., Scahill, L., & Perou, R. (2012). Health care needs of children with Tourette syndrome. *Journal of Child Neurology, 28*, 1626–1636. Available from https://doi.org/10.1177/0883073812465121.

Conelea, C. A., & Woods, D. W. (2008). The influence of contextual factors on tic expression in Tourette's syndrome: A review. *Journal of Psychosomatic Research, 65*, 487–496. Available from https://doi.org/10.1016/j.jpsychores.2008.04.010.

Conelea, C. A., Woods, D. W., Zinner, S. H., Budman, C., Murphy, T., Scahill, L., . . . Walkup, J. (2011). Exploring the impact of chronic tic disorders on youth: Results from the Tourette syndrome impact survey. *Child Psychiatry & Human Development, 42*, 219–242. Available from https://doi.org/10.1007/s10578-010-0211-4.

Cuenca, J., Glazebrook, C., Kendall, T., Hedderly, T., Heyman, I., Jackson, G., ... Hollis, C. (2015). Perceptions of treatment for tics among young people with Tourette syndrome and their parents: A mixed methods study. *BMC Psychiatry*, *15*, 1–12. Available from https://doi.org/10.1186/s12888-015-0430-0.

Freeman, R. D., Fast, D. K., Burd, L., Kerbeshian, J., Robertson, M. M., & Sandor, P. (2000). An international perspective on Tourette syndrome: Selected findings from 3500 individuals in 22 countries. *Developmental Medicine and Child Neurology*, *42*, 436–447. Available from https://doi.org/10.1111/j.1469-8749.2000.tb00346.x.

Ginsburg, G. S., & Kingery, J. N. (2007). Management of familial issues in persons with Tourette syndrome. In D. W. Woods, J. C. Piacentini, & J. T. Walkup (Eds.), *Treating Tourette Syndrome and Tic Disorders* (pp. 225–241). New York: Guilford Press.

Himle, M. B., & Capriotti, M. R. (2016). Behavior therapy for Tourette disorder: An update. *Current Behavioral Neuroscience Reports*, *3*, 211–217.

Himle, M. B., Capriotti, M. R., Hayes, L. P., Ramanujam, K., Scahill, L., Sukhodolsky, D. G., ... Piacentini, J. (2014). Variables associated with tic exacerbation in children with chronic tic disorders. *Behavior Modification*, *38*, 163–183. Available from https://doi.org/10.1177/0145445514531016.

Houghton, D. C., Capriotti, M. R., Conelea, C. A., & Woods, D. W. (2014). Sensory phenomena in Tourette syndrome: Their role in symptom formation and treatment. *Current Developmental Disorders Reports*, *1*, 245–251. Available from https://doi.org/10.1007/s40474-014-0026-2.

Lavee, Y., McCubbin, H. I., & Olson, D. H. (1987). The effect of stressful life events and transitions on family functioning and well-being. *Journal of Marriage and the Family*, *49*(4), 857–873.

Lin, H., Katsovich, L., Ghembremichael, M., Findley, D. B., Grantz, H., Lombroso, P. J., ... Leckman, J. F. (2007). Psychosocial stress predicts future symptom severities in children and adolescents with Tourette syndrome and/or obsessive-compulsive disorder. *Journal of Child Psychology & Psychiatry*, *48*, 157–166. Available from https://doi.org/10.1111/j.1469-7610.2006.-1687.x.

Mol Debes, N. M., Hjalgrim, H., & Skov, L. (2008). Limited knowledge of Tourette syndrome causes delay in diagnosis. *Neuropediatrics*, *39*, 101–105. Available from https://doi.org/10.1055/s-2008-1081457.

Nussey, C., Pistrang, N., & Murphy, T. (2013). How does psychoeducation help? A review of the effects of providing information about Tourette syndrome and attention-deficit/hyperactivity disorder. *Child: Care, health and development*, *39*, 617–627. Available from https://doi.org/10.1111/cch.12039.

O'Hare, D., Helmes, E., Reece, J., Eapen, V., & McBain, K. (2016). The differential impact of Tourette's syndrome and comorbid diagnosis on the quality of life and functioning of diagnosed children and adolescents. *Journal of Child and Adolescent Psychiatric Nursing*, *29*, 30–36. Available from https://doi.org/10.1111/jcap.12132.

Olufs, E., Himle, M. B., & Bradley, A. (2013). The effect of generic versus personally delivered education and self-disclosure on the social acceptability of adults with Tourette syndrome. *Journal of Developmental and Physical Disabilities*, *25*, 395–403.

Peterson, A. L., McGuire, J. F., Wilhelm, S., Piacentini, J., Woods, D. W., Walkup, J. T., ... Scahill, L. (2016). An empirical examination of symptom substitution associated with behavior therapy for Tourette's disorder. *Behavior Therapy*, *47*, 29–41. Available from https://doi.org/10.1016/j.beth.2015.09.001.

Ramanujam, K., Himle, M. B., Hayes, L. P., Woods, D. W., Scahill, L. D., Sukhodolsky, D. G., ... Piacentini, J. C. (2015). Correlates and predictors of caregiver strain in children with chronic tic disorders. *Children's Health Care, 44*, 249–263. Available from https://doi.org/10.1080/02739615.2014.948166.

Rivera-Navarro, J., Cubo, E., & Almazan, J. (2009). The diagnosis of Tourette's syndrome: Communication and impact. *Clinical Child Psychology & Psychiatry, 14*, 13–23. Available from https://doi.org/10.1177/1359104508100127.

Santangelo, S. L., Pauls, D. L., Lavori, P. W., Goldstein, J. M., Faraone, S. V., & Tsuang, M. T. (1996). Assessing risk for the Tourette spectrum of disorders among first-degree relatives of probands with Tourette syndrome. *American Journal of Medical Genetics, Part A, 67*, 107–116.

Scahill, L., Erenberg, G., Berlin, C. M., Budman, C., Coffey, B. J., Jankovic, J., ... Walkup, J. (2006a). Contemporary assessment and pharmacotherapy of Tourette syndrome. *NeuroRx, 3*, 192–206. Available from https://doi.org/10.1016/j.nurx.2006.01.009.

Schoeder, C. E., & Remer, R. (2007). Perceived social support and caregiver strain in caregivers of children with Tourette's disorder. *Journal of Child & Family Studies, 16*, 888–901. Available from https://doi.org/10.1007/s10826-007-9133-6.

Steinberg, T., Shmuel-Baruch, S., Horesh, N., & Apter, A. (2013). Life events and Tourette syndrome. *Comprehensive Psychiatry, 54*, 467–473.

Storch, E. A., Lack, C. W., Simons, L. E., Goodman, W. K., Murphy, T. K., & Geffken, G. R. (2007). A measure of functional impairment in youth with Tourette's syndrome. *Journal of Pediatric Psychology, 32*, 950–959. Available from https://doi.org/10.1093/jpepsy/jsm034.

Woods, D. W., Conelea, C. A., & Himle, M. B. (2010). Behavior therapy for Tourette's disorder: Utilization in a community sample and an emerging area of practice for psychologists. *Professional Psychology: Research and Practice, 41*, 518–525.

Woods, D. W., Piacentini, J. C., Scahill, L., Peterson, A. L., Wilhelm, S., Chang, S., ... Walkup, J. T. (2011). Behavior therapy for tics in children: Acute and long-term effects on psychiatric and psychosocial functioning. *Journal of Child Neurology, 26*, 858–865. Available from https://doi.org/10.1177/0883073810397046.

Woods, D. W., Piacentini, J. C., Chang, S. W., Deckersbach, T., Ginsburg, G. S., Peterson, A. L., ... Wilhelm, S. (2008). *Managing Tourette syndrome: A behavioral intervention for children and adults: Therapist Guide*. New York: Oxford University Press.

Chapter 15

Promoting Healthy Behaviors

Anjali Gera, MD and Katie Kompoliti, MD
Department of Neurological Sciences, Rush University Medical Center, Chicago, IL, United States

INTRODUCTION

Historically, health has been viewed as a state of normal physical and psychological functioning that is interrupted by disease. The World Health Organization (WHO) in 1948 defined health as: "a state of complete physical, mental, and social well-being and not merely the absence of disease or infirmity," thus departing from the definition of health as the absence of disease and introducing the concept of well-being as a crucial component of health (Huber et al., 2011). In the early 1980s, the definition evolved from viewing health not as a state, but as a process, and the movement of health promotion was fostered. In 1984 the WHO amended the definition of health as "the extent to which an individual or group is able to realize aspirations and satisfy needs, and to change or cope with the environment." Thus health became a resource for everyday life, not the objective of living (World Health Organization, 1984). Indeed, beyond biology, health is a determinant of where people live, work, learn, create relations, and pray.

Medical care systems have been historically organized to respond to acute illness or injury, and in this model, the patient is largely passive. When it comes to living with a chronic illness in these systems, patients can struggle with a distinct set of challenges. Indeed, patients with chronic illness often must wrestle with the physical, psychological, and social demands of their illness without consistent help from the medical system. A patient with a chronic illness, independent of whether it is mainly physical or psychological, is presented with a set of challenges in dealing with the symptoms and disability, uncertainty about the future, emotional sequelae, difficult lifestyle adjustments, and navigating through the medical system (Wagner et al., 2001). Effective management of a chronic disease requires more than the medical system typically offers, and health care professionals (no matter how compassionate or caring) are only a small part of it. Wagner et al.

The Clinician's Guide to Treatment and Management of Youth with Tourette Syndrome and Tic Disorders.
DOI: https://doi.org/10.1016/B978-0-12-811980-8.00015-7

(2001) describes his colleague's experience of living with chronic disease, which he compares to flying a small plane:

> *"If it is flown well, one gets where one wants to go with the exhilaration of mastering a complicated set of challenges. If it is flown badly, one either crashes or lands shakily in the wrong airport, reluctant to ever leave the ground again. The patient must be the pilot, because the only other possible pilot, the health care professional is in the plane few hours every year. If chronically ill patients must pilot their own planes, then the role of health care is to ensure skilled pilots, safe planes, flight plans that safely get the pilots to their destination, and air traffic control surveillance to prevent mishaps and keep them on course. Medical care then must assure that persons with chronic illness have the confidence and skills to manage their condition; the most appropriate treatments to assure optimal disease control and prevention of complications; a mutually understood care plan; and careful, continuous follow up."*

More recent models that approach health and health care suggest that broadening the patient-centered approach to one that is wellness-focused and person-centered leads to substantial improvement in health outcomes (Koh, 2016). Thus patient-centered approaches might entirely focus on the patient's goal of reduction of symptom severity and frequency. A patient-centered approach includes understanding treatment preference: observation, medical management, or simply reassurance and confirmation of the patient's diagnosis. Meanwhile, a therapeutic approach that is both wellness-focused and person-centered prioritizes quality of life and outcomes that are tailored to the person. For patients with chronic disease, there is growing interest in "self-management" programs that emphasize the patients' central role in managing his/her illness. A recent randomized clinical trial demonstrated the potential of self-management to improve health status and reduce health care utilization in patients with chronic diseases (Lorig, Sobel, Ritter, Laurent, & Hobbs, 2001). Furthermore, a growing focus on population health, wellness, and prevention is driving improvements in health and quality of life in the US (Dzau, McClellan, & McGinnis, 2016).

Patients with Tourette disorder and other tic disorders (collectively referred to as TD) have to face the multitude of issues common to patients with chronic disease. As with other chronic diseases, it is rare for medications to eliminate all tics. Thus patients with TD have to cope with the functional impact of tic symptoms on different aspects of their life. One study analyzed data from the National Survey of Children's Health to compare the needs of children with TD relative to asthma, another chronic condition (Bitsko et al., 2013). Similar to children with asthma, children with TD and coexisting mental disorders required more comprehensive education about management of their disease, more complex medication regimens, and precautions to take to minimize aggravation of symptoms. Similar to other chronic conditions, patients (and families) with TD often have to make difficult lifestyle adjustments (e.g., making the time to attend doctor's appointments, etc.), and confront practical limitations that symptoms can intermittently cause (e.g., challenges with going to the movies when vocal tics are severe). Therefore children with TD (and parents) need to learn to effectively navigate the health care system to obtain helpful medical care. Moreover, children with TD often have co-occurring emotional, mental, or behavioral conditions that can interfere with and complicate treatment and may require additional educational and medical services. Finally, obtaining comprehensive health care can be complicated for patients and families with chronic health conditions like TD due to limited access to "specialty care." This "specialty care" may include knowledge, access, and availability of care specific to the child's medical conditions and its comorbidities, and specialized therapeutic interventions (e.g., evidence-based behavior therapy and pharmacotherapy, see Chapter 3: Habit Reversal Training for Tics, Chapter 4: Pharmacological Management of Tic Disorders in Youth). While steps are being taken to address the limited access and availability of knowledgeable providers, there is still a need to further disseminate evidence-based knowledge and treatment to clinicians and shift the emphasis to comprehensively support children's (and parents') physical, emotional, academic, and social well-being.

PROMOTING PHYSICAL WELL-BEING

As with any chronic disease, ensuring good health in TD requires optimizing physical well-being. A physically healthy person should be able to cope and respond better when faced with physical, emotional, and social stress that often accompanies chronic disease. Keeping physically fit requires regular exercise, healthy eating habits, and good sleep hygiene.

Regular Exercise

While there are not many studies assessing the effect of exercise on TD, there are reports of tic reduction from maintaining a physically active lifestyle (Nixon, Glazebrook, Hollis, & Jackson, 2014). There are several potential hypotheses to help explain the mechanism of such an effect. First, regular exercise is a great way of minimizing stress and anxiety (Jayakody, Gunadasa, & Hosker, 2014). It stimulates production of endorphins and neurotrophins (including brain-derived neurotrophic factor) that improves mood and increases feelings of optimism (Sleiman et al., 2016). Second, it has been proposed that exercise allows the mind to wander into a meditative state, or essentially serves as a "break" from daily life events (including tics!) that could cause stress. Third, exercise has also been known to increase self-confidence, which in turn could change the patient's attitude towards the tics. Finally, exercise can give a sense of discipline in an otherwise hectic lifestyle in which a patient's symptoms often feel "out of control." While exercise may not directly reduce specific tic symptoms, a patient with TD who regularly exercises will likely feel healthier overall and be able to bear tic and co-occurring symptoms much better relative to a patient who leads a more sedentary lifestyle.

Sports or forms of exercise that involve both mental and physical engagement are thought to be particularly helpful. Many clinicians have shared anecdotal parental reports that children's tics are minimal or absent when participating in a team sports activity. Since there is no body of literature supporting that a specific form of exercise (i.e., aerobic vs anaerobic, stretching vs strengthening, team vs individual, etc.) would be more beneficial for individuals with TD, clinicians should recommend that patients with TD follow his/her preference for an activity that would be easy and enjoyable to incorporate into his/her daily life. It is important to note that the duration and choice of exercise should be chosen carefully. Exercise can be easily overdone to the point of exhaustion, which can worsen tic and co-occurring symptoms. Additionally, participating in competitive sports may increase pressure to perform well, which could potentially increase stress and in turn worsen tic symptoms. Nevertheless, as noted above, anecdotal evidence suggests that few people report tics increase when involved in intense exercise. Despite its many benefits, it is important to be mindful that exercise activities do not become excessive and/or ritualistic, especially for patients who have co-occurring obsessive-compulsive disorder (OCD). In such cases, it may be prudent to set personal limits on time that is dedicated to exercise. Finally, a common side effect of the anti-tic medications is weight gain, which can further affect the youth's self-confidence. Exercise and proper nutrition can be an efficient way to control the weight for individuals on these medications.

When considering promoting a patient's physical well-being in treatment, motivational interviewing strategies have been shown to be an effective approach to inspire a patient to change lifelong unhealthy behaviors (Franklin & Vanhecke, 2008). When employing these strategies, it is important that the clinician communicate a sense of empathy, understanding, and acceptance of the patient. The topic of physical well-being can be introduced by using broad, open-ended questions, such as "*If you wanted to make one change to improve your well-being, what would that be?*" The conversation should move forward with the clinician expressing empathy, particularly during moments that are difficult for the patient (and family) and validating the patient's accomplishments. The clinician should also guide the patient's answers by reflecting the patient's thoughts back to them and help them arrive at their own ideas for change, rather than telling them what to do. Below is an example of this technique applied to a young adult with TD.

Clinician: *"Last time we met, you had questions about possible side effects from the tic medication we started earlier in the year. In particular, you were concerned about your increase in body weight. Are you still concerned about your weight, and have you done anything to try to reduce your weight gain?"*

Patient: *"I'm still overweight, and just don't feel good about myself. I've tried some diets to lose the weight, but haven't really stuck with any of them. They are pretty hard, and I just don't see the results."*

Clinician: *"It can be really hard to make a lifestyle change, no matter who you are. However, your physical well-being is important. If you wanted to make one change to improve your well-being, what would that be?"*

Patient: *"Well...I wish I didn't sit on the couch all the time."*

Clinician: *"You are fairly inactive?"*

Patient: *"Yes on most days. I know I should exercise, but I just don't feel like going to the gym once I get home."*

Clinician: *"Hmm...So it sounds like you want to exercise and be healthy, but making it all the way to the gym is hard."*

Patient: *"Especially after a long day, I just want to rest on the couch for the rest of the evening."*

Clinician: *"So exercise and your health are important to you, but going all the way to the gym is difficult and once you sit down on the couch it's hard to motivate yourself to get up again. Is that right?"*

Patient: *"Yes."*

Clinician: *"Well, what are some exercise activities you would be interested and able to do on a regular basis that don't require going to the gym?"*

Patient: *"Well, I could go the park to play pick-up games of basketball, or just walk around my neighborhood."*

Clinician: *"Those are both great ideas. It might be best to start with 30 minutes of walking daily. Since it's hard to get up once you sit down on the couch, you might consider starting the exercise once you get home, so you don't get distracted by the couch. You could also even consider inviting a friend to join you on the walks, too."*

As demonstrated above, the clinician should summarize the conversation during the visit to help the patient hone in on the important points and then formulate an achievable goal. The goals should be written in the chart and reviewed at the next appointment.

Healthy Eating Habits

In addition to exercise, another important component of physical health is maintaining a healthy diet. This includes (but is not limited to) consuming healthy types of fats, eating plenty of fruits and vegetables, and replacing refined grains with whole grains. Eating a well-balanced diet and timely meals minimizes both mental and physical stress, and has been shown to positively impact chronic disease (Lichtenstein et al., 2006). While some patients and parents may seek to supplement healthy eating with vitamins and supplements, there is limited empirical support for the effect of specific supplements on tic symptom severity. For example, limited literature exists on the effects of omega 3-fatty acids (O3FA) in TD. Although O3FA have not been shown to directly reduce tic symptom severity, one small study suggested that O3FA may improve tic-related impairment for some children and adolescents (Gabbay et al., 2012). This randomized, double-blind, placebo-controlled trial examined the efficacy of O3FA in 33 children and adolescents (ages 6–18) with TD. The patients were given O3FA or placebo and were followed for 20 weeks. While O3FA did not directly reduce tic symptom severity scores ($p > 0.1$), children with TD who were taking O3FA exhibited a tendency toward greater improvement in tic-related impairment compared to children with TD who were taking placebo ($p = 0.06$). While more studies need to further evaluate the preliminary findings of O3FA in children with TD, the use of omega-3 polyunsaturated fatty acids has been associated with small effects for reducing emotional dysregulation, oppositional behavior, and conduct problems in subgroups of children with attention-deficit/hyperactivity disorder (ADHD) (Cooper, Tye, Kuntsi, Vassos, & Asherson, 2016). Additionally, the effects of magnesium and vitamin B6 supplementation on tic reduction have also been investigated in a small study of children with TD ($n = 10$) (Garcia-Lopez et al., 2009). This was a randomized, blinded, placebo-controlled trial that used a combination of 0.5 mEq/kg magnesium and 2 mg/kg vitamin B6 in children aged 7–14. Patients' tic symptom severity was reassessed at 15, 20, 60, and 90 days using the Yale Global Tic Severity Scale (YGTSS). Children receiving the combination of magnesium and vitamin B6 exhibited a 50% improvement from the baseline YGTSS score (mean total number of tics 12.9 ± 11.20 in the experimental group versus 26.7 ± 7.38 in the control group). Based on these promising preliminary findings, a larger randomized controlled trial is currently underway (Garcia-Lopez et al., 2009). Notably, this study did not discuss maximum doses and as such, caution should be used with high-dose vitamin B6 to avoid adverse side effects. Finally, studies have suggested that patients with TD have been found to have low ferritin and iron levels in the serum (Gorman, Zhu, Anderson, Davies, & Peterson, 2006). This study included 63 patients with TD and 44 controls. Serum ferritin and iron levels were measured and found to be in the normal range; however, significantly lower in patients with TD when compared to controls, suggesting that perhaps lower iron levels may play a role in the pathophysiology of TD.

Given the limited evidence on vitamins and supplements for children with TD, it is difficult to draw definitive conclusions at this time. There is no strong empirical evidence that vitamins or supplements dramatically reduce tic symptom severity in children with TD. However, given that vitamins and supplements have minimal side effects in recommended dosages, these over-the-counter items may be useful to promote the child's overall physical health. It is important to note that vitamins and supplements should not be considered a substitute for eating a well-balanced diet that has been shown to positively impact chronic disease (Lichtenstein et al., 2006). As patients, parents, and families may likely inquire about the benefits of vitamins and supplements, clinicians might offer some general guidance, such as the following:

> *"There are several studies that investigate the efficacy of supplements for tic disorders, but positive evidence remains limited and more studies need to be completed to provide definitive guidelines in this area. However, eating a well-balanced diet and timely meals can reduce physical and psychological distress, and has been shown to positively impact chronic disease in studies. So before considering the addition of a vitamin or supplement, it might first be helpful to focus on creating a well-balanced diet."*

The effect of food and drinks was investigated in a survey of German patients with TD. A questionnaire assessing the effect of 32 different foods was sent to 887 people, but only 224 questionnaires could be used for data analysis. Respondents reported tic deterioration with the use of caffeine- and theine-containing drinks, such as coke, coffee, and black tea, as well as preserving agents, refined sugar, and sweeteners (Müller-Vahl, Buddensiek, Geomelas, & Emrich, 2008). However, better-designed studies are needed to confirm these associations since findings were entirely based on self-report and only a quarter of the patients' data was included in analyses. Given the common cooccurrence of other psychiatric conditions with TD, it is also important to consider the impact of healthy eating on common comorbid conditions such as ADHD. There is a body of literature suggesting an inverse correlation between sugar intake and ADHD (Yu et al., 2016). One study followed the effects of sugar-sweetened beverages in 173 children with clinician-diagnosed ADHD and 159 non-ADHD control children between the ages of 4 and 15. After adjusting for covariates (including blood lead levels and dopaminergic-related genetic polymorphisms), a dose-dependent relationship was found between the consumption of sugar-sweetened beverages and ADHD symptoms (Yu et al., 2016). Thus it would be prudent to moderate sugar intake in children with TD who have inattention, hyperactivity, and/or impulsivity (by limiting high sugar foods, such as sugar-sweetened beverages) to prevent worsening of the ADHD symptoms.

Good Sleep Hygiene

Finally, good sleep quality is an integral component of maintaining physical well-being. This can be particularly true for children with TD, as stress and fatigue can exacerbate tic symptoms. Several factors that can disturb sleep quality include artificial light exposure from electronic devices including smartphones, variable sleep, and wake times from day to day with significant swings particularly on weekends, caffeine consumption later in the day, intensive exercise prior to sleep, and stimulant medications dosed late in the day. In particular, for children and adolescents, a significant sleep disturbance factor is the use of electronics close to or at bedtime (Mindell, Sedmak, Boyle, Butler, & Williamson, 2016). However, sleep quality can be optimized by maintaining good sleep hygiene in both children and adults. Several aspects of good sleep hygiene include: waking and sleeping at approximately the same time each day, sleeping approximately 7–8 hours each night, limiting naps during the day, minimizing flashing lights in the bedroom, and reducing noise during bedtime. For instance, a pilot study examined the efficacy of a parent-based sleep education program called "Sleep Well!" that supplemented an outreach program to provide beds to socioeconomically disadvantaged children. Alongside receiving a bed, 152 children (average age of 5.95 years, 57% boys) were randomly assigned to receive either the sleep education intervention that consisted of three text message prompts nightly (bedtime before 9 p.m., no caffeine, and keep electronics out of the bedroom) or a control text message related to dental hygiene education. Children were followed over 4 weeks and received a different text message on a nightly basis each week (e.g., bedtime before 9 p.m. per night on week 1). Relative to the control group, children whose parents received the sleep education intervention showed significant improvement in sleep duration when keeping electronics out of the bedroom. However, there was no significant effect for text message prompts related to caffeine consumption or 9 p.m. bedtime from baseline to follow-up (Mindell et al., 2016). Although these two components are important, the young age of the sample may have minimized the possible effects of these two reminder prompts (e.g., 6-year-old children likely go to bed before 9 p.m., 6-year-old children may already have limited access to caffeine in evening hours). An approach to discussing sleep, sleep hygiene, and sleep interventions is presented below using the same case of a young adult male with TD mentioned earlier in this chapter.

Clinician: *"I know that we have been talking about incorporating physical activity into your daily life, but let's also discuss another important aspect of your physical well-being, sleep. How have you been sleeping lately?"*

Patient: *"It is not that great. I always feel tired."*

Clinician: *"Why do you think that is? For example, do you have trouble falling asleep, or staying asleep, or difficulty getting out of bed in the morning? Or is it that you just never feel fully 'rested' from your sleep?"*

Patient: *"I don't sleep well. I wake up at night and have trouble falling back asleep."*

Clinician: *"It can be very frustrating and tiring to not be able to sleep well. Why do you think you have problems sleeping?"*

Patient: *"I don't know. I just can't sleep."*

Clinician: *"For most people, an important part of getting good sleep is having good sleep hygiene. Tell me a little bit about your bedtime routine? What do you do before bed? Once you get in bed?"*

Patient: *"Well, I usually start to get ready for bed around 11 p.m., and actually get into bed around 11:15 PM. Then I typically watch television shows, or videos on my phone until I start to feel tired, which is usually a little after 12AM. However, I usually wake up at some point in the night and have trouble*

	falling back asleep. So I just watch videos on my phone again until I can fall asleep, which can sometimes be a while."
Clinician:	*"So it sounds like you have a regular bedtime of 11 p.m., which is great! However, you mentioned that you use your phone to watch videos once you're in bed and even when you wake up in the middle of the night. While its normal to want to use electronics to 'wind down', research suggests that the use of electronics like your phone or TV close to or at bedtime can disturb your sleep."*
Patient:	*"I guess that sounds right. Sometimes when I wake up in the middle of the night and watch videos on my phone, it can keep me awake for hours. So you are saying that I shouldn't watch any television or videos on my phone before bed?"*
Clinician:	*"I understand that it might be hard, but it also sounds like your sleep has been suffering. Let's try an experiment to start if you're willing. Let's keep your television remote and phone out of the bedroom at night time over the next two weeks, and monitor your sleep."*
Patient:	*"That's a good idea and then that way I won't be tempted to watch videos or shows if I wake up in the middle of the night."*
Clinician:	*"Is there anything you could do once you are in bed instead of watching shows?"*
Patient:	*"Well, I guess I could try reading a book. There is a science fiction book I have been wanting to read, so this would be a good way to make it happen."*
Clinician:	*"That's a great idea to start, but if it also keeps you up at night, then we might want to remove the book as well."*

While this example is entirely focused on the patient's bedtime routine, it would also be important to assess for other factors that might cause sleep disturbances (e.g., ingesting caffeine at night, noisy environment, etc.). While the aforementioned sleep hygiene strategies are beneficial, it is important to consider that patients with TD have an increased risk for sleep disorders (Ghosh et al., 2014). For instance, in a sample of 31 patients with TD alone (without comorbid ADHD) who were 21 years of age or younger, 10 (32%) reported insomnia irrespective of ADHD or medication use (Ghosh et al., 2014). Therefore if a patient with TD has good sleep hygiene, but continues to exhibit persistent sleep problems, a polysomnogram at a qualified sleep center is advisable.

While this chapter has reviewed several common problems that affect the well-being of patients with TD, there are several other problems that are not covered in this chapter (such as mood disorders including anxiety and depression). TD is also associated with an increased risk of suicide (Fernández de la Cruz et al., 2017). One study found that 1 in 10 youth with chronic tic disorders experiences suicidal thoughts and/or behaviors (Storch et al., 2015). Neurologic complications can also occur in TD particularly in patients with violent motor tics. Such complications include cervical myelopathy, cervical disk herniation, ischemic stroke resulting from arterial dissection, bone fractures, and retinal detachments (Patterson et al., 2016). This is a detailed assessment of the physical health of a patient with TD that is encouraged at the start of treatment, with evidence-based approaches utilized to address any impairing concerns.

PROMOTING EMOTIONAL WELL-BEING

There are several key elements for the successful adjustment of a chronic diagnosis, which include the use of adequate adaptive techniques, such as adjustment to the specific functional sequelae of the disease (e.g., coping with physical pain due to tics), maintaining emotional balance (e.g., managing frustration and practicing mindfulness when tics worsen), and preserving healthy relationships (e.g., developing and maintaining supportive friendship with peers). Accordingly, interventions that focus on promoting adaptive techniques can help patients achieve emotional well-being and promote emotional health. This section describes the impairments in emotional well-being that many individuals with TD experience, and review the empirical evidence to enhance emotional well-being in TD.

Impairments in Emotional Well-Being in TD

While tics are the hallmark symptom of TD, children with TD often experience psychiatric comorbidities that can cause more emotional and social adjustment problems than the tics themselves (Bernard et al., 2009; Carter et al., 2000; Pringsheim, Lang, Kurlan, Pearce, & Sandor, 2009). For instance, a study examined social-emotional and family functioning of 72 children between 8 and 14 years of age who either had TD (n = 16), TD + ADHD (n = 33), or no psychiatric disorders (n = 23) (Carter et al., 2000). Tic symptom severity was not associated with social, behavioral, or emotional functioning among children with TD, even after stratifying by medication status. However, ADHD diagnosis, obsessive symptom severity, and family functioning were significantly associated with social and emotional adjustment among children with TD. Meanwhile, family functioning was associated with social and emotional well-being, even after controlling for TD and ADHD diagnostic status (Carter et al., 2000). These findings underscore that health care professionals should closely consider the impact of comorbidity on social and emotional functioning in children with TD, tailor treatments to the specific manifestations with the greatest impact on functioning, and also take into account the family situation.

Self-esteem is another major factor in the emotional well-being of patients with TD. Previous studies have shown that adolescents with higher self-esteem are better able to cope with problems compared to those with lower self-esteem (Dumont & Provost, 1999). Tic disorders can lower self-esteem, which can generalize into other aspects of life including adapting to social settings and performing well in school (Leckman & Cohen, 1988). For example, 57 patients (aged 6–16 years) with TD and 57 unaffected children and adolescents in the control group participated in a study that investigated self-esteem in children with TD using the Rosenberg Self-esteem Scale (Hesapçıoğlu, Tural, & Kandil, 2014). There was a significant difference in self-esteem between children with TD (M = 2.3, SD = 1.5) and unaffected control children (M = 1.2, SD = 1.0), with a logistic regression revealed that there was a 6.5 fold increased risk of low or moderate self-esteem in children with TD compared to unaffected children. Additionally, the risk of low or moderate self-esteem was increased 6.7-fold among girls with TD. Furthermore, when comparing age groups among children with TD, children below 12 years of age (M = 2.7, SD = 1.4) had a significantly higher self-esteem compared to children older than 12 years of age (M = 1.5, SD = 1.4). As this study found low self-esteem to be correlated with low quality of life among children with TD, this suggests that interventions to improve self-esteem in patients with TD may positively impact their quality of life.

In addition to self-esteem, self-competence can also influence the quality of life for patients with TD. One study examined the role of self-competence on health-related quality of life and behavioral functioning in 39 children with TD (aged 8–17 years) and 72 caregivers (Gutierrez-Colina, LaMotte, Eaton, Kardon, & Blount, 2015). Although children with TD were not found to have lower self-competence compared to unaffected samples on the Perceived Competence Scale for Children, social and general self-competence domains were positively correlated with most emotional outcomes (e.g., separation anxiety, social anxiety, and depression). Interestingly, social (but not general) self-competence was associated with health-related quality of life. Taken together, findings suggest that promoting children's perceived self-competence can be protective for emotional well-being and may lead to an improved quality of life. While strategies to target self-competence are discussed further in Chapter 5, Cognitive Restructuring About Tics and Chapter 6, Improving Self-Esteem for Youth With Tourette Syndrome and Tic Disorders, helping patients with TD set goals and focus on career, academics, and extracurricular activities (e.g., hobbies, sports) can build self-competence, rechannel tic-related energy, as well as cultivate a sense of autonomy and a feeling of control over one's life.

Beyond quantitative studies of social functioning, self-esteem, and quality of life, qualitative studies can offer important insight into promoting the emotional well-being of patients with TD. For example, a qualitative, phenomenological research study of 12 adolescents with TD in Taiwan investigated the self-experience of having TD in the context of peer interactions (Lee, Mu, Wang, & Wang, 2016). Adolescents responded to open-ended questions in one-on-one in-depth interviews that lasted 60 to 90 minutes. Adolescents with TD reported that tolerance, respect, and support of parents and teachers sparked their courage for self-acceptance. Additionally, these youth endorsed that receiving recognition from and being accepted by their peers allowed them to identify themselves as people living their lives just like their peers and thus easing their coexistence with TD (Lee et al., 2016). Indeed, healthy peer relationships can help patients with TD achieve a sense of unity and social identity, and be closer to self-acceptance. Additionally, friendships can become more intimate and supportive as children with TD and their peers mature and navigate adolescence (Lee et al., 2016). Thus positive relationships with parents, teachers, and peers can be protective on both a personal (e.g., reducing anxiety and stress, improving self-esteem) and environmental level (e.g., minimizing peer teasing) (Lee et al., 2016).

Similarly, another qualitative study explored the perceived impact of TD on self and relationships with others through the psychosocial experiences of six adolescents with TD (14–16 years old) (Wadman, Tischler, & Jackson, 2013). While interviews with adolescents revealed that TD was a constant presence in their lives, they reportedly had learned to cope with it well. Although it was a small sample, these adolescents reported developing supportive relations and felt most comfortable within their close friends, but less comfortable within a wider network (Wadman et al., 2013). While demonstrating the resilience of some youth with TD, this raises an interesting point. Patients with TD report some ability to consciously suppress tics based on situational factors. Thus patients would typically attempt to suppress tics in order to appear as "normal" as best as possible with peers. However, when the patient with TD discloses the TD diagnosis, this may create some confusion amongst peers as tics may have been largely suppressed during prior peer interactions. The presentation of appropriate psychoeducation and practice of disclosure to peers (covered in Chapter 7: Talking About Tics With Peers and Coping in Social Interactions) is essential to cultivate peer understanding, acceptance, and empathy, all of which provide the foundation for long-lasting friendships. Therefore clinicians should consider using the strategies outlined in this book to help patients develop and maintain close friendships, which can help the patient cope and feel comfortable with his/her chronic condition.

Interventions to Improve Emotional Well-Being in TD

Various approaches have been proposed to help reduce stress and anxiety and thereby enhance psychological and emotional well-being. These include therapeutic techniques, such as progressive relaxation, guided imagery, deep breathing exercises, biofeedback, meditation/mindfulness, and self-hypnosis. However, to date, there are few empirical studies investigating the impact of these practices on the well-being of patients with TD. Systematic literature reviews of psychosocial interventions and expert consensus concluded that while there are randomized studies looking into the behavioral treatments for tics, treatments, such as contingency management and relaxation training, are not backed by well-designed studies. Furthermore, interventions such as neurofeedback should be considered experimental since there are only case studies or small case series reported in the literature (Verdellen, Van De

Griendt, Hartmann, Murphy, & Group, 2011; Zhuo & Li, 2014). As a result of the limited evidence for these techniques in TD populations, this section draws from other chapters in this book and the available literature to offer strategies that improve the psychological and emotional well-being of patients with TD. Given the above-mentioned impairments in patients with TD, the psychological and emotional well-being in patients with TD can be advanced by using a multidimensional approach that includes (but is not limited to): self-esteem and self-acceptance (see Chapter 5: Cognitive Restructuring About Tics and Chapter 6: Improving Self-Esteem for Youth With Tourette Syndrome and Tic Disorders), forming positive relations with others (see Chapter 7: Talking About Tics With Peers and Coping in Social Interactions), environmental adjustment (see Chapter 9: Managing Avoidance and Accommodation of Tics and Related Behaviors and Chapter 14: Family Issues Associated with Tic), achieving purpose in life, autonomy, and personal growth.

Beyond these therapeutic techniques, there is some evidence for interventions that can directly improve the quality of life among children with TD. For instance, one study applied a 12 to 14 week manualized treatment for TD named "Facotik" in a case series of children (aged 8–12 years) (Leclerc, O'connor, J-Nolin, Valois, & Lavoie, 2016). Participants met with clinicians for 90 minute weekly sessions, which included 20 minutes of training of parents as well. Session content included awareness training, strategies to improve motor control, modifying style of planning, cognitive and behavioral training, and relapse prevention. Specifically, cognitive training focuses on the judgmental and perfectionistic styles of thinking and behavior including over-planning and over-preparation, anticipation, rigid beliefs of organization and actions, to name a few (Leclerc, O'Connor, J-Nolin, Valois, & Lavoie, 2016). After treatment, all participants were found to have either maintained and/or reached medium-to-high levels of self- esteem on the Culture-Free Self-Esteem Inventory. Meanwhile, another study investigated the efficacy of cognitive behavioral intervention (called "Living with Tics" or LWT) to reduce tic-related impairment and improve quality of life in children with TD aged 7–17 years (McGuire et al., 2015). In this randomized controlled trial of 24 children with TD, patients were randomly assigned to receive 10 weekly sessions of LWT or a 10-week waitlist control period. Children who received LWT experienced a significant reduction in tic-related impairment and improved quality of life relative to the waitlist condition. Importantly, the treatment gains were maintained at a 1-month follow-up visit. Taken together, these studies demonstrate that psychosocial interventions can improve self-esteem and quality of life among children with TD—key components of emotional well-being.

In addition to these cognitive behavioral interventions, mindfulness meditation can be a useful adjunctive intervention. Mindfulness meditation can be used to manage a range of psychological and emotional symptoms (e.g., stress), and teach patients better self-regulation techniques in response to psychological and emotional distress (Perry-Parrish, Copeland-Linder, Webb, & Sibinga, 2016) (see Chapter 13: Mindfulness for Tics for mindfulness skills). Indeed, preliminary functional neuroimaging studies suggest that mindfulness improves emotional regulation by enhancing cortical regulation of limbic circuits and attentional control (Sipe & Eisendrath, 2012). Although helpful as an adjunctive intervention, the evidence of the efficacy for reducing tic symptom severity is scarce. One small pilot study examined a form of mindfulness-based stress reduction (MBSR)-tics for reducing tic symptom severity in 18 patients with TD (aged 16–67) (Reese et al., 2015). In this open-label study, participants received 8 weekly 2-hour classes and one 4-hour retreat in the fifth or sixth week of the program. The MSBR-tics intervention resulted in a 20.2% reduction in tic symptom severity, with 58.8% of participants rated as treatment responders at the post-treatment assessment. These therapeutic gains were maintained at a 1-month follow-up assessment. Although not currently empirically evaluated, other techniques that enhance mindfulness and have been attempted by patients with TD include meditation, yoga, *tai chi*, mental healing, prayer, and *qi gong*.

Finally, hypnosis has been used to address symptom control and well-being in numerous medical disorders. Unfortunately, most of the literature in TD consists of case studies. One case series examined a standardized method of training 33 children with TD in self-hypnosis using a videotape series of a boy undergoing self-hypnosis training for tic control (Lazarus & Klein, 2010). Improvement of tic control was recorded per subjective patient report. Interestingly, 79% of patients trained in this technique self-reported a positive treatment response, with most achieving this response after three sessions. Although appearing promising, these preliminary results warrant replication in a more rigorously designed study that uses a control group, random assignment, and a psychometrically validated outcome measure like the YGTSS. Thus when patients inquire about the efficacy of self-hypnosis and other mind-body interventions for reducing tic symptom severity, clinicians might respond with the following explanation:

> *"While there are several treatments such as self-hypnosis, neurofeedback deep breathing exercises, and guided imagery, to name a few, there is no definitive evidence that these treatments reduce tic symptom severity and/or improve quality of life for patients with TD. However, these interventions can be attempted as an adjunctive treatment, but should not be relied upon as a sole form of management of tic disorders."*

PROMOTING ACADEMIC WELL-BEING

Academic well-being is another important aspect of children's lives. In an academic setting, children with TD can have significant difficulties due to tics and common co-occurring neuropsychiatric conditions, such as ADHD, anxiety, and learning disabilities. Indeed, all of these conditions can have a direct impact on lowering self-esteem and/or have consequences that lead to poorer psychosocial functioning and quality of life. An international multisite study of patients with TD found that 60% of patients with TD experienced co-occurring ADHD (Freeman et al., 2000). Additionally, patients also reported frequently experiencing anxiety disorders (18%) and learning disorders (23%). Tics and comorbid ADHD can cause problems in the classroom by impairing a child's ability to focus on academic lessons (due to tics) and lead to further inattention, distractibility, and impulsivity associated with ADHD. In social situations at school, co-occurring anxiety can further fuel the social exclusion, discrimination, and bullying that often accompanies TD. For example, a study of 53 patients with TD (aged 17–72 years) found that patients who had higher relationship anxiety were more likely to have an insecure attachment, which thereby leads them to avoid creating relationships (Dehning et al., 2015). Therefore both ADHD and anxiety can negatively impact children's academic well-being both in and outside the classroom.

Alongside comorbid ADHD, the prevalence of learning disabilities is increased in patients with TD (Burd, Freeman, Klug, & Kerbeshian, 2005) and can occur even in the absence of ADHD (Scahill, Sukhodolsky, Williams, & Leckman, 2005). Even though cognitive deficits in patients with TD are specific for executive function, fine motor skills, and visual-motor problems, learning disabilities in TD can affect the whole gamut of learning activities. Learning disabilities often go undiagnosed early on in patients with TD. Lack of awareness of a learning disability in a patient with TD creates more difficulty in educating the patient, with regards to not only learning in school, but also therapeutic interventions for the TD itself. Thus when evaluating patients with TD, the presence of learning disabilities should always be a consideration.

In order to optimize academic performance and academic well-being, it is important to consider TD and co-occurring conditions in the contexts within which children primarily spend the majority of their time: the school and the family system. If a patient's academic performance is compromised (see Chapter 8: Tourette's in the Classroom: Support and Guidance on Education Issues for Clinicians), it may be beneficial for children with TD to undergo educational, intelligence, and/or neuropsychological testing. This can help school personnel, parents, and child understand the child's specific learning challenges and develop individualized educational programs to make learning and the child's overall school experience less cumbersome and more pleasant (see Chapter 8: Tourette's in the Classroom: Support and Guidance on Education Issues for Clinicians for a more detailed discussion of Coping with Tics at School).

When considering other school-related interventions, it is important to remember that tics follow a waxing and waning pattern of frequency and intensity. Additionally, tics tend to worsen when a child is fatigued, stressed, or put in certain environmental situations. For example, one-third of children reported tic reduction during holidays, and up to 50% reported improved tics when engaged in artistic or creative activities (e.g., playing, dancing, taking photographs, music) (Lee et al., 2016). Similarly, several reports note that children's tics decrease when engaged in goal-directed behavior (e.g., fine motor or vocal movements, movements that require increased attention) (Eapen, Fox-Hiley, Banerjee, & Robertson, 2004). However, 40%–70% of patients identified nonstressful situations, such as social gatherings, celebrations, and watching television that appeared to worsen tic symptoms (Caurín, Serrano, Fernández-Alvarez, Campistol, & Pérez-Dueñas, 2014). Indeed, television and video games ("screen time") have been associated tic aggravation and problems with attention in some youth (Weiss, Baer, Allan, Saran, & Schibuk, 2011). Therefore any intervention or plan that is created needs to be flexible and should take into consideration the environmental and situational factors that influence tic expression.

In addition to the school system, children spend a considerable portion of time in "the family system." Therefore a stable and healthy home atmosphere with a strong support network can improve a child's academic functioning (as well as enhance functioning in other domains). Stable family functioning enables the child to have a routine at home to facilitate the completion of academic assignments/projects, as well as encourages out-of-school socialization with peers. Comparatively, a stressed family system can contribute to and/or exacerbate psychosocial difficulties. While there may be many reasons for a stressed family system, psychoeducation and effective communication can address some aspects of family functioning (see Chapter 14: Family Issues Associated With Tics for further discussion). For example, some parents (and other family members) may not understand the diagnosis of TD and struggle to recognize why the patient can control tics in some circumstances but not others (i.e., believing tic symptoms to be volitional). Meanwhile, other family members may feel frustrated by the attention directed toward the affected child. Accordingly, clinicians can provide appropriate psychoeducation to the parents and family members (with consent) to help educate those individuals about TD and its related conditions (see Chapter 2: Psychoeducation About Tic Disorders and Treatment). This same information may be useful for school personnel, who often do not have specialized training or experience working with children with TD. In regards to effective communication, the clinicians can help parents become effective communicators of this information and advocate for the affected child with TD. In particular, parents often reported that the lack of understanding of TD by teachers and peers causes difficulties at school. Therefore promoting the well-being of children with TD requires parents (and older adolescents) to educate those around them about TD and become active advocates for the child in and outside of the school system. However, as family systems can be stressful for many other reasons, it may be worthwhile to consider if a referral for family therapy would be beneficial to address larger family systems issues.

CONCLUSION

As is the case in all patients with chronic disease, patients with TD have to face and adapt to many issues and limitations in various aspects of their life. While patient-centered approaches to health care focus on symptom reduction, a therapeutic approach that is wellness-focused and person-centered is important in chronic disease. In collaboration with their health care team, patients with TD have to craft an individualized treatment regimen that is best addressed to their specific needs. Thus treatment goals often include both reductions in tic symptom severity and improving the patient's quality of life. Promoting healthy behaviors can help alleviate the impact tics have on the daily life. Optimizing nutrition, regular exercise, and tailoring the patient's environment are a few of the many changes that a clinician can help make in the lifestyle of a patient with TD. Although optimizing physical, emotional, social, and academic well-being can be strenuous and effort-dependent, this time is well-spent in allowing the patient to journey toward living a fully functional and independent life. At the health care provider's level, promoting health and well-being encompasses having knowledge of the patient's perspectives, helping them set goals, applying relevant clinical and behavioral interventions, and ensuring continuous follow up. Finally, at the policy level, promoting healthy behaviors involves making healthy behavioral choices easier, less expensive and more socially normative.

REFERENCES

Bernard, B. A., Stebbins, G. T., Siegel, S., Schultz, T. M., Hays, C., Morrissey, M. J., ... Goetz, C. G. (2009). Determinants of quality of life in children with Gilles de la Tourette syndrome. *Movement Disorders, 24*, 1070–1073.

Bitsko, R. H., Danielson, M., King, M., Visser, S. N., Scahill, L., & Perou, R. (2013). Health care needs of children with Tourette syndrome. *Journal of Child Neurology, 28*, 1626–1636.

Burd, L., Freeman, R. D., Klug, M. G., & Kerbeshian, J. (2005). Tourette syndrome and learning disabilities. *BMC Pediatrics, 5*, 34.

Carter, A. S., O'Donnell, D. A., Schultz, R. T., Scahill, L., Leckman, J. F., & Pauls, D. L. (2000). Social and emotional adjustment in children affected with Gilles de la Tourette's syndrome: associations with ADHD and family functioning. *Journal of Child Psychology and Psychiatry and Allied Disciplines, 41*, 215–223.

Caurín, B., Serrano, M., Fernández-Alvarez, E., Campistol, J., & Pérez-Dueñas, B. (2014). Environmental circumstances influencing tic expression in children. *European Journal of Paediatric Neurology, 18*, 157–162.

Cooper, R. E., Tye, C., Kuntsi, J., Vassos, E., & Asherson, P. (2016). The effect of omega-3 polyunsaturated fatty acid supplementation on emotional dysregulation, oppositional behaviour and conduct problems in ADHD: A systematic review and meta-analysis. *Journal of Affective Disorders, 190*, 474–482.

Dehning, S., Burger, M. B., Krause, D., Jobst, A., Yundina, E., Müller, N., ... Buchheim, A. (2015). Tourette syndrome is associated with insecure attachment and higher aggression. *International Journal of Neuroscience, 125*, 521–525.

Dumont, M., & Provost, M. A. (1999). Resilience in adolescents: Protective role of social support, coping strategies, self-esteem, and social activities on experience of stress and depression. *Journal of Youth and Adolescence*, *28*, 343–363.

Dzau, V. J., McClellan, M., & McGinnis, J. M. (2016). Vital directions for health and health care: An initiative of the National Academy of Medicine. *JAMA*, *316*, 711–712.

Eapen, V., Fox-Hiley, P., Banerjee, S., & Robertson, M. (2004). Clinical features and associated psychopathology in a Tourette syndrome cohort. *Acta Neurologica Scandinavica*, *109*, 255–260.

Fernández de la Cruz, L., Rydell, M., Runeson, B., Brander, G., Rück, C., D'Onofrio, B. M., ... Mataix-Cols, D. (2017). Suicide in Tourette's and chronic tic disorders. *Biological Psychiatry*, *82*, 111–118.

Franklin, B. A., & Vanhecke, T. E. (2008). Counseling patients to make cardioprotective lifestyle changes: strategies for success. *Preventive Cardiology*, *11*, 50–55.

Freeman, R. D., Fast, D. K., Burd, L., Kerbeshian, J., Robertson, M. M., & Sandor, P. (2000). An international perspective on Tourette syndrome: selected findings from 3500 individuals in 22 countries. *Developmental Medicine and Child Neurology*, *42*, 436–447.

Gabbay, V., Babb, J. S., Klein, R. G., Panzer, A. M., Katz, Y., Alonso, C. M., ... Coffey, B. J. (2012). A double-blind, placebo-controlled trial of omega-3 fatty acids in Tourette's disorder. *Pediatrics*, *129*, 1493–1500.

Garcia-Lopez, R., Perea-Milla, E., Garcia, C. R., Rivas-Ruiz, F., Romero-Gonzalez, J., Moreno, J. L., ... Diaz, J. C. R. (2009). New therapeutic approach to Tourette Syndrome in children based on a randomized placebo-controlled double-blind phase IV study of the effectiveness and safety of magnesium and vitamin B6. *Trials*, *10*, 16.

Ghosh, D., Rajan, P. V., Das, D., Datta, P., Rothner, A. D., & Erenberg, G. (2014). Sleep disorders in children with Tourette syndrome. *Pediatric Neurology*, *51*, 31–35.

Gorman, D. A., Zhu, H., Anderson, G. M., Davies, M., & Peterson, B. S. (2006). Ferritin levels and their association with regional brain volumes in Tourette's syndrome. *American Journal of Psychiatry*, *163*, 1264–1272.

Gutierrez-Colina, A. M., LaMotte, J., Eaton, C., Kardon, P., & Blount, R. L. (2015). The Role of self-competence in health-related quality of life and behavioral functioning of children with Tourette syndrome. *Journal of Developmental & Behavioral Pediatrics*, *36*, 743–751.

Hesapçıoğlu, S., Tural, M., & Kandil, S. (2014). Quality of life and self-esteem in children with chronic tic disorder. *Turkish Archives of Pediatrics*, *49*, 323–332.

Huber, M., Knottnerus, J. A., Green, L., van der Horst, H., Jadad, A. R., Kromhout, D., ... van der Meer, J. W. (2011). How should we define health? *British Medical Journal*, *343*, d4163.

Jayakody, K., Gunadasa, S., & Hosker, C. (2014). Exercise for anxiety disorders: systematic review. *British Journal of Sports Medicine*, *48*, 187–196.

Koh, H. K. (2016). Improving health and health care in the United States: Toward a state of complete well-being. *JAMA*, *316*, 1679–1681.

Lazarus, J. E., & Klein, S. K. (2010). Nonpharmacological treatment of tics in Tourette syndrome adding videotape training to self-hypnosis. *Journal of Developmental & Behavioral Pediatrics*, *31*, 498–504.

Leckman, J. F., & Cohen, D. J. (1988). Descriptive and diagnostic classification of tic disorders. In R. D. B. D. J. Cohen, & J. F. Leckman (Eds.), *Wiley Series in Child and Adolescent Mental Health. Tourette's Syndrome and Tic Disorders: Clinical Understanding and Treatment* (pp. 3–19). Oxford, England: John Wiley.

Leclerc, J., O'Connor, K., J-Nolin, G., Valois, P., & Lavoie, M. (2016). The effect of a new therapy for children with tics targeting underlying cognitive, behavioral, and physiological processes. *Frontiers in Psychiatry*, *7*, 135–135.

Lee, M. Y., Mu, P. F., Wang, W. S., & Wang, H. S. (2016). 'Living with tics': Self-experience of adolescents with Tourette syndrome during peer interaction. *Journal of Clinical Nursing, 25*, 463–471.

Lichtenstein, A. H., Appel, L. J., Brands, M., Carnethon, M., Daniels, S., Franch, H. A., ... Howard, B. (2006). Diet and lifestyle recommendations revision 2006. *Circulation, 114*, 82–96.

Lorig, K. R., Sobel, D. S., Ritter, P. L., Laurent, D., & Hobbs, M. (2001). Effect of a self-management program on patients with chronic disease. *Effective Clinical Practice, 4*, 256–262.

McGuire, J. F., Arnold, E., Park, J. M., Nadeau, J. M., Lewin, A. B., Murphy, T. K., & Storch, E. A. (2015). Living with tics: Reduced impairment and improved quality of life for youth with chronic tic disorders. *Psychiatry Research, 225*, 571–579.

Mindell, J. A., Sedmak, R., Boyle, J. T., Butler, R., & Williamson, A. A. (2016). Sleep well!: A pilot study of an education campaign to improve sleep of socioeconomically disadvantaged children. *Journal of Clinical Sleep Medicine: JCSM: official publication of the American Academy of Sleep Medicine, 12*, 1593–1599.

Müller-Vahl, K. R., Buddensiek, N., Geomelas, M., & Emrich, H. M. (2008). The influence of different food and drink on tics in Tourette syndrome. *Acta Paediatrica, 97*, 442–446.

Nixon, E., Glazebrook, C., Hollis, C., & Jackson, G. M. (2014). Reduced Tic symptomatology in tourette syndrome after an acute bout of exercise: An observational study. *Behavior Modification, 38*, 235–263.

Patterson, A. L., Choudhri, A. F., Igarashi, M., McVicar, K., Shah, N., & Morgan, R. (2016). Severe neurological complications associated with Tourette syndrome. *Pediatric Neurology, 61*, 99–106.

Perry-Parrish, C., Copeland-Linder, N., Webb, L., & Sibinga, E. M. (2016). Mindfulness-based approaches for children and youth. *Current Problems in Pediatric and Adolescent Health Care, 46*, 172–178.

Pringsheim, T., Lang, A., Kurlan, R., Pearce, M., & Sandor, P. (2009). Understanding disability in Tourette syndrome. *Developmental Medicine & Child Neurology, 51*, 468–472.

Reese, H. E., Vallejo, Z., Rasmussen, J., Crowe, K., Rosenfield, E., & Wilhelm, S. (2015). Mindfulness-based stress reduction for Tourette syndrome and chronic tic disorder: A pilot study. *Journal of Psychosomatic Research, 78*, 293–298.

Scahill, L., Sukhodolsky, D. G., Williams, S. K., & Leckman, J. F. (2005). Public health significance of tic disorders in children and adolescents. *Advances in Neurology, 96*, 240–248.

Sipe, W. E., & Eisendrath, S. J. (2012). Mindfulness-based cognitive therapy: theory and practice. *The Canadian Journal of Psychiatry, 57*, 63–69.

Sleiman, S. F., Henry, J., Al-Haddad, R., El Hayek, L., Haidar, E. A., Stringer, T., ... Ratan, R. R. (2016). Exercise promotes the expression of brain derived neurotrophic factor (BDNF) through the action of the ketone body β-hydroxybutyrate. *eLife, 5*, e15092.

Storch, E. A., Hanks, C. E., Mink, J. W., McGuire, J. F., Adams, H. R., Augustine, E. F., ... Lewin, A. B. (2015). Suicidal thoughts and behaviors in children and adolescents with chronic tic disorders. *Depression and Anxiety, 32*, 744–753.

Verdellen, C., Van De Griendt, J., Hartmann, A., Murphy, T., & Group, E. G. (2011). European clinical guidelines for Tourette syndrome and other tic disorders. Part III: Behavioural and psychosocial interventions. *European Child & Adolescent Psychiatry, 20*, 197–207.

Wadman, R., Tischler, V., & Jackson, G. (2013). 'Everybody just thinks I'm weird': A qualitative exploration of the psychosocial experiences of adolescents with Tourette syndrome. *Child: Care, Health and Development, 39*, 880–886.

Wagner, E. H., Austin, B. T., Davis, C., Hindmarsh, M., Schaefer, J., & Bonomi, A. (2001). Improving chronic illness care: Translating evidence into action. *Health Affairs, 20*, 64–78.

Weiss, M. D., Baer, S., Allan, B. A., Saran, K., & Schibuk, H. (2011). The screens culture: Impact on ADHD. *ADHD Attention Deficit and Hyperactivity Disorders, 3*, 327–334.

World Health Organization. (1984). Health promotion: A discussion document on the concept and principles: summary report of the Working Group on Concept and Principles of Health Promotion, Copenhagen, 9–13 July 1984.

Yu, C.-J., Du, J.-C., Chiou, H.-C., Feng, C.-C., Chung, M.-Y., Yang, W., ... Chen, M.-L. (2016). Sugar-sweetened beverage consumption is adversely associated with childhood attention deficit/hyperactivity disorder. *International Journal of Environmental Research and Public Health, 13*, 678.

Zhuo, C., & Li, L. (2014). The application and efficacy of combined neurofeedback therapy and imagery training in adolescents with Tourette syndrome. *Journal of Child Neurology, 29*, 965–968.

Chapter 16

Relapse Prevention Strategies and Guidance on Refractory Cases

Robert R. Selles[1,2], Tara Jukes[2], Melanie McConnell[1,2] and S. Evelyn Stewart[1,2,3,4]

[1]University of British Columbia, Vancouver, BC, Canada, [2]British Columbia Children's Hospital, Vancouver, BC, Canada, [3]Massachusetts General Hospital, Boston, MA, United States, [4]Harvard Medical School, Boston, MA, United States

The treatment descriptions provided in the previous chapters of this book are designed to provide clinicians with tools for effectiveness; however, treatment is associated with varying levels of response across patients. With consistent strategy implementation and tic management abilities as markers of treatment success (rather than elimination of tics), treating clinicians should be prepared to encounter youth who demonstrate exceptional improvement at first intervention, as well as those who continue to struggle despite multiple appropriate treatment attempts. As such, clinicians face complex decisions regarding treatment termination, modification, extension, and/or the pursuit of alternative treatments. The purpose of the present chapter is to explore the various needs, considerations, and decisions related to response and nonresponse to both pharmaceutical and/or psychosocial approaches. In particular, this chapter will address questions that are faced regularly by clinicians treating tic disorders, namely, "*Is this as good as it gets?*," "*What else can we try?*," "*How do we keep tics from coming back?*," and "*How can we further improve functioning?*"

As these decisions are complex, available evidence should be used to inform decisions. For one, given that tics have a waxing and waning course that is independent from treatment response, clinicians are recommended to implement, at repeated time points, evidence-based assessment measures to closely evaluate the varying success of treatments (see Chapter 1: Introduction to Treatment and Management of Youth With Tourette Disorders and Tic Disorders for discussion on evidence-based assessments). As outlined in Chapter 1, Introduction to Treatment and Management of

The Clinician's Guide to Treatment and Management of Youth with Tourette Syndrome and Tic Disorders.
DOI: https://doi.org/10.1016/B978-0-12-811980-8.00016-9

Youth With Tourette Disorders and Tic Disorders, these assessments should include measures of tic symptom severity, tic-related impairment, and the quality of life. It is important to include both youth and parents in the assessment process because tics may cause more distress or irritation to parents than tic-affected youth. Similarly, when contextualizing these ratings as measures of therapeutic response, a joint focus on the child's quality of life and performance in home, school, and other settings is strongly recommended. While tics and tic-related impairment are likely the predominant focus of treatment, it is also important to consider factors, such as comorbid disorders, social difficulties, behavioral difficulties, and emotional challenges that can also contribute to impairment. Based on these assessments and clinical judgment, treatment decisions related to psychosocial or pharmaceutical interventions should be collaboratively discussed with the affected youth and parents. Ideally, this will include an active discussion of risks, benefits, and alternatives. Tic symptom severity, functional impact of tics, and quality of life must be weighed against adverse effects, accessibility, cost, and other possible consequences associated with ongoing evidence-based treatment. Keeping this in mind, this chapter will first present guidance on treatment decisions when youth continue to have problematic tics and/or tic-related impairment, followed by a discussion of relapse prevention strategies to implement when treatment discontinuation is being considered.

GUIDANCE ON REFRACTORY CASES

Contributors to treatment nonresponse can differ across patients and treatments. As a result, clinicians require flexibility in determining appropriate next steps. In general, clinicians should consider which factors have contributed to nonresponse, whether response to the same treatment can be improved by addressing these factors, and whether alternative treatment options are available.

Returning to the Beginning of the Book

As the present book has outlined, effective treatment of tic disorders involves a comprehensive application of a number of treatment interventions that engage youth in a variety of domains and skills. These interventions may be used flexibly depending on individual needs and presentations, and youth may differ in which components produce the largest benefit. For example, specific treatment components may be easier to understand and implement, may more directly target the mechanisms that contribute to symptoms, or may have a greater impact due to their relationship with impairment for some youth versus others. Conducting thorough assessment, closely monitoring treatment progress, soliciting feedback from youth and their families, and observing extraneous variables that may moderate patients' ability to respond to treatment components provide the basis for making decisions about which components may be useful to return to or emphasize in the face of initial nonresponse.

Some children have challenges engaging with or benefiting from habit reversal training (HRT), but may benefit from emphasis on alternate aspects of behavior therapy. In particular, utilizing function-based assessment and intervention pertaining to triggers and consequences for tics can have benefit for many individuals (see Chapter 14: Family Issues Associated with Tics). In fact, recent meta-analytic findings have highlighted this contingency management portion of treatment as having an important role in treatment outcomes (Theule, Ward, Cheung, & Lee, 2016). Although this is often employed by modifying activities or circumstances to reduce environmental triggers for tics, it can also be adapted to focus on emotion regulation or anxiety management to address emotion states that negatively impact tics. For example, a 12-year-old boy with tics causing marked impairment in addition to comorbid attention deficit hyperactivity disorder (ADHD) and oppositional defiant disorder (ODD) eagerly attended treatment sessions. However, he experienced significant challenges engaging in awareness training and competing response practice due to issues with oppositional behavior and low sustained attention. Given these challenges, the treatment approach was revised to focus on practice and implementation of emotion regulation strategies using a contingency management approach. Specifically, identifying triggers for negative emotion states (e.g., not understanding session content, being given negative feedback, disagreeing with parents) and implementing appropriate calming strategies (e.g., taking a 5-minute break, using a deep breathing exercise, sharing feelings with a caregiver or group leader) proved particularly beneficial in the moment for this individual. In addition, ongoing practice of relaxation, visualization, and mindfulness strategies during times of low distress (e.g., after school, before bed) was reported as helpful by the family. Following these changes, the patient's treatment engagement and adherence improved and a subsequent reduction in tics were observed.

As discussed throughout the book, the frequency and intensity of tics are not always reliably associated with tic-related impairment/distress. For instance, children with mild tics may present as extremely self-conscious, anxious, and distraught about their tics (e.g., to the point of avoiding school and extracurricular activities). In particular, many youth with tics demonstrate social deficits and these deficits predict, beyond tic severity, poorer functioning, and quality of life (McGuire, Hanks, Lewin, Storch, & Murphy, 2013). In contrast, children experiencing almost constant motor and vocal tics that significantly interfere with verbal communication and purposeful movements may be only mildly bothered by their tics. Consequently, in attempting to identify a treatment that may be beneficial for a nonresponsive youth, clinicians should consider looking to factors that may produce improvements in the quality of life, even if they may not impact tic severity.

Addressing Poor Adherence

Poor treatment adherence represents a significant barrier to outcomes across a variety of pediatric behavioral health and mental health interventions. Estimates vary greatly, with multiple studies reporting that over half of all families are nonadherent with recommended treatment plans (e.g., Duncan, Mentrikoski, Wu, & Fredericks, 2014 Morgan et al., 2013; Nock & Ferriter, 2005). While reported attrition rates for behavior therapy are low, ranging from 8% to 14% (Piacentini et al., 2010; Wilhelm et al., 2012), there has been some speculation that the demands of certain elements of HRT (i.e., awareness training and competing response practice) may present a barrier to treatment engagement and success, due to the degree of effort and attention required (Dopfner & Rothenberger, 2007). Given that treatment outcome has been linked to both adherence to behavioral intervention (Olatunji et al., 2015; Park et al., 2014) and to compliance with medication (Horwitz & Horwitz, 1993; LaRosa, 2000; Misdrahi, Llorca, Lancon, & Bayle, 2002), addressing issues of nonadherence is important to ensure sufficient opportunity to benefit from treatment. While families may not volunteer their noncompliance, it is helpful to ask about who manages the treatment delivery, such as ensuring homework compliance or providing medication reminders and distribution.

Considerable effort has been made to identify and address factors contributing to poor adherence to pediatric behavioral/mental health interventions (e.g., Duncan et al., 2014; Morgan et al., 2013; Olatunji et al., 2015). A wide variety of factors have been identified that affect treatment adherence more generally, including *patient-related* features (e.g., age, gender, education level, beliefs about therapy/medication), *treatment-related* considerations (e.g., treatment complexity, adverse effects, duration of treatment, degree of behavioral change required), and *social/economic* issues (e.g., time commitment, social support, cost of therapy; Jin, Sklar, Min Sen oh, & Chuen li, 2008). Motivational interviewing (MI) strategies are particularly well suited to the task of identifying and addressing underlying contributors to nonadherence or poor adherence (Dean, Britt, Bell, Stanley, & Collings, 2016; Gold & Kokotailo, 2007; Sibley et al., 2016). In essence, MI involves enhancing patients' motivation to change by exploring potential reasons for nonadherence, supporting patients to resolve ambivalence about making changes (i.e., following treatment recommendations), and strengthening their commitment to change (Miller & Rollnick, 2012). Though less applicable to younger children due to parental involvement in treatment, MI strategies are particularly beneficial when working with adolescents and parents (Dean et al., 2016; Gold & Kokotailo, 2007; Pakpour, Gellert, Dombrowski, & Fridlund, 2015; Sibley et al., 2016). For example, MI techniques may benefit a youth who is bothered by their tics, but expresses low desire to engage in treatment, or a parent who believes treatment is important, but struggles to find time to complete home practice with their child. (Recommended MI resources include Naar-King and Suarez (2011) and Rollnick, Miller, and Butler (2008)). In addition to—or arising from—MI, practical strategies, and solutions may be needed to address issues contributing to poor adherence with treatment. From helping patients to identify barriers or impediments to taking their medication or following through with homework tasks can be a useful tool. The following tables (see Tables 16.1–16.3) outline common reasons for nonadherence to interventions for children along with recommended interventions for clinical management. Where available, relevant, or related empirical support for these strategies is provided. Of note, there is limited research on many of these aspects of nonadherence specifically for youth with tic disorders, so literature from treatment for other childhood psychological disorders has been included where appropriate. As a clinical example of applying MI strategies in behavioral therapy, let us consider a teenager who consistently neglects to complete his home practice and as a result is seeing minimal gains:

Clinician: How did your competing response practice go this week?

Patient: I didn't do it. I was too busy.

Clinician: You had a really busy week and you weren't able to get your home practice done.

Patient: Yeah. And my tics were really bad this week, so it just felt like there was a lot going on.

Clinician: So on top of having a busy week, it sounds like your tics were really bothering you.

Patient: Yeah—they make things so much worse. I had a soccer game and I couldn't even keep up with the pace of the game because every time I tried to kick the ball my leg tic happened.

Clinician: So because of your tics you weren't able to participate how you wanted in something that you really enjoy—your soccer game.

Patient: Yeah—it's so unfair. And then I feel mad at myself because I let down my teammates. So the last thing I wanted to do after that was go home and practice strategies from session—I just needed a break.

Clinician: So it sounds like it was really difficult to find time and energy to practice tic management strategies this week, but you're also finding that the tics are becoming a really big barrier to doing things that are important to you, like playing soccer.

Patient: Yeah—I wish they would just go away, or at least not interfere with the things I want to do.

Clinician: You wish there was something that could help with your tics so they wouldn't get in the way of the things that really matter to you.

Patient: Yeah. I do want to be able to use those strategies if they will make things better, I just find it really hard to practice them at home.

Clinician: So it sounds like working on tic management strategies is actually something that is pretty important to you, but it's been really difficult to find opportunities to do it. I wonder if it might be helpful for you and I to talk together about how you might be able to make that happen during these really busy weeks, given how important it is to you?

[*From here, the clinician can move into some collaborative problem solving and realistic goal setting using MI-based skills to help develop a plan for ongoing practice that the patient feels comfortable and confident about.*]

TABLE 16.1 Interventions for Patient- and Family-Related Factors Affecting Treatment Adherence

Reason for Nonadherence	Recommended Interventions	Empirical Support
Low motivation/ engagement in treatment	Use motivational interviewing (MI) with adolescents and/or parents	MI has been effectively used to increase motivation and behavior change among adolescents in various health care settings (Brown et al., 2003; Channon, Smith, & Gregory, 2003; Pakpour et al., 2015, Spirito et al., 2004)
	Create a "tic inconvenience review" to highlight aspects of tics that are distressing/impairing (Woods et al., 2008)	MI has effectively been used to foster participation in exposure therapy among adults with OCD (Simpson, Zuckoff, Page, Franklin, & Foa, 2008; Simpson et al., 2010)
	If tic-related impairment is low, discontinue treatment and resume if/when motivation and/or impairment increases	Positive reinforcement strategies can significantly improve treatment outcomes, particularly for children with comorbid attention challenges [see Dopfner and Rothenberger, 2007].
	If tic-related impairment is moderate to severe, utilize external reinforcements as needed (e.g., rewards for treatment adherent behaviors)	
Parent-child conflict/ disruptive child behavior	For mild concerns, utilize problem-solving strategies or collaborative and proactive solutions (CPS) to address any interference with treatment	Growing evidence supports the use of CPS for parenting/child behavior concerns (Epstein and Saltzman-Benaiah, 2010, Ollendick et al., 2016)
	For more severe concerns, recommend an *initial* course of parent management training (PMT) or collaborative and proactive solutions (CPS)	Children with OCD and co-morbid disruptive behaviors had poorer treatment responses (Geller et al., 2003a, Storch et al., 2008), although disruptive behaviors improved following CBT (Selles et al., 2017)
		PMT is a highly effective intervention for parent-child conflict/disruptive behavior (e.g., Ollendick et al., 2016)
		A case study examining PMT prior to treatment for OCD showed improvements in both OCD and disruptive behavior posttreatment (Lehmkuhl et al., 2009)
Challenges with parental mental health or cognitive functioning	Identify additional or alternate support person(s) to attend treatment, administer medications and/or support between-session practice	
	Provide recommendations on emotional support for parents as needed	

TABLE 16.2 Interventions for Treatment-Related Factors Affecting Adherence

Reason for Nonadherence	Recommended Interventions	Empirical Support
Low expectations for success/ skepticism about treatment	Provide additional psychoeducation about the treatment model; review empirical support for assigned treatment	Parents' positive treatment expectations were associated with better treatment outcomes in pediatric depression (Stevens et al., 2009) and pediatric OCD (Lewin, Peris, Lindsey Bergman, Mccracken, & Piacentini, 2011)
	Directly address any concerns or myths about treatment. Specific resources to help with this discussion include:	Parent perceived effectiveness and confidence in treatment were significantly associated with adherence to behavioral treatment for children with ASD (Moore and Symons, 2011)
	Information from Tourette Association of America (TAA)[a,b]	Parent knowledge and opinion of intervention facilitated treatment engagement for children with ADHD (Corkum, Rimer, & Schachar, 1999)
	Journal article: *Current controversies on the role of behavioral therapy in Tourette Syndrome* (Scahill et al., 2013)	
	Journal article: AACAP Practice Parameters (Murphy et al., 2013)	
	Connect patients/families with willing successful treatment "graduates" (with consideration to confidentiality issues)	
No awareness or limited awareness of premonitory urge	General awareness training to start (e.g., awareness of bodily sensations)[c]	Greater interoceptive awareness, or recognition of internal bodily processes, was associated with higher awareness of premonitory urge in adults (Ganos et al., 2015)
	Additional support and practice with awareness training	

(*Continued*)

TABLE 16.2 (Continued)

Reason for Nonadherence	Recommended Interventions	Empirical Support
	Greater emphasis on functional assessment/ intervention	
Perceived stigma	Consider treatment options in non-traditional settings	CBIT has been associated with positive treatment outcomes when administered in primary care settings (Shim and Rust, 2013) and when delivered online (Himle et al., 2012; Ricketts et al., 2016)
	Connect patients with other youth who have tics/ Tourette's to provide social support	
	Review video: "I have Tourette's But Tourette's Doesn't Have Me" (Kent, 2005)	
Insufficient therapeutic skill or alliance	Obtain additional case supervision from experienced clinicians	Clinician skill and therapeutic alliance have been implicated as important factors that contribute to the efficacy of treatments (e.g., Davidson et al., 2004, Martin, Garske, & Davis, 2000, Podell et al., 2013)
	Consider referral to specialized treatment centers or providers	
	Consider transfer to an alternative clinician if efforts to develop rapport have been unsuccessful	

[a] *www.tourette.org/resource/cbit-brochure (paper copies available on request).*
[b] *www.tourette.org/research-medical/cbit-for-patients.*
[c] *www.Anxietybc.com (MindShift App).*

Medication Adverse Effects

Adverse effects may necessitate discontinuation of treatment or lead to poor and nonadherence to prescribed regimens, limiting the opportunity to reach optimal dose and response. Inquiring about both common and rare-but-serious adverse effects at each follow-up assessment will permit an opportunity to openly address this concern (see Chapter 4: Pharmacological Management of Tic Disorders in Youth regarding medication management). Given that multiple factors may contribute to reported physical symptoms at any given time, use of a standard side-effect checklist at baseline (prior to starting the medication) and at follow-up visits will allow for examination of temporal effects.

TABLE 16.3 Interventions for Social/Economic Factors Affecting Adherence

Reasons for Non-Adherence	Recommended Interventions	Empirical Support
Transportation issues for attending treatment	Explore practical solutions, if relevant and available (e.g., options for transportation funding)	Distance and scheduling have been identified as major barriers to treatment adherence in pediatric OCD (Lewin, Mcguire, Murphy, & Storch, 2014)
	Consider more accessible treatment options such as internet- or video conference-based treatment (Himle et al., 2012; Ricketts et al., 2016)	
	Consider online self-guided intervention (e.g., www.tichelper.com)	
Scheduling issues/lack of time	Revisit motivational interviewing to address any ambivalence preventing families from prioritizing treatment	See above empirical support regarding perceived stigma and transportation issues
	Consider more accessible treatment options (see above)	
Child living in two households	Encourage one support person from each household to attend, if appropriate	
	Develop a communication plan for sharing information between households	

In a recent study examining parent experiences and clinical effectiveness of specific pharmacologic tic treatments for youth, risperidone, clonidine, aripiprazole, and haloperidol were the most frequently reported medication treatments (Hollis et al., 2016). Aripiprazole had the highest rates of reported helpfulness (69%) and the lowest rates (25%) of reported moderate to severe adverse effects in a sample of nearly 300 parents and caregivers. Risperidone and clonidine were reported to be helpful by approximately 40% of those taking these medications, although 47%–63% also reported moderate to severe adverse effects (Cuenca et al., 2015; Hollis et al., 2016). Haloperidol is associated with many adverse effects and has low acceptance among families (Hollis et al., 2016). In comparison with perspectives of tic medications, nearly 50% found behavioral interventions, such as HRT helpful, with only

11% reporting associated adverse effects (Hollis et al., 2016). This reinforces the need to carefully consider and weigh risks and benefits associated with tic treatments.

In addressing adverse effects, a few potential solutions exist. Complaints of fatigue and sedation can be addressed by replacing shorter-acting medications with longer acting ones, or by prescribing a larger dose at bedtime than in the morning. Alpha-agonist induced sedation may self-resolve after 6 weeks. However, excessive daytime sedation may outweigh the benefits of tic improvement. As such, dose decrease may be advisable, which typically results in amelioration of this adverse effect. Complaints of dizziness should be addressed by monitoring orthostatic vitals and advising against rapid shifts from lying to standing, as occurs when getting out of bed in the morning. Regarding antipsychotic adverse effect management, an approach of slow gradual dose increases is advised to reduce risk for emergent extrapyramidal symptoms. Weight and abdominal circumference should be regularly monitored in addition to metabolic markers. Moreover, regular assessments for early signs of tardive dyskinesia should take place with a scale, such as the Abnormal Involuntary Movement Scale (AIMS; Guy, 1976).

Problematic Comorbid Symptoms

The presence of psychiatric comorbidities is the rule rather than the exception in tic disorders, with comorbidity rates of 80%–90% (Scahill, Bitsko, Visser, & Blumberg, 2009). The most common comorbidities include ADHD (60%–70%), learning disorders (23%), obsessive-compulsive disorder (OCD) (20%–60%), depression and autism spectrum disorders (ASD) (5%; Burd, Freeman, Klug, & Kerbeshian, 2005; Burd, Li, Kerbeshian, Klug, & Freeman, 2009; Freeman and Tourette Syndrome International Database, 2007; Lebowitz et al., 2012; Robertson, 2006; Murphy, Lewin, Storch, Stock, & The American Academy of Child and Adolescent Psychiatry Committee on Quality Issues, 2013). Moreover, comorbid conditions often cause greater functional impact and quality-of-life impairment than tics. In addition, as discussed above, resolution or improvement of comorbid symptoms may indirectly lead to tic improvement due to associated reductions of triggering states and stress. A particularly challenging combination, sometimes known as the "triple threat," includes comorbid tics, OCD, and ADHD. This is associated with poorer quality of life compared to tics alone or tics plus either OCD or ADHD (Eddy et al., 2012).

Attention Deficit Hyperactivity Disorder

Medication options may be particularly helpful in addressing comorbid ADHD and tics. In particular, the strongest support for alpha-2 agonists (e.g., clonidine) in reducing tics relates to youth with comorbid ADHD, where it has demonstrated a large to medium effect, in comparison to an absence of tic improvement in youth without comorbid ADHD (Weisman, Qureshi, Leckman, Scahill, & Bloch, 2012). Beyond alpha-2 agonists, methylphenidate, as monotherapy or combined with clonidine, atomoxetine, or guanfacine, may also be beneficial in reducing both ADHD- and tic-related impairment (Allen et al., 2005; Tourette Syndrome Study Group, 2002).

Since certain elements of behavior therapy (i.e., awareness training and competing response practice) make considerable demands in terms of concentration and impulse control, it follows that the presence of ADHD may pose a barrier to treatment engagement, adherence, and outcomes (Dopfner & Rothenberger, 2007). In fact, a recent meta-analysis demonstrated that higher levels of ADHD were associated with attenuated behavior therapy outcomes across studies (McGuire et al., 2014). Thus treating ADHD with medication and behavioral interventions prior to initiating behavior therapy can be useful. Despite best efforts to treat comorbid ADHD, many children presenting for behavior therapy will remain symptomatic or show subclinical symptoms of ADHD. In these cases, it may be necessary to modify the behavior therapy protocol to minimize the impact of ADHD-related attentional and behavioral difficulties. Table 16.4 offers several recommended strategies for modifying treatment in the face of comorbid ADHD (for a more comprehensive overview of behavioral management strategies for ADHD see "Attention Deficit Hyperactivity Disorder, Third Edition: A Handbook for Diagnosis and Treatment" by Dr. Russell A. Barkley).

Obsessive-Compulsive Disorder

The presence of tics and OCD has been shown to impact medication response and may influence clinicians' decisions to pursue specific treatment options. Specifically, in youth with OCD, comorbid tics appear to decrease OCD response rates to SSRIs (Garcia et al., 2010), while adult OCD response rates to antipsychotic augmentation are increased by the presence of tics (Bloch et al., 2006a). Given the poorer response to SSRI, clinicians could consider the use of clomipramine for OCD treatment, which has been shown to have superior efficacy than SSRIs despite its less favorable adverse effect profile (Geller et al., 2003b; Varigonda, Jakubovski, & Bloch, 2016).

Empirical evidence suggests that comorbid OCD does not negatively impact outcomes of behavioral treatment for tics in children (McGuire et al., 2014) and comorbid tics have not been found to interfere in CBT for OCD in children and adolescents (Conelea et al., 2014; Himle, Fischer, Van Etten, Janeck, & Hanna, 2003). While difficulties can arise in distinguishing between symptoms of OCD and tics (e.g., "evening up" or "just right" behaviors, repetitive movements that appear to neutralize obsessive thoughts), this may not be particularly concerning from a behavioral treatment perspective. Exposure and response prevention has gained widespread research

TABLE 16.4 Modifications for Comorbid ADHD

Intervention Type	Suggested Modifications
Behavioral Treatment	Emphasize aspects of treatment that require less focused attention – particularly functional assessment/intervention.
	Conduct awareness training and competing response practice while children participate in moderately engaging activities such as board games (highly-engaging tasks may be too demanding in terms of attention).
	Use hands-on activities to explain and practice concepts whenever possible (e.g., videos and apps for relaxation strategies).
	Utilize a visual schedule to outline all tasks to be completed in session and check them off as completed.
	Spend time with parents discussing how to help structure home practice activities to maximize the child's attention capabilities (e.g., short duration, scheduled breaks, frequent praise).
	Support families in developing a clear and consistent reinforcement system, emphasizing traits of effective reinforcement.
	Provide simple fidget toys to engage with during didactic aspects of treatment (assess on a case-by-case basis, as fidget toys increase focus for some children but distract others).
	Schedule brief, frequent breaks into sessions.
	Utilize in-session incentives to support on-task behavior (Dopfner and Rothenberger, 2007).
Medications	Alpha-2 agonists may be particularly helpful in treating comorbid tics and ADHD.
	Stimulant treatment of ADHD has not been proven to cause or worsen tics, although this was historically a controversy (perhaps related to the natural history of tics, which are more likely to emerge following the typical onset of ADHD, regardless of treatment)

support as an effective intervention for treating pediatric OCD (Freeman et al., 2014) and has some preliminary support for use in tics (Verdellen, Keijsers, Cath, & Hoogduin, 2004). Thus for children who meet criteria for *both* disorders, or where it is difficult to distinguish between compulsions and tics, ERP or a combination of ERP and HRT may be most effective in targeting the greatest number of symptoms. However, if OCD is considered as the primary issue or is interfering with successful treatment (e.g., unwilling to engage in competing response due to associated obsessional content), treatment of OCD symptoms prior to engaging in further treatment for tics may be warranted (see Bloch & Storch, 2015; Freeman et al., 2014 for more information on evidence-based treatment of OCD).

Mood Instability

Among youth with tics, common disruptions in mood include irritability/anger, as well as depressive symptoms. Frequently, these symptoms stem from tics/tic-impairment and can be managed through the effective use of strategies for addressing tics. If these concerns require additional focus, other strategies also included in the book may help clinicians address these concerns, including use of parent training (Chapter 11: Brief Trans-Diagnostic Parent Training: A Strengths-Based, Parent-Centered Treatment for Youth With Tourette Syndrome), anger management (Chapter 12: Assessing and Treating Emotion Dysregulation and Anger Management), emotion regulation (Chapter 12: Assessing and Treating Emotion Dysregulation and Anger Management), and mindfulness (Chapter 13: Mindfulness for Tics). If these strategies continue to be ineffective, topiramate may be considered as an option when tics and mood instability cooccur. In a meta-analysis of 14 studies ($n = 1003$), there were mixed findings with reported improvement on the YGTSS, although the 50% improvement cutoff was not reached (Yang, Zhang, Zeng, Huang, & Liu, 2013). It is also noteworthy that atypical antipsychotics may have a dual role in these circumstances, given their efficacy in the treatment of mood disorders and tics. Finally, should mood concerns be primary, unrelated to tics, and/or interfering with treatment motivation and adherence, evidence-based treatment for the mood symptoms should be considered as a first-line support.

High Tic Severity

Individuals with tics of high frequency and/or severity may experience unique challenges with treatment. Treatment options may lose credibility for individuals who continue to experience a high degree of symptoms and associated impairment despite implementation of appropriate management strategies. For such individuals, considering pharmacological treatment approaches may be helpful as medication may initially reduce tics to a level more amenable to behavioral intervention. When behavioral treatment is appropriate, it is worth beginning with a tic of lower frequency and severity that will be more easily managed through HRT; this can help increase confidence and adherence with treatment prior to progressing to more challenging tics.

Considering Alternative Conceptualizations

For youth who appear continuously resistant to evidence-based intervention, one may wish to consider the conceptualization of the presentation and whether or not the diagnosis is accurate. While tics are described as sudden, rapid, recurrent, and nonrhythmic, these may closely resemble other repetitive movements in childhood that are not necessarily responsive to the same treatment modalities (Murphy et al., 2013). This may be particularly confusing in cases when the youth has clear, classic symptoms of tic disorders and a comorbid illness. For example, tic disordered youth with ASD may exhibit stereotypies (which occur more during times of excitement; see Freeman, Soltanifar, & Baer, 2010) and, as discussed above, OCD rituals and tics can present as indistinguishable. Further, habit behaviors, such as nail biting and impulsive volitional movements, frequently observed in ADHD and ODD, may be tic-like in appearance. Medication-induced tics may also be hard to differentiate from idiopathic tics. As previously mentioned, akathisia is an adverse effect of antipsychotic medications that may mimic tics and the potential of medication-induced tics should also be considered. Examining the temporal course and response of tics to dose changes can clarify this question. In complex cases, with ongoing symptoms that are hard to disentangle, neurological consultation and a further medical work-up should be considered. A second opinion may also be helpful to examine for previously unidentified factors contributing to treatment nonresponse. The following list is an example of how a clinician may approach discussing these concerns with a patient who has been nonresponsive to traditional treatments:

Clinician: Unfortunately, despite our efforts, it seems that the tics have not improved with what we would consider "first-line" treatments. When we started, we discussed how these treatments have been shown to be helpful for tics on average; however, we also discussed how there is no guarantee that they will work for any one individual and there can be a variety of reasons why these treatments may not have been helpful. One step we'll take is to try and identify what those reasons may have been and if it is something we can adjust to make things work. If not, there are still a number of possible treatment options that exist that we can explore.

Alternative Treatment Options

Experimental Pharmacotherapy

Once it is established that the prescribed medications are being taken as planned, that adverse effects are not overwhelming, that comorbid conditions and other relevant factors are being addressed, if response remains lacking, other first-line or second-line agents should be considered. Several clinical treatment guidelines have been established, including those in the US (Murphy et al., 2013), Canada (Pringsheim et al., 2012), and Europe (Roessner et al., 2011). Once a decision is made to begin a medication, it is best to set clear parameters including the expected trial length, and factors that will be weighed in future decisions to shift the dosage, change medications, continue, or discontinue use. It is also important to establish an agreement around treatment goals.

Efficacy differences between typical and atypical antipsychotics have not been clearly demonstrated for tic disorders. Meta-analysis has identified no efficacy differences between haloperidol, pimozide, risperidone, and ziprasidone (Weisman et al., 2012). In a more recent meta-analysis, aripiprazole demonstrated similar efficacy to haloperidol, with fewer movement side effects (1.5% vs 43.5%; Zheng et al., 2016). According to a Cochrane review, the efficacy of cannabinoids is undetermined (Curtis, Clarke, & Rickards, 2009). Other medications with studies underway include D1 antagonist ecopipam and H3 antagonist AZD5213. A critical aspect in weighing risks and benefits of a medication trial involves consideration of risks related to treatment inaction.

Botox

Dangers related to self-injurious tics should be seriously considered, especially those such as "whiplash" tics with the potential for resultant paralysis. In the presence of specific focal motor tics, such as above-mentioned tics, and for impairing vocal tics, Botulinum toxin has been recommended for adults. This has demonstrated efficacy in an adult randomized double-blind placebo control trial (Marras, Andrews, Sime, & Lang, 2001). If considering utilizing Botox, the potential adverse effect of hypophonia should be considered in a risk/benefit assessment.

Deep Brain Stimulation

A comprehensive review and set of recommendations regarding deep brain stimulation (DBS) for tic disorders were recently compiled and released on behalf of the Tourette Syndrome Association (Schrock et al., 2015). The review elucidates that while evidence has emerged supporting the efficacy of DBS in treating severe treatment-refractory tic cases, it remains an invasive and risky procedure without clear optimal surgical targets. Therefore these recommendations note that while, in contrast to prior reviews, individuals under 18 may be considered for DBS, local ethics committees should be involved in the case. These recommendations also set forth a number of additional criterion that should be met before DBS is considered including high levels of severity and impairment, stable treatment of comorbid disorders, failure of all other empirically supported treatments, stable medical functioning, and active social, and psychological support. If a clinician has a patient who they feel meets these requirements and is in need of DBS, they should refer that patient for a comprehensive evaluation by a multidisciplinary team at an experienced DBS center (Schrock et al., 2015).

Interventions Lacking Empirical Evidence

While treatments including repetitive transcranial magnetic stimulation (rTMS), IVIG, plasma exchange, or acupuncture have been studied, these are not deemed sufficiently safe and effective to warrant use in children and youth (Hollis et al., 2016). Beyond behavior therapy, a broad range of nonpharmacological approaches to reducing tics have been examined, with preliminary evidence for improvement with musical performance and exposure (Bodeck, Lappe, & Evers, 2015). Approaches that have not been clearly proven as beneficial for reducing tic symptom severity include relaxation therapy, parent training, and omega-3 fatty acids.

RELAPSE PREVENTION STRATEGIES

In support of the potential for eventual termination of treatments, unlike other mental illnesses with a more chronic long-term course, the natural history of tic disorders is characterized by waxing and waning periods and, in many cases, a dramatic decrease in the number, frequency, and intensity of tics around early adulthood. Typical onset of tics occurs around 5–10 years of age with the subsequent marked reduction over the following decade, such that only 20% report ongoing moderate to severe impairment by 20 years of age (Bloch et al., 2006b). This indicates that treatment is not necessarily a long-term endeavor and, when impairment is low, clinicians should consider whether the opportunity to discontinue treatment exists. Prior to terminating, clinicians can implement relapse prevention strategies, which are designed to cement existing treatment progress, encourage continued symptom improvement, and minimize the risk of a return in symptoms (Marlatt & George, 1984).

Maintaining Behavior Management Gains

If a patient (and family) have successfully learned and applied therapeutic skills (e.g., HRT, cognitive restructuring, exposure therapy, distress tolerance) over the course of treatment, relapse prevention primarily focuses on how to continue to use those skills without clinician support. Often, at the end of treatment, a child may still demonstrate residual symptoms and will benefit from the continued application of strategies posttreatment to manage tics, minimize related functional impairment, and continue to improve quality of life. However, even if a child is symptom free at treatment end, relapse prevention skills are important to prepare a patient for symptom relapse should it occur. In particular, relapse prevention techniques for behavioral management strategies primarily focus on providing psychoeducation, ensuring mastery over learned strategies, and building self-treatment plans.

Psychoeducation

As discussed in other chapters, psychoeducation represents an important component of comprehensive treatment for tics. A thorough understanding of both tics (e.g., presentation, etiology, course) and behavioral treatment (e.g., strategies, mechanisms) allows youth to better understand their condition and, as a result, helps them be more flexible and adept in their application of the techniques. Specific to relapse prevention, psychoeducation should include a discussion of potential problem areas, a review of tic management strategies, realistic goal setting, and a discussion of how to handle symptom/impairment reemergence, whether temporary/minor or considerable. Many youth, particularly those who have made significant progress, may experience periods of tic symptom exacerbations, believing them to be indicators of a return to a pretreatment state. Clinicians can help youth and parents normalize the occurrence of periods of symptom exacerbation, and help youth understand that if they apply the skills learned over the course of treatment during these exacerbations, they can minimize/mitigate the reemergence of associated impairment. As with other domains of treatment, families play an important role in relapse prevention and should be included in psychoeducation sessions. As with children, it is important that families understand the distinction between lapses and relapses so that they can help and support the child in using learned strategies when a lapse occurs rather than catastrophizing a perceived return in symptoms. Altogether, a family that has a comprehensive knowledge of tics and their treatment will be more capable of independently and flexibly addressing lapses and preventing relapses.

Ensuring Mastery Over Techniques

Once an understanding of tics and tic treatment has been established, clinicians should ensure that the child/family is fully competent in the therapeutic skills and can apply them with flexibility. Given that future symptom exacerbations may not mirror tics/impairment previously exhibited, it is important that patients understand the fundamental concepts of the skills and how they would apply them to variety situations. Ultimately, the goal is to ensure that the child (and parent) has sufficient skills to implement the techniques without therapeutic support. This skill is generally developed by testing youth with a variety of scenarios and having them propose appropriate response plans. For example, let us consider a scenario for a child who has had only facial tics in treatment:

Clinician: You've learned a lot and worked really hard to gain more control over your facial tics! Like we discussed, tics can come and go, and sometimes new tics are quite different than the ones that occurred before. Let's imagine a few weeks from now you begin to experience an abdominal tensing tic. What would our first step be in taking back control from the tic?

Child: Figuring out when it's happening?

Clinician: That's right and how have you learned to do that?

Child: Recognize the physical sensations or urge that happen right before.

Clinician: Excellent, improving awareness of the premonitory urge is a really important step. What else might you want to know about when it's happening?

Child: Things that make it more or less likely.

Clinician: Right, paying attention to factors like emotions, locations, and other situational factors that make tics worse. Okay, so you've developed a better sense of when the tic is likely to happen and how it feels before it occurs. What's the last big step?

Child: Using a competing response.

Clinician: That's right, and what sort of competing response could you use in this situation?

Child: Holding your abs tight?

Clinician: Awesome! That would likely be an excellent competing response to try as if you're flexing your abs, it is likely not possible for the tic to occur.

Scheduling Self-Sessions

A large portion of youth will continue to demonstrate ongoing symptoms despite improvement over the course of treatment. In these cases, it is important that a system is developed in which they can continue to implement the treatment without clinician support. Without appropriate discussion, youth may equate termination of treatment sessions to termination of implementing treatment skills. In addition, the success youth have obtained over treatment and the excitement of no longer needing to attend sessions, can lead to complacency regarding skill use. This can be particularly problematic, as the families also lose the accountability and related motivation that comes with regularly scheduled therapy sessions. As a result, part of the relapse prevention focus should be on identifying a continued treatment plan that families can implement. Important skills that should be included are as follows: identifying when specific practices may be completed, identifying a specific parent or rotating schedule regarding confirmation of homework completion, setting up family meetings in which progress can be discussed and problem solving can occur, and identifying a tic-priority plan to help families progress through remaining treatment targets in a realistic manner. The relapse prevention skills discussed above (psychoeducation, ensuring mastery) will have provided families with all the necessary tools to continue treatment, but having a well-developed outline for implementation will help to ensure that they use those tools. The following list is an example of how a clinician might introduce the concept of scheduling self-sessions to a patient:

Clinician: Today is our last session together, are you nervous about continuing on your own?

Patient: A little bit, but I know how to do everything and I'm excited not to have to come anymore.

Clinician: Awesome! It's great that you're ready to end treatment. Do you think ending treatment means you should stop practicing these skills?

Patient: No

Clinician: Why not?

Patient: Because I might forget how to use them and things might get worse again.

Clinician: Exactly, so let's come up with a specific plan about when you are going to keep practicing these skills and how your parents will help.

Supplemental Options

While the previous sections outline the essential components of relapse prevention strategies, variations in their delivery and the inclusion of additional posttreatment supports can further bolster the likelihood of treatment maintenance. Rather than following a consistent time schedule, staggering sessions toward the end of treatment (i.e., treatment fading) provides an opportunity for families to develop, practice, and implement strategies for managing new tics more independently. For example, treatment may begin with weekly sessions to coach families through each step of treatment for a number of tics, tic-related impairment, and the quality of life. Following this, treatment can fade to bi-weekly (or less frequent) sessions with home practice focused on implementing strategies between sessions. With the added benefit of more at-home and independent experience, staggered sessions can then focus on the topics discussed above with a better understanding of how to: (1) support families to develop greater confidence carrying out therapeutic skills independently, (2) fine-tune skills and strategies to support increased mastery, and (3) problem solving around any barriers to treatment progress while families work more independently.

The provision of booster sessions (i.e., family returns to see clinician at a later date) can also be helpful in maintaining treatment gains, as has been shown with CBT for other youth mental health concerns (Gearing, Schwalbe, Lee, & Hoagwood, 2013; Kolko & Lindhiem, 2014). Scheduling a booster session approximately 1 month following the treatment, with specific goals and self-sessions for families to complete in the interim, may promote treatment maintenance and provide some additional accountability to continue implementing treatment skills. This follow-up session provides an opportunity to reevaluate families' therapeutic skills and provide additional psychoeducation, modeling, and/or supported practice, as needed. In addition, this session allows for additional problem solving, when necessary, around any barriers to continued progress with tic management.

For a long-term support, telephone or video conference check-ins may be helpful when families encounter challenges applying skills to a new tic and/or other handling tic-related challenges. These check-ins have been especially beneficial when families are attempting to manage a particularly complex or challenging tic as clinicians can help identify potential competing responses for specific tics. However, these check-ins can also be extremely helpful when tics have resulted in new or returning tic-related impairment. Clinicians can help the parents to design a function-based intervention to address this impairment, such as reviewing cognitive restructuring for self-esteem, and/or discuss an exposure plan to address tic-related avoidance.

Postresponse Medication Management

Once tics have decreased and functioning optimized, families may begin to ask about whether and when medications will be stopped. Family perspectives vary greatly on this, depending on perceived risks of long-term medication use compared to that related to tic reemergence.

Deciding to Discontinue

In situations where tic history is severe and debilitating, it may be tempting to continue rather than attempting to taper and discontinuation pharmacotherapy. Other factors that may influence a decision to continue a medication regime include a history of self-injurious tics that have ameliorated during the trial, past failed discontinuation trials, and the presence of comorbidities that worsen with tic severity. Factors that may influence a decision to discontinue medications following tic improvement include the presence of bothersome or serious adverse effects, concerns regarding long-term adverse effects (especially for antipsychotics), financial costs, and medication-associated stigma and embarrassment.

When to Discontinue

As mentioned elsewhere, several guidelines exist that support the management of patients with tic disorders. While these are fairly consistent in their recommendations for acute and short-term treatment, they are uniformly lacking in detailed recommendations for the long-term medication management for tics. As such, it is challenging for clinicians to make informed decisions regarding when to discontinue medications trials.

Canadian guidelines point out that evidence for the long-term efficacy of antipsychotics in treating tics is lacking, and state that treatment benefit should be weighed against risks and side effects for long-term use (Pringsheim et al., 2012). European guidelines also identify the paucity of long-term outcome studies of atypical antipsychotic use in Tourette syndrome (Roessner et al., 2011). These guidelines also remind clinicians to ensure that medication dosages are being appropriately adapted with patient growth and weight gain over time. The most specific guidance identified on a review of the literature is provided by Scahill et al. (Scahill, King, Lombroso, Sukhodolsky, & Leckman, 2011) who recommended that, if tics are stable, dose reduction should be considered on an annual basis. While Canadian guidelines suggest that dosage should be tapered "periodically" due to the natural history of tic remission (Pringsheim et al., 2012), the frequency implied by "periodically" was not clearly identified.

How to Discontinue

Regardless of the above, efforts should be made to optimize chances of success for a discontinuation trial. As such, advance selection and planning for a period with low "tic-ogenic" social and environmental factors is advisable. Tics are sensitive to stress, fatigue, heat, and illness (Murphy et al., 2013). Other tic-exacerbating factors have also been identified including caffeine (Müller-Vahl, Buddensiek, Geomelas, & Emrich, 2008) and screen time (Himle et al., 2014). Minimization of life stressors and ensuring regular and adequate amounts of sleep during discontinuation are concrete actions that may improve chances of success. In addition, focus on the importance of resilience and strengths rather than on the presence of tics as identity-defining factors is helpful in decreasing the importance of residual and lingering tics. As a clinical example of discussing medication discontinuation, let us consider Luca, a 16-year-old boy whose eye blinking, throat clearing, and shoulder shrugging tics have been under good control for over a year, following stabilization on guanfacine:

Clinician:	It's been awhile since I've seen you, how are things going related to your tics?
Patient:	I've been doing great— I don't think I have tics at all anymore!
Mother:	Well actually, I do notice some of Luca's sounds and eye blinking when he is tired or stressed, but that only happens every now and then.
Clinician:	So it sounds like things are much better, and that the tics have stopped getting in the way of Luca's life and activities over a year now. Is that right?
Patient and Mother:	Yes, totally.
Clinician:	Are you still feeling tired during the daytime after taking your medication?
Patient:	Yeah—I usually take a nap after school. Sometimes I doze off in class—even in the ones I really like! I'm so pumped that this is the last week before summer.
Clinician:	It sounds like now is a good time to talk about whether to decrease or stop your meds. Do you remember when we discussed this possibility before?
Patient:	Sort of, I guess.
Clinician:	That's true—it was a while ago when we started guanfacine! We talked about the need to weigh the positives of taking meds against the possible negatives. I also told you how tics often go away on their own during adolescence.
Mother:	Yes, I remember that.
Clinician:	Well it seems that the tics haven't been a problem for a year now, but Luca is still dealing with the sleepiness that the meds cause. Are either of you interested in stopping them?
Patient:	Yes, totally!
Mother:	Well, what if they come back?
Clinician:	That is an excellent point. We would want to pick a low stress time when Luca's tics have typically been under better control, such as this summer. We will also decrease the dose gradually and check-in regularly to make sure the tics haven't become a problem again. If that is the case, we can increase the dose.

[From here, the clinician can move on to discuss specific indicators of when the planned medication decreases should continue or stop, or when doses should be re-increased. Reminders of non-pharmacologic approaches to tic management should also be reinforced at this time.]

Maintaining Quality-of-Life Gains

Beyond maintaining progress in regards to reductions in severity, relapse prevention can also be beneficial in ensuring a child's overall functional impairment and quality of life remain improved. For example, a child can progress through treatment and reduce the severity of many tics, but still have one tic that significantly bothers them and impairs them socially, reducing their functioning, and the quality of life. As a result, in addition to helping children continue addressing tics posttreatment, relapse prevention strategies can help to ensure that treatment remains beneficial for more general domains important to the child's overall well-being.

Prioritizing Treatment Targets

While clinicians do classify the severity of tics by evaluating factors, such as their frequency and complexity, an equally severe tic may create different levels of impairment across individuals. Further, beyond the most extreme tics, which can risk physical injury, the primary problematic nature of tics is the impairment they can create within the child's life. As a result, in order to maximize and maintain quality-of-life gains, clinicians should build a post-treatment plan with patients around the ways in which tics interfere in their lives. For example, when helping families plan self-sessions, clinicians can ensure that the tics they choose to address first will be those are associated with the most impairment and/or whose improvement will most greatly improve the quality of life. Below provides an example:

John and Nancy have identical tics: a right-arm extension and a throat clearing. John is able to manage his arm tic during school hours and is not overly bothered by it at home; however, he hates when he repeatedly clears his throat during conversations with friends and his siblings often get annoyed with him. Nancy, has explained her throat clearing tic to her friends and her family finds it minimally invasive; however, she often injures herself when her arm extension leads her to hit objects. Given this scenario, John may benefit from working on his throat clearing tic prior to the arm extension tic, while Nancy would benefit from addressing her arm extension tic prior to the throat clearing tic.

In maintaining quality-of-life gains, it may be advisable for clinicians to advise patients to focus energy on alternative concerns to tics if they present more impairment. This may include encouraging continued efforts to manage social challenges, hierarchy planning to continue addressing tic-related avoidance, or provision of referrals to provide support in addressing other psychological symptoms.

CONCLUSIONS AND AREAS OF CONTINUED RESEARCH

The materials presented in this book provide clinicians with a comprehensive guide to treating youth with tics and the present chapter offers clinicians guidance on making end-of-treatment decisions. While evidence continues to grow and support a variety of intervention strategies for youth with tics, research on youth after completing treatment is minimal. In particular, additional examination of factors associated with nonresponse, as well as interventions aimed at addressing these factors, is needed. Continued research in this area would aid clinicians in their initial selection and structure of treatments and could result in treatment modifications that increase the likelihood of response. In addition, there is a paucity of studies exploring treatment-discontinuation strategies, such as levels or timing of fading for behavioral treatments or varying dose decreases for pharmacological treatments. These studies would be extremely valuable in helping clinicians and patients make informed decisions regarding treatment termination. Finally, interventions (such as this book) should continue to expand their scope of treatment targets, aiming to improve not only outcomes for tic frequency/severity, but also more global domains, such as impairment, social functioning, and comorbid symptoms, which significantly contribute to youths' overall quality of life.

REFERENCES

Allen, A. J., Kurlan, R. M., Gilbert, D. L., Coffey, B. J., Linder, S. L., Lewis, D. W., ... Spencer, T. J. (2005). Atomoxetine treatment in children and adolescents with ADHD and comorbid tic disorders. *Neurology*, *65*, 1941–1949.

Bloch, M. H., Landeros-Weisenberger, A., Kelmendi, B., Coric, V., Bracken, M. B., & Leckman, J. F. (2006a). A systematic review: Antipsychotic augmentation with treatment refractory obsessive-compulsive disorder. *Molecular Psychiatry*, *11*, 622–632.

Bloch, M. H., Peterson, B. S., Scahill, L., Otka, J., Katsovich, L., Zhang, H., & Leckman, J. F. (2006b). Adulthood outcome of tic and obsessive-compulsive symptom severity in children with Tourette syndrome. *Archives of Pediatrics and Adolescent Medicine*, *160*, 65–69.

Bloch, M. H., & Storch, E. A. (2015). Assessment and management of treatment-refractory obsessive-compulsive disorder in children. *Journal of the American Academy of Child & Adolescent Psychiatry*, *54*, 251–262.

Bodeck, S., Lappe, C., & Evers, S. (2015). Tic-reducing effects of music in patients with Tourette's syndrome: Self-reported and objective analysis. *Journal of the Neurological Sciences*, *352*, 41–47.

Brown, R. A., Ramsey, S. E., Strong, D. R., Myers, M. G., Kahler, C. W., Lejuez, C. W., ... Abrams, D. B. (2003). Effects of motivational interviewing on smoking cessation in adolescents with psychiatric disorders. *Tobacco Control*, *12*(Suppl 4), IV3–IV10.

Burd, L., Freeman, R. D., Klug, M. G., & Kerbeshian, J. (2005). Tourette syndrome and learning disabilities. *BMC Pediatrics*, *5*, 34.

Burd, L., Li, Q., Kerbeshian, J., Klug, M. G., & Freeman, R. D. (2009). Tourette syndrome and comorbid pervasive developmental disorders. *Journal of Child Neurology*, *24*, 170–175.

Channon, S., Smith, V. J., & Gregory, J. W. (2003). A pilot study of motivational interviewing in adolescents with diabetes. *Archives of Disease in Childhood*, *88*, 680–683.

Conelea, C. A., Walther, M. R., Freeman, J. B., Garcia, A. M., Sapyta, J., Khanna, M., & Franklin, M. (2014). Tic-related obsessive-compulsive disorder (OCD): Phenomenology and treatment outcome in the Pediatric OCD Treatment Study II. *Journal of the American Academy of Child & Adolescent Psychiatry*, *53*, 1308–1316.

Corkum, P., Rimer, P., & Schachar, R. (1999). Parental knowledge of attention-deficit hyperactivity disorder and opinions of treatment options: Impact on enrollment and adherence to a 12-month treatment trial. *Canadian Journal of Psychiatry*, *44*, 1043–1048.

Cuenca, J., Glazebrook, C., Kendall, T., Hedderly, T., Heyman, I., Jackson, G., ... Hollis, C. (2015). Perceptions of treatment for tics among young people with Tourette syndrome and their parents: A mixed methods study. *BMC Psychiatry*, *15*, 46.

Curtis, A., Clarke, C. E., & Rickards, H. E. (2009). Cannabinoids for Tourette's Syndrome. *Cochrane Database of Systematic Reviews*, CD006565.

Davidson, K., Scott, J., Schmidt, U., Tata, P., Thornton, S., & Tyrer, P. (2004). Therapist competence and clinical outcome in the Prevention of Parasuicide by Manual Assisted Cognitive Behaviour Therapy trial: the POPMACT study. *Psychological Medicine*, *34*, 855–863.

Dean, S., Britt, E., Bell, E., Stanley, J., & Collings, S. (2016). Motivational interviewing to enhance adolescent mental health treatment engagement: A randomized clinical trial. *Psychological Medicine*, *46*, 1961–1969.

Dopfner, M., & Rothenberger, A. (2007). Behavior therapy in tic-disorders with co-existing ADHD. *European Child & Adolescent Psychiatry*, *16*(Suppl 1), 89–99.

Duncan, C. L., Mentrikoski, J. M., Wu, Y. P., & Fredericks, E. M. (2014). Practice-based approach to assessing and treating nonadherence in pediatric regimens. *Clinical Practice in Pediatric Psychology*, *2*, 322–336.

Eddy, C. M., Cavanna, A. E., Gulisano, M., Cali, P., Robertson, M. M., & Rizzo, R. (2012). The effects of comorbid obsessive-compulsive disorder and attention-deficit hyperactivity disorder on quality of life in Tourette syndrome. *Journal of Neuropsychiatry and Clinical Neurosciences*, *24*, 458–462.

Epstein, T., & Saltzman-Benaiah, J. (2010). Parenting children with disruptive behaviours: Evaluation of a collaborative problem solving pilot program. *Journal of Clinical Psychology Practice*, *1*, 27–40.

Freeman, J., Garcia, A., Frank, H., Benito, K., Conelea, C., Walther, M., & Edmunds, J. (2014). Evidence base update for psychosocial treatments for pediatric obsessive-compulsive disorder. *Journal of Clinical Child and Adolescent Psychology Journal of Clinical Child & Adolescent Psychology*, *43*, 7–26.

Freeman, R. D., Soltanifar, A., & Baer, S. (2010). Stereotypic movement disorder: Easily missed. *Developmental Medicine and Child Neurology*, *52*, 733–738.

Freeman, R. D., & Tourette Syndrome International Database, C. (2007). Tic disorders and ADHD: answers from a world-wide clinical dataset on Tourette syndrome. *European Child & Adolescent Psychiatry*, *16*(Suppl 1), 15–23.

Ganos, C., Asmuss, L., Bongert, J., Brandt, V., Munchau, A., & Haggard, P. (2015). Volitional action as perceptual detection: Predictors of conscious intention in adolescents with tic disorders. *Cortex*, *64*, 47–54.

Garcia, A. M., Sapyta, J. J., Moore, P. S., Freeman, J. B., Franklin, M. E., March, J. S., & Foa, E. B. (2010). Predictors and moderators of treatment outcome in the Pediatric Obsessive Compulsive Treatment Study (POTS I). *Journal of the American Academy of Child & Adolescent Psychiatry*, *49*, 1024–1033, quiz 1086.

Gearing, R. E., Schwalbe, C. S., Lee, R., & Hoagwood, K. E. (2013). The effectiveness of booster sessions in CBT treatment for child and adolescent mood and anxiety disorders. *Depression and Anxiety*, *30*, 800–808.

Geller, D. A., Biederman, J., Stewart, S. E., Mullin, B., Farrell, C., Wagner, K. D., ... Carpenter, D. (2003a). Impact of comorbidity on treatment response to paroxetine in pediatric obsessive-compulsive disorder: Is the use of exclusion criteria empirically supported in randomized clinical trials? *Journal of Child and Adolescent Psychopharmacology, 13* (Suppl 1), S19–S29.

Geller, D. A., Biederman, J., Stewart, S. E., Mullin, B., Martin, A., Spencer, T., & Faraone, S. V. (2003b). Which SSRI? A meta-analysis of pharmacotherapy trials in pediatric obsessive-compulsive disorder. *American Journal of Psychiatry, 160*, 1919–1928.

Gold, M. A., & Kokotailo, P. K. (2007). Motivational interviewing strategies to facilitate adolescent behavior change. *Adolescent Health Update, 20*, 1–9.

Guy, W. (1976). Abnormal involuntary movement scale (AIMS). *ECDEU Assessment Manual for Psychopharmacology, 338*, 534–537.

Himle, J. A., Fischer, D. J., Van etten, M. L., Janeck, A. S., & Hanna, G. L. (2003). Group behavioral therapy for adolescents with tic-related and non-tic-related obsessive-compulsive disorder. *Depression and Anxiety, 17*, 73–77.

Himle, M. B., Capriotti, M. R., Hayes, L. P., Ramanujam, K., Scahill, L., Sukhodolsky, D. G., ... Piacentini, J. (2014). Variables associated with tic exacerbation in children with chronic tic disorders. *Behavior Modification, 38*, 163–183.

Himle, M. B., Freitag, M., Walther, M., Franklin, S. A., Ely, L., & Woods, D. W. (2012). A randomized pilot trial comparing videoconference versus face-to-face delivery of behavior therapy for childhood tic disorders. *Behaviour Research Therapy, 50*, 565–570.

Hollis, C., Pennant, M., Cuenca, J., Glazebrook, C., Kendall, T., Whittington, C., ... Stern, J. (2016). Clinical effectiveness and patient perspectives of different treatment strategies for tics in children and adolescents with Tourette syndrome: A systematic review and qualitative analysis. *Health Technology Assessment, 20*, 1–450, vii–viii.

Horwitz, R. I., & Horwitz, S. M. (1993). Adherence to treatment and health outcomes. *Archives of Internal Medicine, 153*, 1863–1868.

Jin, J., Sklar, G. E., Min Sen oh, V., & Chuen li, S. (2008). Factors affecting therapeutic compliance: A review from the patient's perspective. *Therapeutics and Clinical Risk Management, 4*, 269–286.

Kent, E. G. (2005). (Producer, Director) *I have Tourette's but Tourette's doesn't have me*. USA: HBO/Tourette Syndrome Association.

Kolko, D. J., & Lindhiem, O. (2014). Introduction to the special series on booster sessions and long-term maintenance of treatment gains. *Journal of Abnormal Child Psychology, 42*, 339–342.

LaRosa, J. C. (2000). Poor compliance: the hidden risk factor. *Current Atherosclerosis Reports, 2*, 1–4.

Lebowitz, E. R., Motlagh, M. G., Katsovich, L., King, R. A., Lombroso, P. J., Grantz, H., ... Leckman, J. F. (2012). Tourette syndrome in youth with and without obsessive compulsive disorder and attention deficit hyperactivity disorder. *European Child & Adolescent Psychiatry, 21*, 451–457.

Lehmkuhl, H. D., Storch, E. A., Rahman, O., Freeman, J., Geffken, G. R., & Murphy, T. K. (2009). Just say no: Sequential parent management training and cognitive-behavioral therapy for a child with comorbid disruptive behavior and obsessive compulsive disorder. *Clinical Case Studies, 8*, 45–58.

Lewin, A. B., Mcguire, J. F., Murphy, T. K., & Storch, E. A. (2014). The importance of considering parent's preferences when planning treatment for their children—the case of childhood obsessive-compulsive disorder. *Journal of Child Psychology and Psychiatry, 55*, 1314–1316.

Lewin, A. B., Peris, T. S., Lindsey Bergman, R., Mccracken, J. T., & Piacentini, J. (2011). The role of treatment expectancy in youth receiving exposure-based CBT for obsessive compulsive disorder. *Behaviour Research and Therapy, 49*, 536–543.

Marlatt, G. A., & George, W. H. (1984). Relapse prevention: Introduction and overview of the model. *British Journal of Addiction, 79*, 261–273.

Marras, C., Andrews, D., Sime, E., & Lang, A. E. (2001). Botulinum toxin for simple motor tics: a randomized, double-blind, controlled clinical trial. *Neurology, 56*, 605–610.

Martin, D. J., Garske, J. P., & Davis, M. K. (2000). Relation of the therapeutic alliance with outcome and other variables: a meta-analytic review. *Journal of Consulting and Clinical Psychology, 68*, 438–450.

McGuire, J. F., Hanks, C., Lewin, A. B., Storch, E. A., & Murphy, T. K. (2013). Social deficits in children with chronic tic disorders: Phenomenology, clinical correlates and quality of life. *Comprehensive Psychiatry, 54*, 1023–1031.

McGuire, J. F., Piacentini, J., Brennan, E. A., Lewin, A. B., Murphy, T. K., Small, B. J., & Storch, E. A. (2014). A meta-analysis of behavior therapy for Tourette Syndrome. *Journal of Psychiatric Research, 50*, 106–112.

Miller, W. R., & Rollnick, S. (2012). Meeting in the middle: Motivational interviewing and self-determination theory. *International Journal of Behavioral Nutrition and Physical Activity, 9*, 25.

Misdrahi, D., Llorca, P. M., Lancon, C., & Bayle, F. J. (2002). [Compliance in schizophrenia: predictive factors, therapeutical considerations and research implications]. *Encephale, 28*, 266–272.

Moore, T. R., & Symons, F. J. (2011). Adherence to treatment in a behavioral intervention curriculum for parents of children with autism spectrum disorder. *Behavior Modification, 35*, 570–594.

Morgan, J., Caporino, N. E., De nadai, A. S., Truax, T., Lewin, A. B., Jung, L., . . . Storch, E. A. (2013). Preliminary predictors of within-session adherence to exposure and response prevention in pediatric obsessive-compulsive disorder. *Child & Youth Care Forum, 42*, 181–191.

Müller-Vahl, K. R., Buddensiek, N., Geomelas, M., & Emrich, H. M. (2008). The influence of different food and drink on tics in Tourette syndrome. *Acta Paediatrica, 97*, 442–446.

Murphy, T. K., Lewin, A. B., Storch, E. A., Stock, S., & The American Academy of Child and Adolescent Psychiatry Committee on Quality Issues. (2013). Practice parameter for the assessment and treatment of children and adolescents with tic disorders. *Journal of the American Academy of Child & Adolescent Psychiatry, 52*, 1341–1359.

Naar-King, S., & Suarez, M. (2011). *Motivational interviewing with adolescents and young adults*. New York, NY: Guilford Press.

Nock, M. K., & Ferriter, C. (2005). Parent management of attendance and adherence in child and adolescent therapy: A conceptual and empirical review. *Clinical Child and Family Psychology Review, 8*, 149–166.

Olatunji, B. O., Rosenfield, D., Monzani, B., Krebs, G., Heyman, I., Turner, C., . . . Mataix-Cols, D. (2015). Effects of homework compliance on cognitive-behavioral therapy with D-Cycloserine augmentation for children with obsessive compulsive disorder. *Depression and Anxiety, 32*, 935–943.

Ollendick, T. H., Greene, R. W., Austin, K. E., Fraire, M. G., Halldorsdottir, T., Allen, K. B., . . . Wolff, J. C. (2016). Parent Management Training and Collaborative & Proactive Solutions: A Randomized Control Trial for Oppositional Youth. *Journal of Clinical Child & Adolescent Psychology, 45*, 591–604.

Pakpour, A. H., Gellert, P., Dombrowski, S. U., & Fridlund, B. (2015). Motivational interviewing with parents for obesity: An RCT. *Pediatrics*, *135*, e644–e652.

Park, J. M., Small, B. J., Geller, D. A., Murphy, T. K., Lewin, A. B., & Storch, E. A. (2014). Does d-cycloserine augmentation of CBT improve therapeutic homework compliance for pediatric obsessive-compulsive disorder? *Journal of Child and Family Studies*, *23*, 863–871.

Piacentini, J., Woods, D. W., Scahill, L., Wilhelm, S., Peterson, A. L., Chang, S., ... Walkup, J. T. (2010). Behavior therapy for children with Tourette disorder: A randomized controlled trial. *JAMA*, *303*, 1929–1937.

Podell, J. L., Kendall, P. C., Gosch, E. A., Compton, S. N., March, J. S., Albano, A. M., ... Piacentini, J. C. (2013). Therapist Factors and Outcomes in CBT for Anxiety in Youth. *Professional Psychology Research and Practice*, *44*, 89–98.

Pringsheim, T., Doja, A., Gorman, D., Mckinlay, D., Day, L., Billinghurst, L., ... Sandor, P. (2012). Canadian guidelines for the evidence-based treatment of tic disorders: Pharmacotherapy. *Canadian Journal of Psychiatry*, *57*, 133–143.

Ricketts, E. J., Goetz, A. R., Capriotti, M. R., Bauer, C. C., Brei, N. G., Himle, M. B., ... Woods, D. W. (2016). A randomized waitlist-controlled pilot trial of voice over Internet protocol-delivered behavior therapy for youth with chronic tic disorders. *Journal of Telemedicine and Telecare*, *22*, 153–162.

Robertson, M. M. (2006). Mood disorders and Gilles de la Tourette's syndrome: An update on prevalence, etiology, comorbidity, clinical associations, and implications. *Journal of Psychosomatic Research*, *61*, 349–358.

Roessner, V., Plessen, K. J., Rothenberger, A., Ludolph, A. G., Rizzo, R., Skov, L., ... Group, E. G. (2011). European clinical guidelines for Tourette syndrome and other tic disorders. Part II: pharmacological treatment. *European Child & Adolescent Psychiatry*, *20*, 173–196.

Rollnick, S., Miller, W. R., & Butler, C. C. (2008). *Motivational interviewing in health care: Helping patients change behavior*. New York, NY: Guilford Press.

Scahill, L., Bitsko, R. H., Visser, S. N., & Blumberg, S. J. (2009). Prevalence of diagnosed Tourette syndrome in persons aged 6–17 years—United States, 2007. *Morbidity and Mortality Weekly Report*, *58*, 581–585.

Scahill, L., King, R. A., Lombroso, P., Sukhodolsky, D. G., & Leckman, J. F. (2011). Tourette Syndrome and other tic disorders. In A. Martin, L. Scahill, & C. Kratochvil (Eds.), *Pediatric Psychopharmacology* (2nd ed.). USA: Oxford University Press.

Scahill, L., Woods, D. W., Himle, M. B., Peterson, A. L., Wilhelm, S., Piacentini, J. C., ... Mink, J. W. (2013). Current controversies on the role of behavior therapy in Tourette syndrome. *Movement Disorders*, *28*, 1179–1183.

Schrock, L. E., Mink, J. W., Woods, D. W., Porta, M., Servello, D., Visser-Vandewalle, V., ... Registry study, G. (2015). Tourette syndrome deep brain stimulation: a review and updated recommendations. *Movement Disorders*, *30*, 448–471.

Selles, R. R., Belschner, L., Negeiros, J., Lin, S. Y., Schuberth, D., McKenney, K., ... Stewart, S. E. (2017). Group family-based cognitive behavioral therapy for pediatric obsessive compulsive disorder: Global outcomes and predictors of improvement. *Psychiatry Research*, *260*, 116–122.

Shim, R., & Rust, G. (2013). Primary care, behavioral health, and public health: Partners in reducing mental health stigma. *American Journal of Public Health*, *103*, 774–776.

Sibley, M. H., Graziano, P. A., Kuriyan, A. B., Coxe, S., Pelham, W. E., Rodriguez, L., ... Ward, A. (2016). Parent-teen behavior therapy + motivational interviewing for adolescents with ADHD. *Journal of Consulting and Clinical Psychology*, *84*, 699–712.

Simpson, H. B., Zuckoff, A., Page, J. R., Franklin, M. E., & Foa, E. B. (2008). Adding motivational interviewing to exposure and ritual prevention for obsessive-compulsive disorder: an open pilot trial. *Cognitive Behavioural Therapy, 37*, 38–49.

Simpson, H. B., Zuckoff, A. M., Maher, M. J., Page, J. R., Franklin, M. E., Foa, E. B., ... Wang, Y. (2010). Challenges using motivational interviewing as an adjunct to exposure therapy for obsessive-compulsive disorder. *Behaviour Research and Therapy, 48*, 941–948.

Spirito, A., Monti, P. M., Barnett, N. P., Colby, S. M., Sindelar, H., Rohsenow, D. J., ... Myers, M. (2004). A randomized clinical trial of a brief motivational intervention for alcohol-positive adolescents treated in an emergency department. *Journal of Pediatrics, 145*, 396–402.

Stevens, J., Wang, W., Fan, L., Edwards, M. C., Campo, J. V., & Gardner, W. (2009). Parental attitudes toward children's use of antidepressants and psychotherapy. *Journal of Child and Adolescent Psychopharmacology, 19*, 289–296.

Storch, E. A., Merlo, L. J., Larson, M. J., Geffken, G. R., Lehmkuhl, H. D., Jacob, M. L., ... Goodman, W. K. (2008). Impact of comorbidity on cognitive-behavioral therapy response in pediatric obsessive-compulsive disorder. *Journal of the American Academy of Child & Adolescent Psychiatry, 47*, 583–592.

Theule, J., Ward, M. A., Cheung, K., & Lee, J. B. (2016). Psychosocial treatments for tic disorders: A meta-analysis. *Journal of Psychiatric Research, 74*, 8–9.

Tourette Syndrome Study Group. (2002). Treatment of ADHD in children with tics: a randomized control trial. *Neurology, 58*, 526–536.

Varigonda, A. L., Jakubovski, E., & Bloch, M. H. (2016). Systematic review and meta-analysis: early treatment responses of selective serotonin reuptake inhibitors and clomipramine in pediatric obsessive-compulsive disorder. *Journal of the American Academy of Child & Adolescent Psychiatry, 55*, 851–859.e2.

Verdellen, C. W., Keijsers, G. P., Cath, D. C., & Hoogduin, C. A. (2004). Exposure with response prevention versus habit reversal in Tourettes's syndrome: A controlled study. *Behaviour Research and Therapy, 42*, 501–511.

Weisman, H., Qureshi, I. A., Leckman, J. F., Scahill, L., & Bloch, M. H. (2012). Systematic review: Pharmacological treatment of tic disorders—Efficacy of antipsychotic and alpha-2 adrenergic agonist agents. *Neuroscience & Biobehavioral Reviews.*

Wilhelm, S., Peterson, A. L., Piacentini, J., Woods, D. W., Deckersbach, T., Sukhodolsky, D. G., ... Scahill, L. (2012). Randomized trial of behavior therapy for adults with Tourette syndrome. *Archives of General Psychiatry, 69*, 795–803.

Woods, D. W., Piacentini, J., Chang, S., Deckersbach, T., Ginsburg, G. S., Peterson, A. L., ... Wilhelm, S. (2008). *Managing Tourette Syndrome: A Behavioral Intervention for Children and Adults (Therapist Guide)*. New York: Oxford University Press.

Yang, C. S., Zhang, L. L., Zeng, L. N., Huang, L., & Liu, Y. T. (2013). Topiramate for Tourette's syndrome in children: A meta-analysis. *Pediatric Neurology, 49*, 344–350.

Zheng, W., Xiang, Y. T., Xiang, Y. Q., Li, X. B., Ungvari, G. S., Chiu, H. F., & Correll, C. U. (2016). Efficacy and safety of adjunctive topiramate for schizophrenia: A meta-analysis of randomized controlled trials. *Acta Psychiatrica Scandinavica, 134*, 385–398.

Index

Note: Page numbers followed by "f" and "t" refer to figures and tables, respectively.

B

C

F

G

M

N

O

T

U

V

FSC
www.fsc.org
MIX
Papier | Fördert
gute Waldnutzung
FSC® C083411

Kolibri 360 GmbH
Ferdinand-Jühlke-Straße 7
99095 Erfurt, Deutschland
produktsicherheit@kolibri360.de